CANCER:

CAUSES, OCCURRENCE AND CONTROL

INTERNATIONAL AGENCY FOR RESEARCH ON CANCER

The International Agency for Research on Cancer (IARC) was established in 1965 by the World Health Assembly, as an independently financed organization within the framework of the World Health Organization. The headquarters of the Agency are at Lyon, France.

The Agency conducts a programme of research concentrating particularly on the epidemiology of cancer and the study of potential carcinogens in the human environment. Its field studies are supplemented by biological and chemical research carried out in the Agency's laboratories in Lyon and, through collaborative research agreements, in national research institutions in many countries. The Agency also conducts a programme for the education and training of personnel for cancer research.

The publications of the Agency are intended to contribute to the dissemination of authoritative information on different aspects of cancer research. A complete list is printed at the end of this book.

WORLD HEALTH ORGANIZATION

INTERNATIONAL AGENCY FOR RESEARCH ON CANCER

CANCER:

CAUSES, OCCURRENCE AND CONTROL

Editor–in–Chief

L. Tomatis

Co–editors:

A. Aitio, N.E. Day, E. Heseltine, J. Kaldor,
A.B. Miller, D.M. Parkin & E. Riboli

IARC Scientific Publications No. 100

International Agency for Research on Cancer
Lyon, 1990

Published by the International Agency for Research on Cancer,
150 cours Albert Thomas, 69372 Lyon Cedex 08, France

Distributed by Oxford University Press, Walton Street, Oxford OX2 6DP, UK

Distributed in the USA by Oxford University Press, New York

ISBN 92 832 0110 8

ISSN 0300–5085

Printed in the United Kingdom

CONTENTS

PART II. THE CAUSES OF CANCER

PART IV. THE CONTROL OF CANCER THROUGH PREVENTION AND EARLY DETECTION

FOREWORD

The International Agency for Research on Cancer, since its inception in 1965, has devoted most of its activities to research into the etiology of cancer and the prevention of human cancer. A team of epidemiologists, biostatisticians and experimentalists fulfils these aims in a large number of projects, based partly in Lyon but widened considerably through worldwide collaboration with national institutes and with scientists in many countries.

The volume presented here is the Agency's first attempt to present a concise, easily readable description of what is known about the incidence of and mortality from cancer, its causes and the actual possibilities for preventing it. This book is more than a hymn to the progress of science; it is a realistic and perhaps more humble survey of the present state of the art of cancer prevention and control. Cancer research is today advancing at a rapid pace, and in this book we touch only marginally on these exciting new frontiers. As new hopes for the prevention, diagnosis and therapy of cancer arise (and there are good grounds to believe that some of today's expectations may be fulfilled in the not too distant future), we hope that there will soon be reason for substantially updating this volume.

We at the Agency wish to pay tribute to the many scientists in different countries who were willing to put their time, experience and knowledge into producing the collective effort that this book constitutes. Without their help, it would have been impossible to put together the large amount of material at hand and to condense it into a volume of reasonable dimensions. In addition, the book would not have seen the light without the unselfish, dedicated, competent input of many scientists at the Agency. Attribution of authorship is often somewhat arbitrary, and this is so in the present case. The co-editors are those scientists from the Agency and from outside the Agency whose contributions to the end result were clearly substantial; all the other contributors are listed in the Acknowledgements. Our gratitude goes to all of them.

The Editors

ACKNOWLEDGEMENTS

The editors wish to thank the following for drafting or commenting upon parts of the text in its various stages:

Professor B. Armstrong, Commissioner of Health for Western Australia, Perth, Australia

Dr D.F. Austin, Chief, Resource for Cancer Epidemiology, State of California Department of Health Services, Oakland, CA, USA

Dr R. Baserga, Department of Pathology, Temple University School of Medicine, Philadelphia, PA, USA

Dr F. Berrino, Director, Unit of Epidemiology, National Institute for Treatment and Research on Cancer, Milan, Italy

Dr D.A. Boyes, Director, Cancer Control Agency of British Columbia, Vancouver, BC, Canada

Professor L. Breslow, Professor of Public Health and Director, Health Services Research, Division of Cancer Control, University of California, Los Angeles, CA, USA

Dr L.A. Brinton, Chief, Environmental Studies Section, Environmental Epidemiology Branch, National Cancer Institute, Bethesda, MD, USA

Professor J. Cairns, Harvard School of Public Health, Boston, MA, USA

Professor P. Carbone, Chairman, Department of Human Oncology, Wisconsin Clinical Cancer Center, Madison, WI, USA

Dr J. Cohen, Adviser on Health Policy, Director-General's Office, World Health Organization, Geneva, Switzerland

Dr J. Crowley, Southwest Oncology Group – Statistical Center, Fred Hutchinson Cancer Research Center, Seattle, WA, USA

Dr A. Davis, Catcott, Bridgwater, Somerset, UK (formerly Head, Parasitic Diseases Programme, World Health Organization, Geneva, Switzerland)

Dr P.B. Desai, Director, Tata Memorial Centre, Bombay, India

Dr G. Hislop, Department of Epidemiology, Cancer Control Agency of British Columbia, Vancouver, BC, Canada

Professor O.M. Jensen, Director, Danish Cancer Registry, Copenhagen, Denmark

Dr M.S. Kanarek, Associate Professor, Preventive Medicine and Environmental Studies, Department of Preventive Medicine, University of Wisconsin, Madison, WI, USA

Dr P. Karran, Clare Hall Laboratories, Potter's Bar, Hertfordshire, UK

Dr L.J. Kinlen, Cancer Epidemiology Unit, University of Edinburgh, Edinburgh, UK

Professor S. Kramer, Department of Radiation Therapy and Nuclear Medicine, Thomas Jefferson University Hospital, Philadelpia, PA, USA

Professor T. Kuroki, Department of Cancer Cell Research, The Institute of Medical Science, The University of Tokyo, Tokyo, Japan

Dr E. Läärä, Department of Community Health, University of Kuopio, Kuopio, Finland

Dr P. Lawley, The Institute of Cancer Research: Royal Cancer Hospital, Chester Beatty Laboratories, London, UK

Dr D. Leon, Division of Medical Statistics and Epidemiology, London School of Hygiene and Tropical Medicine, London, UK

Dr R.A. Macbeth, National Institute of Canada, Canadian Cancer Society, Toronto, Ontario, Canada

Professor M.G. Marmot, Head, Department of Community Medicine, University College and Middlesex School of Medicine, University College London, London, UK

Dr D. Osoba, Sunnybrook Medical Centre, University of Toronto, Toronto, Ontario, Canada

Dr J.L. Pater, Director, Clinical Trials Group, National Cancer Institute of Canada, Kingston, Ontario, Canada

Dr F.G. Peers, Natal, North Coast, South Africa

Dr O. Pelkonen, Department of Pharmacology, Oulu, Finland

Dr F. Perera, Columbia University School of Public Health, New York, NY, USA

Professor H. Rubin, Department of Molecular Biology, University of California, Berkeley, CA, USA

Dr R. Santella, Columbia University School of Public Health, New York, NY, USA

Dr P. Swann, Courtauld Institute of Biochemistry, The Middlesex Hospital Medical School, London, UK

Dr F. Tejada, Oncology Associates of Miami, Miami, FL, USA

Dr J.M. Vasiliev, Cancer Research Center, USSR Academy of Medical Sciences, Moscow, USSR

Professor M.P. Vessey, Department of Community Medicine and General Practice, University of Oxford, Radcliffe Infirmary, Oxford, UK

Dr P. Vineis, Department of Biomedical Science and Human Oncology, University of Turin, Turin, Italy

Professor A. Wasunna, Department of Surgery, University of Nairobi, Faculty of Medicine, Nairobi, Kenya

Dr H.K. Weir, Division of Epidemiology and Statistics, The Ontario Cancer Treatment and Research Foundation, Toronto, Ontario, Canada

Professor W.C. Willett, Harvard School of Public Health, Channing Laboratory, Boston, MA, USA

Professor G.N. Wogan, Head, Department of Applied Biological Sciences, Massachusetts Institute of Technology, Cambridge, MA, USA

Dr S.H. Yuspa, Chief, Laboratory of Cellular Carcinogenesis and Tumor Promotion, National Cancer Institute, Bethesda, MD, USA

The following who are or were working at the IARC at the time, devoted particular time to preparation of various drafts of this book:

Dr H. Bartsch, Dr P. Boyle, Dr E. Cardis, Dr J. Cheney, Dr J. Estève, Dr M. Kogevinas, Dr G. Lenoir, Dr R. Montesano, Ms S.M. Moss, Dr C.S. Muir, Dr N. Muñoz, Dr S.A. Narod, Dr S. Preston–Martin, Dr R. Saracci, Dr A. Sasco, Dr L. Simonato, Professor R. Sohier, Dr H. Vainio, Dr J.P. Velema, Mr J. Wilbourn and Dr H. Yamasaki.

Invaluable technical help in the preparation of the manuscript was given by Mrs H. Biehe, Ms B. Fischer, Mrs A. Romanoff and Mrs J. Thévenoux.

INTRODUCTION

Aims of this book

The aims of this book are to present the available evidence on the preventability of human cancer, to describe its occurrence, to give information about the agents and risk factors that have been causally associated with the development of human cancer and about those for which there is reasonable suspicion of a causal relationship, and to give estimates of the extent to which deaths from cancer at some specific anatomical sites can actually be prevented.

The book addresses the causes, occurrence, primary prevention and early detection of cancer and concentrates on providing current information that could lead to practicable preventive intervention at the population level. Because of this focus, the entire field of genetics and cancer, currently undergoing major, innovative developments which may yield applications in the future, is touched upon only tangentially. We also do not discuss the very important issues of diagnosis and treatment of cancer, beyond the concise historical description given below. A first-class, detailed account of currently available means of cancer therapy is given in the exhaustive volume *Cancer Principles and Practice of Oncology* by V.T. DeVita, S. Hellman and S.A. Rosenberg (1985) and, more recently, by Frei *et al.* (1986). We also do not expand on the mechanisms by which cancer occurs, as several excellent books have been published on the subject; in addition, many easily available scientific journals provide up-to-date information on this particularly fast-moving area. Among the books that can be recommended are *The Biology of Cell Reproduction* by R. Baserga (1985); *Molecular Biology of the Cell* by B. Alberts, D. Bray, J. Lewis, R. Raff, K. Roberts and J.D. Watson (1989); and *Introduction to the Cellular and Molecular Biology of Cancer*, edited by L.M. Franks and N. Teich (1986).

This general introduction is followed by a section on the occurrence of cancer throughout the world (Part I). The frequency (incidence) of and number of deaths (mortality) from cancer are described, and geographical and other differences in occurrence are shown both for cancer as a whole and for cancers at particular body sites. Such descriptive epidemiology provides the global dimension to the cancer problem. It indicates which organs of the body are the most frequent targets, points to possible priorities for intervention and, by showing geographical and temporal trends in cancer incidence and mortality, provides the basis for hypotheses about the etiology of cancer.

Part II begins with a discussion of how causes of cancer are identified. Inherent to this aspect is knowledge of the mechanisms underlying the development of cancer – the carcinogenic process; and a very brief account is given, with a discussion of individual ('host') factors that alter susceptibility to tumour development, including genetic predisposition. The major part of this section of the book deals with known environmental determinants of cancer. We describe agents that are recognized as being causally related to human cancer, as well as those for which a causal relationship is not yet firmly established and factors that appear to modify risk but are at present only partially understood.

In Part III, we review the potential benefits of early detection – that is, the screening of individuals who have no overt symptom of the disease. In the final part (Part IV), we attempt to quantify the extent to which primary prevention and early detection are feasible for the most common cancers.

Conceptions and misconceptions about cancer

The term 'cancer' derives from the Latin *cancer* and from the Greek *karkinos*, both meaning 'crab'. Some types of malignant tumours were so described because swollen veins within them look like the claws of a crab, and, like a crab, a tumour has a central core and 'limbs', through which the disease spreads to the rest of the body. It is perhaps unfortunate that this disease, or rather this group of diseases, which is highly complex and which is today the second most frequent cause of death in many parts of the world, is still defined by a very vague descriptive term.

The definition of what constitutes a cancer has changed over the centuries, as the number and types of lesions that are grouped under this term have expanded. Today's glossaries tell you that a cancer is a malignant tumour, but there was for a long time confusion over whether nonmalignant lesions should be included in the term 'cancer'. Galen, in the second century AD, wrote a book in which he described 61 different kinds of what he called 'tumours contrary to nature' (*Tumores Praeter Naturam*), including among the cancerous lesions some that were not neoplasias, such as erysipelas and oedema (Galen, cited by Sigerist, 1956). Galen's ideas remained largely unchallenged for over a millenium.

The way in which cancer has been considered in different historical periods generally determined the practical measures taken to control it. Grouping nonmalignant tumours under this heading permitted the periodic rise of 'cancer cures' and of quacks specializing in curing 'cancers'. Uncertainties about its definition contributed to placing the stigma on cancer of being an incurable disease. The ancient, deeply rooted fear of cancer, for long seen as a curse of the gods, prevails, in spite of the fact that many of the misconceptions on which it was based have been eliminated. As we demonstrate in this book, several different causes of cancer have been identified, primary prevention can be implemented to a considerable extent, and therapy, aided by early diagnosis, can be efficiently used to cure several types of cancer.

The first known reference to human cancer, or at least to a disease which was probably cancer, goes back between 5300 and 4500 years (Grmek, 1975–76; Shimkin, 1977; Cassileth, 1983), but it is reasonable to assume that the human species was never completely sheltered from some form of deregulation of the biological control of cellular growth that may have, as its end point, malignant tumours.

The remains of animals that lived on this planet at the same time as primitive hominids or even earlier, and certainly much before *Homo sapiens*, bear traces of what have been interpreted as benign tumours, including signs of an osteoma and a haemangioma in a dinosaur that lived during the Cretaceous period, many million years ago. It is at least possible, therefore, that cancerous disease is older than the human species. Cancer can occur in all animal species that have been thoroughly studied. In a nonexhaustive list prepared in 1959 (Graffi & Bielka, 1959), tumours were reported to occur in 13 types of invertebrates, 16 types of birds, ten amphibians and 11 types of reptiles. More recently, it has been shown that malignant and benign tumours can be induced in all species that have been adequately tested. For instance, all of 39 species, ranging from insects to fish, reptiles and mammals, were susceptible to the carcinogenic activities of a group of chemicals known as *N*-nitroso compounds (Bogovski & Bogovski, 1981). Similarly, viruses can produce tumours in a variety of animal species, and uncontrolled growth with certain characteristics of malignancy occurs in plants, too. Cancer is therefore far from being a curse of the gods brought down only on human beings.

Cancer, although not unknown in childhood, is rare in people under the age of 30, but its frequency increases with age. The only exception to this trend with age (and which does not apply entirely to the area of the world where the childhood cancer, Burkitt's lymphoma, is common) is children between six and nine years of age, among whom the frequency appears to be slightly lower than that during the first few years of life. More than 60% of all cancer deaths in developed countries, however, occur in people over 65 years; the proportion in developing countries is about 40%, the difference being due largely to different age distributions in the two populations. But is the ageing process a sufficient explanation for the increasing frequency of cancer with age?

On the surface, it certainly is, since the older one becomes, at least until 75, the greater is one's risk for dying from cancer. In this sense, age is indeed the most important risk factor for cancer, but only because the older one becomes, the longer one is exposed to the factors that, directly or indirectly, increase the risk for developing a clinical cancer. Although predisposition to some cancers can be inherited, there is, in fact, no evidence that cancer is normally inscribed in the programme of our cells, and thus no evidence that most cancers are unavoidable (Cairns, 1978). With growing knowledge of the factors that cause cancer, there are more possibilities for avoiding it.

A large body of data points to the very important role of environmental factors in the causation of human cancer. As is discussed in detail in Chapter 1, the risk for cancer varies widely among different populations, with over 100-fold differences for the occurrence of certain tumours in adults, like cancers of the oesophagus and of the liver. Much smaller geographic variations in incidence occur for cancers of childhood, although for the commoner cancers, such as acute lymphocytic leukaemia and Wilms' tumour, differences certainly exist (Parkin *et al.*, 1988). These differences may result in part from genetic variations in risk, but they nevertheless provide some evidence that environmental factors also play a role in the origin of at least some tumours occurring in early life.

It is also relevant that the incidence of cancer remains particularly low in children and young adults. This would imply two things. Firstly, in the large majority of cases, the environmental risk factors to which people can be exposed at 'ordinary' levels (not the unusually high levels that have occurred and may occur in certain working environments, in cancer chemotherapy or during a catastrophic event like an atomic bomb explosion) exert their carcinogenic effect after several decades. The long period that in many instances elapses between what is usually thought to be the first event (often called 'initiation') of carcinogenesis and the clinical appearance of cancer can be considerably shortened, however, when the carcinogenic factors interact with predisposing genetic factors, in which case the role of 'ordinary' levels may be magnified by increased susceptibility. This might occur for a fraction of the tumours that appear within the first decade of life. Secondly, cancer incidence is low among people in their most active reproductive period, and thus does not interfere with the survival of the species. Cancer would thus appear to be predominantly a disease of individuals, and in particular of individuals who are well advanced into reproductive age or older; it does not have the characteristics of certain infectious diseases which can spread pandemically among people of all ages and could thus wipe out the human species.

Another misconception about cancer is that it is a disease of the rich, or at least of well-off people. This belief is probably rooted in the fact that since, in general, rich people used to live longer than the poor, they managed to reach the ages at which there is a higher risk for developing cancer. Analysis of data on mortality among people of different socioeconomic classes, however, clearly indicates that mortality rates, not only from all causes but also specifically from many types of cancer, are higher among the less favoured socioeconomic classes (Logan, 1982; Desplanques, 1984; Marmot & McDowall, 1986; Whitehead, 1987). Cancer is thus not a typical disease of affluence; when living conditions are raised above a minimal level, life expectancy is long enough to permit the majority of individuals to reach the age groups at which there is the greatest risk of cancer. However, even if this basic condition is satisfied, it is clear that more of the least favoured people die of cancer than the more favoured.

A great contribution to attempts to distinguish environmental from genetic causes of cancer has been studies of groups who have migrated from one country to another, and these studies are described in Part I. For several types of cancer, the incidence among migrants tends to diverge from that in their country of origin to become similar to that of the inhabitants of the host country. Since, in such studies, comparisons are made between groups that, although not necessarily identical in terms of social stratification, are genetically relatively similar, they provide good circumstantial evidence that migrants adapt to new environmental situations to the point that certain characteristics of a disease in which environmental factors play an important role are modified.

The identification of causative agents

The important changes in our view of cancer came about in conjunction with the introduction of the microscope for use in morbid anatomy, and subsequently with the discovery of the cellular origin of most pathological processes. The scientist who probably contributed the most to this revolution was Rudolph Virchow. Until his time, cancer had been thought to be the result of an imbalance in the humours, or vital body fluids. He was a great scientist and at the same time a strenuous supporter of the idea that diseases are determined by social, cultural and environmental factors (Rosen, 1958).

During the period when the new science of microbiology was expanding rapidly, much research was devoted to a search for the cancer germ, or bacterium. The failure to find such an organism probably contributed to the final disappearance of the belief that cancer is contagious. In fact, the conviction that it is not contagious became so well established that any association with transmissible agents became unacceptable. This may be the reason that the discovery by Peyton Rous of the viral origin of a certain sarcoma in birds (Rous, 1911) attracted very little attention. Rous was awarded the Nobel Prize for this discovery 55 years later, in 1966; and in the past few decades, evidence has accrued that infectious agents may play a substantial role in the causation of certain human cancers.

The observations that cancer can occur in all species studied and that it occurred in species that became extinct before the human species appeared on this planet suggest that the diseases grouped under the term 'cancer' are probably related to a deregulation of cellular division and growth, possibly linked to the evolutionary step from unicellular to multicellular organisms. However, a universal component of this kind is unlikely to be the sole cause of cancer: it is more likely that some factor increases the susceptibility of cells to other inherent (endogenous) and external (exogenous) factors (environmental, cultural and socioeconomic) and may push cells one or several steps towards malignancy.

The first agent to be described as carcinogenic was tobacco snuff (Hill, 1762); then chimney soot was found to be related to the scrotal cancer seen in chimney sweeps (Pott, 1775). During the nineteenth century, several chemicals to which people were exposed occupationally were found to be causally related to cancer, including aromatic amines (Rehn, 1895), which caused bladder cancer in workers in dye factories. Next came X-rays, which were reported to be carcinogenic less than ten years after their discovery by Roentgen (Frieben, 1902; Sick, 1902; Hesse, 1911, quoted by Hayward, 1965). It is of some interest to note that the much celebrated observation of Percival Pott on chimney sweeps is not mentioned in the entry under his name in the 11th edition of the *Encyclopaedia Britannica* (Anon., 1910), while his brilliant achievements as a surgeon are fully acknowledged. Similarly, there is no mention of the observation of Rehn on the frequency of bladder cancer in dye factory workers.

Less well defined risk factors were described even earlier. For example, an increased risk for breast cancer among nuns was reported by Ramazzini in 1713 and by Rigoni-Stern in 1842, with the hypothesis that the increase in risk could be related to the absence of an active reproductive life, in particular pregnancy and lactation.

To date, more than 50 agents or exposures have been identified as causes of human cancer. Most of these are defined chemicals or complex chemical mixtures (IARC, 1988), but they also include ionizing and nonionizing radiation and certain parasites and viruses. Several different agents may be at the origin of similar lesions; for example, although tobacco smoke is by far the most important cause of human lung cancer, exposure to about a dozen other distinct chemical agents is also causally related to the occurrence of lung cancer. Similarly, skin cancer can be induced by ionizing radiation and by ultra-violet light, as well as by a variety of chemicals. Such environmental agents are the cause, or probable cause, of a considerable, but so far ill defined, proportion of cases of human cancer (Wynder & Gori, 1977; Higginson & Muir, 1979; Doll & Peto, 1981). The difficulty of quantifying accurately the portion of risk that can be attributed to exposure to environmental agents is increased by the possibility that exposure to a carcinogenic agent may result in an increased risk for cancer, not only in the individual who is directly exposed, but also in progeny, as a consequence of prenatal exposure (Tomatis, 1988). It should be noted that the causes of some common cancers are as yet unknown.

The preponderance of chemicals among the recognized human carcinogens appears clearly to be related to industrial development, and in particular that of the chemical industry which began in the second half of the last century and has grown steadily since, with a spectacular leap forward after the Second World War. It is also related to the facility with which carcinogens are recognized in occupational groups exposed to high levels – situations sometimes referred to as 'natural experiments'. Industrial development took place initially with little if any concern for possible health effects. This was due partly to genuine ignorance, especially about long-term adverse effects such as cancer; later, however, adverse health effects were dismissed, either as unavoidable evils or as of too little importance to justify expensive modifications to production procedures. It is interesting that the industrial production of cigarettes began at the same time as the expansion of the chemical industry. The first cigarette factories were built in 1853 in Havana, in 1856 in London and in 1860 in Virginia. The human species has therefore been confronted only since the middle of the last century with both a massive increase in the amounts of man-made chemicals in the environment and expansion of the most carcinogenic cultural habit known. With the exception of ionizing radiation, ultra-violet light, combustion products, mycotoxins, *N*-nitroso compounds and certain viruses, the etiological agents of cancer that have so far been identified have been with us for only a relatively short time. To this list of recent human carcinogens can be added asbestos and certain metals, since their massive, systematic exploitation began only in the last century. It would be illusory to pretend that cancer could be prevented solely by controlling these relatively new carcinogenic agents, but it would be similarly deceptive to deny the usefulness of attempts to control their production and use: the industrial exploitation of natural resources and the synthesis of new chemicals have indeed generated new hazards and new carcinogens, to join the older ones.

Some of the chemicals and chemical mixtures that have so far been identified as carcinogenic to humans are widespread, such as tobacco smoke, asbestos, certain industrial chemicals and medical drugs, but there is no compelling evidence that we have yet identified all of the most important chemical carcinogens (Cairns, 1981). The great majority of tests used for the identification of carcinogenic agents are designed to identify agents that are assumed to act by direct interaction with DNA. Such tests are much less likely to assist us in identifying agents that contribute to subsequent phases of carcinogenesis or that act by mechanisms such as the amplification, deletion or recombination of genes.

The evolution of therapy

Cancer was considered by Hippocrates to be incurable, and he even discouraged attempts to operate on cancer patients, since he felt that surgical intervention would make the lesions worse. Celsus discouraged the cauterization of breast and skin cancers; however, he recommended surgery for cancer of the lip and a combination of surgery and cauterization with an arsenic ointment for cancer of the penis (Ackerknecht, 1965). Cancer of the breast, in spite of the opinion of Hippocrates, is the cancer for which the most numerous attempts at surgical intervention can be counted. Galen in the second century AD apparently successfully operated on a case of breast cancer, and, later, attempts were made by others, including Paul of Egina (seventh century) and Lanfranco (fourteenth century).

Generally, however, cancer was considered to be incurable. What is worse, in the seventeenth century the view became widespread that cancer (like leprosy) was contagious; this misconception was reinforced by the then famous clinicians Zacutus Lusitanus and Daniel Sennert (Ackerknecht, 1965; Cassileth, 1983). Every disease of which the origin is unknown, and which is therefore mysterious, evokes primitive fears, and such fears have often led to the conviction that a disease is both physically and morally contagious. Because of this view, cancer patients were refused admission to many hospitals. The first special hospital for cancer patients was created in Reims, France, in 1740, at the initiative of the canon Jean Godinot (D'Argent, 1965). In 1792, at the suggestion of the surgeon John Howard (a student of Percival Pott), a ward was opened at the Middlesex Hospital in London, for the express benefit of persons suffering from cancer (Hayward, 1965).

It was about a century more before a laboratory devoted specifically to cancer research was created, the first probably being that established in Buffalo, New York, in 1899, under the direction of Dr Roswell Park. In 1900, a Deutsches Komitee für Krebsforschung was created, which began its activities by making a census of cancer patients in Germany; what was probably the first international cancer congress was held in Heidelberg and Frankfurt in 1906 (Anon., 1910).

Substantial progress was made in the surgical therapy of cancer during the last part of the nineteenth century and the beginning of the twentieth. Of note are the advances in the surgery of abdominal cancer made by the great Austrian surgeon Christian Billroth in the 1870s, those by Wertheim in surgery of the uterus and those by William Hallsted in 1902 for cancer of the breast. Radiation was introduced as therapy for breast cancer at the end of the nineteenth century, just one year after Roentgen's discovery of it in 1895. In about the same period, the first journals devoted to cancer research were published – in France in 1896, in Germany in 1903, in Japan in 1907 and in Italy in 1911.

The youngest branch of cancer therapy is chemotherapy, if we disregard some of the older, mainly local treatments, such as arsenic ointment, used during the time of Celsus and Galen for cancers of the penis and of the skin. Chemotherapy was introduced in clinical oncology after the Second World War as a result of the extensive studies carried out during the War on the pharmacology of the nitrogen mustards and chloroethylamines, and the declassification of certain war-time experimental findings, in particular those concerning nitrogen mustard (Boyland & Horning, 1949; Cassileth, 1983).

It might be claimed, however, that the first time chemicals were used in cancer therapy, in a modern sense, was the use of oestrogens in the therapy of prostatic cancer (Huggins & Hodges, 1941; Hayward, 1965; Huggins, 1967). Huggins' contribution stemmed from the observation of White in 1894 that prostatic hypertrophy is hormone-dependent (Hayward, 1965) and from the experimental demonstration in the 1930s (Lacassagne, 1932, 1938) of the role of oestrogens in the causation of cancer.

The treatment of most forms of cancer still relies largely on surgery, combined for certain sites with radiotherapy and chemotherapy. Chemotherapy is also sometimes used alone. The adoption of elaborate chemotherapy protocols has resulted in considerably higher rates of durable regression or complete recovery for many of the tumours that appear early in life and those occurring before 30 years of age. The role of chemotherapy in extending survival from cancers or contributing to a durable remission of tumours occurring at later ages has been variously interpreted, and the percentage of cancer cases that can be successfully treated has been the subject of some controversy (Cairns *et al.*, 1983; DeVita *et al.*, 1985; Bailar & Smith, 1986; Frei *et al.*, 1986). The different estimates result, at least in part, from the fact that each author measured the effect of therapy in a different patient population. It may be that results obtained for a patient population treated in major institutions in countries where the most advanced therapeutic approaches are readily available provide a more optimistic estimate than results obtained for a less selected population. If current therapy for cancer were available throughout the world, it could reduce the number of deaths from cancer considerably.

It is a sad reality that in most parts of the world, including large areas of developed countries and most, if not all, developing countries, standards of health care and cancer treatment are far from optimal. Furthermore, it is very unlikely that the necessary funds for improving facilities and equipment and for training personnel will be available everywhere in the world in the near future. It is clear, therefore, that an increased effort should be made to *prevent* cancer whenever possible.

Cancer policy and priorities

Although there has probably never been a period when too much money was correctly spent on research devoted to protecting or improving health, the initiatives taken in the recent past to allocate large amounts of money specifically for the conquest of cancer have not been as successful as one might have wished.

Scientists have always been reminded periodically that funds for research are limited and that priorities must be established. This is often a very painful operation, which has a semi-random component and contains an unavoidable bias. The semi-random component is that scientists have a limited capacity to predict accurately which of several projects will succeed in producing meaningful results. The unavoidable bias is that projects that fall in line with the preferred orientations of granting agencies and contract makers are favoured. An equally unavoidable consequence is that some scientists, consciously or unconsciously, bend part of their intellectual capacity to satisfying requirements which guarantee the availability of funds. If pushed to an extreme, this behaviour may result in a situation in which the obtaining of funds is a conditioning and limiting factor in the design and development of research projects. The competition among scientists of different disciplines within the health sciences may purposely have been stimulated beyond a reasonable limit to divert attention from the true competition – between military expenditures (defense, as it is called) and expenditures to satisfy artificially created needs, and funds allocated for education and health.

The notion of multidisciplinarity is penetrating even the most impervious strongholds of pure science. It would be most beneficial if it were clear to all scientists that, not only are the various areas of research not mutually exclusive or incompatible, but, on the contrary, cross-fertilization may ensure greater possibilities of success. Thus, (i) basic and applied research, studies on the mechanisms of carcinogenesis and research on etiology and prevention are neither opposite nor separate areas of scientific activity; they must be, and indeed are, closely interrelated; and (ii) the assumption that only basic research is 'true' science, and that all other approaches to the primary prevention of cancer are not, is not justified and may reflect a certain degree of intellectual snobbery. There is a clear continuity between studies of the mechanisms of disease, epidemiological and laboratory-based investigations on etiology, and the implementation of primary prevention. To consider basic and applied research as separate and competing areas is a grave error which can only serve the purpose of preventing scientists from forming a common front in spending the available resources rationally and efficiently and perhaps in obtaining more of them.

References

Ackernecht, E.H. (1965) *History and Geography of the Most Important Diseases*, New York, Hufner

Alberts, B., Bray, D., Lewis, J., Raff, R., Roberts, K. & Watson, J.D. (1989) *Molecular Biology of the Cell*, New York, Garland Publishing

Anon. (1910) *Encyclopaedia Britannica*, 11th ed., Cambridge, Cambridge University Press

Bailar, J.C., 3rd & Smith, E.M. (1986) Progress against cancer? *New Engl. J. Med.*, *314*, 1126-1132

Baserga, R. (1985) *The Biology of Cell Reproduction*, Cambridge, MA, Harvard University Press

Bogovski, P. & Bogovski, S. (1981) Animal species in which N-nitroso compounds induce cancer. *Int. J. Cancer*, *27*, 471-474

Boyland, E. & Horning, E.S. (1949) The induction of tumours with nitrogen mustards. *Br. J. Cancer*, *3*, 118-123

Cairns, J. (1978) *Cancer: Science and Society*, San Francisco, W.H. Freeman

Cairns, J. (1981) The origin of human cancers. *Nature*, *289*, 353-357

Cairns, J., Boyle, P. & Frei, E., 3rd (1983) Cancer chemotherapy [Letter]. *Science*, *220*, 252-256

Cassileth, B.R. (1983) The evolution of oncology. *Perspect. Biol. Med.*, *26*, 362-374

D'Argent, M. (1965) Une dissertation académique sur le cancer, à Lyon, en 1773. *L'Ouest Méd.*, *8*, 455-477

Desplanques, G. (1984) L'inégalité sociale devant la mort en France (1975-1980): une étude longitudinale. *Soz. Präventivmed.*, *29*, 268-272

DeVita, V.T., Hellman, S. & Rosenberg, S.A. (1985) *Cancer Principles and Practice of Oncology*, New York, Lippincott

Doll, R. & Peto, R. (1981) The causes of cancer. Quantitative estimates of avoidable risks of cancer in the United States today. *J. Natl Cancer Inst.*, *66*, 1192-1307

Franks, L.M. & Teich, N., eds (1986) *Introduction to the Cellular and Molecular Biology of Cancer*, Oxford, Oxford University Press

Frei, E., 3rd, Miller, D., Clark, J.R., Fallon, B.G. & Ervin, T.J. (1986) Clinical and scientific considerations in preoperative (neoadjuvant) chemotherapy. *Recent Results Cancer Res.*, *103*, 1-5

Frieben, A. (1902) Demonstration eines Cancroids der rechten Handruckens, das sich nach langdauernder Einwirkung von Röntgenstrahlen entwickelt hat. *Fortschr. Roentgenstr.*, *6*, 106-111

Graffi, A. & Bielka, H. (1959) *Probleme der Experimentellen Krebsforschung*, Bd. 6, Leipzig, Akademische Verlagsgesellschaft

Grmek, M.D. (1975-1976) La paléopathologie des tumeurs osseuses malignes. Proposition d'une classification à l'usage de l'ostéo-archéologie, revue des exemples publiés et présentation de deux cas inédits. *Hist. Sci. Med.*, *9*, 21-50

Hayward, O.S. (1965) The history of oncology. *Surgery*, *58*, 460-468, 586-599

Higginson, J. & Muir, C.S. (1979) Environmental carcinogenesis: misconceptions and limitations to cancer control. *J. Natl Cancer Inst.*, *63*, 1291-1298

Hill, J. (1762) Tobacco cancers: Hill and Soemmering. In: Shimkin, M.B., ed. (1977) *Contrary to Nature. Being an Illustrated Commentary on Some Persons and Events of Historical Importance in the Development of Knowledge Concerning Cancer*, Washington DC, Department of Health, Education, and Welfare, pp. 93-94

Huggins, C. (1967) Endocrine-induced regression of cancers. *Science*, 156, 1050-1054

Huggins, C. & Hodges, C.V. (1941) Studies on prostatic cancer. I. The effect of castration, of estrogen and of androgen injection on serum phosphatase in metastatic carcinoma of the prostate. *Cancer Res.*, *1*, 293-297

IARC (1988) *IARC Monographs on the Evaluation of Carcinogenic Risks to Humans*, Vol. 44, *Alcohol Drinking*, Lyon

Lacassagne, A. (1932) Apparition de cancers de la mamelle chez les souris males, soumis à des injections de folliculine. *Comp. Rend. Acad. Sci.*, *195*, 630-632

Lacassagne, A. (1938) Apparition d'adénocarcinomes mammaires chez les souris males, traitées par une substance oestrogène synthétique. *Comp. Rend. Soc. Biol.*, *229*, 641-643

Logan, W.P.D. (1982) *Cancer Mortality by Occupation and Social Class, 1851-1971* (IARC Scientific Publications No. 36; Studies on Medical and Population Subjects No. 44), Lyon, IARC

Marmot, M.G. & McDowall, M.E. (1986) Mortality decline and widening social inequalities. *Lancet*, *ii*, 247-276

Parkin, D.M., Stiller, C.A., Draper, G.J. & Bieber, A. (1988) International incidence of childhood cancer. *Int. J. Cancer*, *42*, 511-520

Pott, P. (1775) Chimney sweeps' cancer. In: Shimkin, M.B., ed. (1977) *Contrary to Nature. Being an Illustrated Commentary on Some Persons and Events of Historical Importance in the Development of Knowledge Concerning Cancer*, Washington DC, Department of Health, Education, and Welfare, pp. 95-96

Rehn, L. (1895) Aniline bladder cancer. In: Shimkin, M.B., ed. (1977) *Contrary to Nature. Being an Illustrated Commentary on Some Persons and Events of Historical Importance in the Development of Knowledge Concerning Cancer*, Washington DC, Department of Health, Education, and Welfare, pp. 165-166

Rosen, G. (1958) *A History of Public Health*, New York, MD Publications

Rous, P. (1911) Chicken sarcomas. In: Shimkin, M.B., ed. (1977) *Contrary to Nature. Being an Illustrated Commentary on Some Persons and Events of Historical Importance in the Development of Knowledge Concerning Cancer*, Washington DC, Department of Health, Education, and Welfare, pp. 217-218

Shimkin, M.B., ed. (1977) *Contrary to Nature. Being an Illustrated Commentary on Some Persons and Events of Historical Importance in the Development of Knowledge Concerning Cancer*, Washington DC, Department of Health, Education, and Welfare

Sick, H. (1902) Karzinom der Haut das auf dem Boden eines Röntgenulcus entstanden ist. *Münch. Med. Wochenschr.*, *50*, 1445

Sigerist, H.E. (1956) *Landmarks in the History of Hygiene*, Oxford, Oxford University Press

Tomatis, L. (1988) Prenatal carcinogenesis. In: Kakunaga, T., Sugimura, T., Tomatis, L. & Yamasaki, H., eds, *Cell Differentiation, Genes and Cancer* (IARC Scientific Publications No. 92), Lyon, IARC, pp. 121-132

Whitehead, M. (1987) *The Health Divide: Inequalities in Health in the 1980s*, London, Health Education Authority

Wynder, E. & Gori, G.B. (1977) Contribution of the environment to cancer incidence: an epidemiological exercise. *J. Natl Cancer Inst.*, *58*, 825-832

PART I

THE OCCURRENCE OF CANCER

Chapter 1. Measuring the burden of cancer

Descriptive epidemiology is used to investigate the occurrence of cancer in different population groups. The objective may be simply to enumerate the size of the problem that cancer poses to health (how many cases, how many deaths) or, more often, to investigate how the *risk* for developing cancer varies in relation to different attributes of the populations studied, such as their place of residence, ethnicity, social status or occupation. Studies of changes in the risk for developing cancer can be made by measuring the risk in the same population at different periods of time.

Variations in incidence rates between different population groups, as defined by personal ('demographic') variables or by place of residence, may suggest the importance of environmental factors in the causation of a particular cancer. Therefore, descriptive epidemiological data are often described as 'hypothesis generating'. It may sometimes be possible to obtain quantitative data on the exposure of populations to environmental factors – for example, the level of an atmospheric pollutant, or the average intake of a dietary item. Then, so-called 'ecological studies' are possible, in which the strength of an association between disease risk and the level of exposure is tested – but always at the level of a population rather than for individuals. The study of exposure in relation to disease risk in individuals is the domain of analytical epidemiology.

In this chapter, we review the measures that are used to define both the burden of and the risk for disease in human populations, and we illustrate the way in which studies of risk in relation to geography, personal variables and time can provide important information on etiology. Finally, the descriptive epidemiology of the major types of cancer is reviewed systematically.

Measurement

Measuring the risk for cancer

In studies in which the aim is to elucidate the etiology of cancer, the risk for disease must be estimated. At the level of a population, this is most conveniently expressed as the incidence rate. When data on incidence are not available, surrogate measures such as rates of mortality or relative frequency (proportions) of different cancers must be used.

The increase in risk associated with a given exposure, measured in terms of an observed increase in the rate of incidence of the cancer in question, as discussed below, can be expressed either in absolute terms – the extra number of cases per head of population per year – or in proportional terms – the proportional increase over the observed background incidence rate. For certain practical reasons, the latter is often the more convenient measure: background rates of cancer incidence vary very widely by age and, to a lesser extent, among populations, but, empirically, for many exposures, the excess risk has been shown to be approximately proportional to the background risk. Therefore, the proportional increase can be expressed simply in quantitative terms, often by a single number. The absolute excess risk often varies more widely with age and between populations, and is poorly expressed by a single figure.

Proportional increase in risk is usually expressed by the *'relative risk'*, defined simply as the ratio of the incidence rate in the exposed population to that in the unexposed population. Relative risks are sometimes defined in terms of mortality rather than incidence rates, but the difference between them should be small.

When the cancer in question is very rare in the unexposed population, the absolute rather than relative risk is a better measure of effect. For example, associations usually described in terms of absolute risk include those between asbestos and mesothelioma, vinyl chloride and angiosarcoma of the liver, and diethylstilboestrol and adenocarcinoma of the vagina.

Incidence

Incidence refers to the new cases of cancer that occur in a defined population, and the incidence *rate* is the number of such events in a specified period of time referred to a standard unit of population. Since incidence rates relate to a period of time, it is necessary to define the exact date of onset of disease. In cancer epidemiology, this is usually taken as the date of definitive diagnosis.

The 'instantaneous rate' or 'force of morbidity' (the true 'risk for disease') is given by the incidence rate for an infinitely short time period. In practice, since cancer is a relatively rare event, quite large populations must be observed over a period of several years. Incidence rates are conventionally expressed in terms of annual rates (per year) per 100 000 population, and when data are collected over several years the denominator is converted to an estimate of person-years of observation (number of years of observation multiplied by the average size of the population under observation).

As discussed later (p. 37), the most powerful determinant of an individual's risk for cancer is age: the incidence of most cancers rises sharply with age. Thus, comparisons of incidence rates in different populations must be made between groups of the same age, by calculating age-specific rates, rather than by using rates for the whole population calculated without regard to age (crude rates). The crude rate is strongly influenced by the age structure of the population.

Comparisons of large tables of rates are time-consuming and sometimes difficult to interpret. For this reason, 'standardization' procedures are often employed – in which summary figures are produced with the aim of retaining important information about the comparison of interest (Doll & Cook, 1967; Inskip *et al.*, 1983). In the *direct method*, age-specific rates for the group under study are applied to a hypothetical standard population, the number of cases of cancer to be expected in the standard population is determined and the corresponding standardized rate calculated. The most commonly used standard population for this purpose is the 'World Standard Population' (Doll & Smith, 1982), and, in this book, all of the age-standardized rates presented are standardized to this population and are hence comparable. Cancer risk can also be expressed in terms of the risk that a person has of developing, or dying from, a specific cancer during his lifespan or a defined portion thereof, by use, for example, of the 'cumultive risk' derived from the 'cumulative rate' (Day, 1976).

While rates are the most commonly used measure of cancer occurrence, it may be convenient to express the risk of a particular group relative to that of some other population. For this purpose, the standardized incidence ratio (SIR) may be calculated. This is the number of cases of cancer in a given group expressed as a percentage of the number that would have been expected in that group on the basis of the age- and sex-specific rates for the comparison population (usually the general population). This method is referred to as 'indirect standardization'. The SIR (or the analogous standardized mortality ratio (SMR)) is widely used for comparing population groups within a single country – for example, from different provinces, social classes or occupational groups. However, the values are meaningful only in comparison to a standard population, and the values for subgroups cannot be compared directly with each other, as they can using directly standardized rates (Rothman, 1986).

It must be remembered that age-standardized rates, although convenient, are summary figures, and like all summaries they may hide important detail.

Mortality

Mortality rates are calculated and interpreted in precisely the same way as incidence rates, except that the event being measured is, of course, death from cancer rather than its diagnosis. The fact of death from cancer is rarely of interest in cancer epidemiology (except in studies of survival and of cancer burden), but, because data on mortality are generally more readily available than those on incidence, they are widely used as proxy measures of cancer occurrence. For cancers for which there is a high fatality rate, such as those of the oesophagus, pancreas, lung and liver, the measurement of death rates gives a good indication of risk for the disease. For cancers from which only a proportion of patients die, such as those of the breast and colon, mortality rates provide an underestimation of the incidence to an equivalent extent; however, since most epidemiological studies are concerned with comparisons (between population groups), comparisons of mortality rates can indicate the size of a difference in risk, provided that the fatality rate in the two groups is more or less the same. This is usually the case, although there have been exceptions. On the basis of a case-control study of prevalent cases of leukaemia, Rogentine *et al.* (1972) originally drew the conclusion that the risk for acute leukaemia was associated with the presence of certain human histocompatibility locus antigens (HLA); however, they later found that this factor influenced survival rather than incidence (Rogentine *et al.*, 1973).

For those tumours with improved prognosis due to modern treatment, such as childhood leukaemia, Hodgkin's disease and testicular cancer, mortality rates have declined with time, with no corresponding decrease in incidence. In such circumstances, time trends in mortality rates are a useless guide to changing risk for the disease. Mortality rates are also of little value for the study of cancers with low fatality rates, such as skin tumours.

Relative frequency

In many parts of the world, data are not available on incidence or mortality rates, and all that can be obtained is information on series of patients seen in one or more hospitals or studied in pathology laboratories. Since the characteristics of the population from which cases were drawn is not known, rates cannot be calculated, and the series can be compared only in terms of the proportional distribution of different types of cancer – the relative frequency. Comparisons can then be made between different series – from different areas, different ethnic groups or different time periods.

Such comparisons pose several problems. The first is that the ratio of two relative frequencies does not represent the ratio of incidence rates. Since the relative frequencies of the cancers in different series must always total 100%, the ratio between two percentages will be the same as the ratio between their incidence rates only if the overall incidence rates (for all cases) are also the same. A more serious problem is that case series almost always represent a biased sample of the tumours that are actually occurring in the population and may differ from the true situation in various ways, including tumour type, sex, age and socioeconomic group, depending on the source of the cases. In series from pathology departments, for example, easily accessible tumours may be overrepresented in comparison with those at internal sites which are diagnosed by other means (see Parkin, 1986).

Despite these drawbacks, data on relative frequency are often all that is available for many parts of the world, for which they provide the only information on cancer patterns.

Availability of data

The data on which descriptive epidemiology is based are statistics from different countries and international organizations, such as the World Health Organization, on mortality from and incidence and relative frequency of cancer. In order that such statistics can be put together, and so that statistics from different regions can be compared, an International Classification of Diseases (ICD; in full, the International Statistical Classification of Diseases, Injuries and Causes of Death) was established by the World Health Organization and is revised regularly. In this huge classification, codes are given for each entity, with several subdivisions for greater precision. In this volume, when ICD codes are mentioned to define a cancer site, they are those of the ninth revision (ICD-9; World Health Organization, 1977, 1978).

Mortality statistics

Data on mortality are produced through the vital statistics systems of many countries, in which not only the fact of death and some personal details about each person who dies are recorded, but also the cause of death, frequently as determined by a medical practitioner. The format of the part of the death certificate on which the cause of death is recorded has now been standardized (World Health Organization, 1977), so that statistics of deaths by cause can be produced.

In some countries, death certificates are completed by non-medical personnel; this inevitably results in inaccurate statements of 'cause of death', ranging from defects in precision (e.g., simply 'cancer' as the underlying cause) to inability to specify any diagnosis. However, even when death certificates are signed by physicians, there is no guarantee that the quality of the statements on cause of death will be good; many studies have shown that the registered cause of death may differ from the 'true' diagnosis, as judged at autopsy or by review of clinical records (Moriyama *et al.*, 1958; Heasman & Lipworth, 1966). In a study of over 43 000 deaths in ten Latin American cities (plus Bristol and San Francisco), Puffer and Wynn-Griffith (1967) found that of the 8800 deaths that were finally ascribed to cancer, 92% had been recorded as 'cancer' on the death certificate; however, there were marked variations in the accuracy with which the correct body site had been identified. A common finding was lack of specificity in certification, e.g., assigning carcinoma of both the cervix and corpus uteri to 'uterus'. Almost half of the deaths assigned to 'benign and unspecified neoplasms' proved to be due to malignant tumours. A further problem arises in that different rules may be used for selecting 'underlying' cause of death from the certificate in statistical offices in different countries, which can lead to quite wide divergences between countries in the numbers of deaths allocated to a specific type of cancer, even when the same certificates are being interpreted (Percy & Dolman, 1978). A certain amount of caution is therefore required in using mortality rates as indirect indicators of cancer risk or occurrence.

Data on mortality from cancer in many countries are collected by the World Health Organization and presented in tabular form in the *World Health Statistics Annual*. In some countries, mortality statistics have been published for over 100 years; the data of the World Health Organization start from 1950–55. Cancer mortality statistics are available for almost all of the 'developed' countries but for relatively few countries in Asia and Africa (Table 1). The quality of the data is far from uniform, however, and in many countries, particularly in the developing world, there is clear under-enumeration of deaths from cancer (with mortality rates far below what might reasonably be expected), and a large proportion of deaths are ascribed to the category 'senility and ill defined conditions'.

The material available from the World Health Organization is for entire national populations; however, in most countries data can be provided for much smaller geographic subdivisions and can be categorized by other demographic variables. These data are an invaluable resource in studies on the descriptive epidemiology of cancer.

Incidence statistics

Rates of the incidence of cancer can be derived only from population-based cancer registries. The number of such registries in the world has increased steadily over the last 50 years, but, in comparison with the availability of data on mortality, the population so covered remains relatively limited (Table 1). Furthermore, the populations served by cancer registries are often not representative of a country as a whole, comprising only the inhabitants of a major city, for example.

Cancer registration is quite a complex undertaking, and careful quality control is essential to ensure that the resulting data on incidence are valid and reliable. The major problem, however, is ensuring that every new case of cancer is identified. The ease with which this can be done depends on the extent of the medical facilities available and the quality of the statistical and recording systems already in place (e.g., pathology request forms, hospital discharge abstracts, treatment records). A further difficulty is identifying individuals and ascertaining that they do in fact come from the population under study. These problems are

Table 1. Availability (1980) of data on mortality from and incidence of cancers by United Nations area

Area	Population (millions)	% of population for which data are available	
		Mortality data	Incidence data
World	4453	37.5	14
Developed countries	1136	100	58
Less developed countries	3317	16	2.3
Africa	476	9	0.5
Eastern Africa	137	0.7	(0.5)[a]
Middle Africa	55	0	0
Northern Africa	108	38	0
Southern Africa	33	0	0
Western Africa	144	0.2	(1)[b]
Latin America	362	97	9.6
Caribbean	30	80	46
Central America	92	100	2.5-4.7[c]
Temperate South America	42	100	1.7
Tropical South America	198	97[d]	9
Northern America	252	100	34[e]
Asia	2591	10	3.3
China	1003	0 (100)[f]	1
Japan	117	100	43[g]
Other eastern Asia	63	8	8
South eastern Asia	362	27	2.4
Southern Asia	949	1.5	1
Western Asia	98	14	53
Europe	484	99	26 (38)
Eastern Europe	110	100	27-80[h]
Northern Europe	82	100	95
Southern Europe	139	98	9
Western Europe	154	100	6
Oceania	23	81	81
Australia/New Zealand	18	100	100
Melanesia	4	14	20
Micronesia/Polynesia	0.8	0	0
USSR	265	100[i]	100[i]

[a] Estimated rates, Kilimanjaro Registry, 1975-79
[b] Estimated rates, Ibadan Registry, 1970-76
[c] Figure of 4.7 includes histologically verified cases only from the Panamanian Registry
[d] Rates for Brazil based on a sample only
[e] Canada, Delaware, Los Angeles, CA, New Jersey, New Orleans, LA, New York, Rhode Island, Virginia and the Surveillance, Epidemiology and End Results (SEER) programme of the USA
[f] Available from a mortality survey, 1973-75, but not routinely
[g] 13 prefectures and two cities (Research Group for Population-based Cancer Registration in Japan, 1981)
[h] 20% represents those registries contributing to *Cancer Incidence in Five Continents* (see Napalkov & Eckhardt, 1982)
[i] A few sites only

more difficult to surmount in developing countries, which explains why relatively few registries have succeeded in surviving for long.

Incidence statistics from cancer registries around the world are published in the series of compilations *Cancer Incidence in Five Continents* (Doll *et al.*, 1966, 1970; Waterhouse *et al.*, 1976, 1982; Muir *et al.*, 1987), which also contain a description of the methods used to measure the validity of registry data.

In general, the accuracy of data on diagnosis recorded in cancer registries is superior to that of death certificates, although review of registration often reveals the presence of errors (West, 1976). An additional advantage is that information from histological examinations may be available. Changes in the completeness of registration over time, and in the definition of what constitutes an 'incident' case of cancer, may, however, complicate interpretation of series of cases from cancer registries over time (see discussion by Doll & Peto, 1981).

Relative frequency statistics

These data are readily generated from information on series of cancer patients, such as those attending one or more hospitals, treated in a particular service, or diagnosed in one or more laboratories. As discussed above, interpretation of such data is much less straightforward than the interpretation of population-based incidence and mortality statistics. However, they may be all that is available from many parts of the world and can yield useful information on probable differences in risk by place, time or personal variables.

Measuring the burden of cancer

'Burden' is a concept without formal definition but which implies the quantity of a particular disease in a community – hence, its importance as a challenge to health and related services, and to society as a whole.

Burden can be expressed simply as the number of new cases of a disease (incidence) or as a number of deaths (mortality), and comparisons can be made between the different diseases (or causes of death) or between different cancers. The world burden of cancer has been estimated in terms of new cases by Parkin *et al.* (1988) and as numbers of deaths by Hakulinen *et al.* (1986).

The prevalence of cancer is defined as the proportion of a population alive at a given time who have cancer; it is proportional to the incidence of the disease multiplied by its average duration. Prevalence is often advanced as a useful measure of cancer burden, since it indicates the number of patients who are alive and require medical care. However, there is no standard definition of a prevalent case of cancer: it can refer to all persons currently alive who were ever diagnosed as having 'cancer'; it might exclude patients considered to be 'cured' – that is, those still alive in the first three to five years after diagnosis; or it can refer only to patients being followed-up actively. It is probably easier to estimate the needs for health care services from knowledge about incidence and about the average resources required for each patient.

A further measure of burden is the person-years of life lost (PYLL) due to cancer. This calculation takes into account not only the number of deaths from different cancers but also the *age* at death, so that deaths occurring in young people – who might have been expected to live for many more years – receive a much greater weighting than deaths in the elderly. This measure has been used for defining priorities for health care, and particularly for preventive services.

Several methods can be used to calculate the PYLL due to a given cause (Romeder & McWhinnie, 1977), the main difference being the definition of the age to which persons might have been expected to live if they had not died from the disease in question – in this case, cancer. In practice, the simplest solution is to choose an arbitrary upper age (usually between 65 and 75) to which everyone would be expected to live. Although this assumption does not take into account the probability of dying from other causes, for comparative purposes this makes little difference to the results. In this chapter, PYLL before the age of 70 have been calculated for different populations. When comparisons are made between populations of different sizes, PYLL must be compared in relation to that of a population at risk of fixed size.

The number of PYLL is influenced not only by the number of deaths, but by their distribution by age. This, in turn, is the result of the interplay of two factors – the age-specific death rates and the age structure of the population. In young populations, such as those in the developing countries, a larger proportion of deaths will occur among young people, so that causes of death that predominate among the young will result in a number of PYLL that is relatively large in relation to the size of the population. If one is interested in making comparisons in which the effect of population structure is excluded, this can be done using the World Standard Population (see p. 16). This produces a standardized rate of PYLL, calculated as the years of life that would be lost if the population under study had the same age structure as the standard population.

Counts of cases, deaths or PYLL are objective measures of the size of the cancer problem. Programmes of primary prevention aim to reduce the number of cases of cancer occurring. Early detection and treatment aim to reduce the number of deaths and, more optimally, the number of PYLL, since it is generally agreed that preventing a 'young' death is more valuable than preventing a death in old age. Cancer therapy may also have objectives related to improving the quality of life of cancer patients, even though death is not deferred, for example by the relief of pain or by the maintenance of independence. The difficulties in agreeing upon objective measures of 'quality of life' in no way detract from the importance of trying to do so.

The burden of cancer in the world

Numbers of cases

The burden of cancer in the world in terms of numbers of cases of cancer of 16 types in each of 24 geographical areas has been estimated for the year 1980 by Parkin *et al.* (1988). A wide variety of sources was used to make these estimations. The primary source was information on cancer incidence rates derived from population-based cancer registries – such data were used whenever they were available. When incidence data were not available, rates were estimated statistically on the basis of rates of mortality. For many countries and for some entire areas for which neither incidence rates nor mortality data were available, the frequency of different tumours was used together with estimates of the crude incidence rate for cancers at all sites.

It was estimated that approximately 6.35 million cases of cancer occurred in 1980, of which 3.25 million were in men and 3.10 million in women. These figures exclude skin cancer (other than melanoma), which, although very common, is generally not fatal; it is also poorly recorded in incidence statistics and not reflected in mortality statistics. When data for people of each sex were combined, stomach cancer was seen to be the most common cancer in 1980 (10.5% of the total; see Table 2). However, with the world-wide incidence of stomach cancer estimated to be declining at a rate of 2.2% each year, and with the rising frequency of lung cancer, the latter would have become the most frequent tumour in the world by the end of 1981. The second most striking feature seen in Table 2 is the frequency of the two specifically female cancers – breast cancer and cancer of the uterine cervix. These together account for one-third of cancers in females, and breast cancer is the third most frequent cancer in the world, even when people of each sex are considered together. Colorectal cancer is almost exactly as frequent in men as in women; it is fourth in frequency overall, and, like lung cancer, appears to be increasing in incidence.

Figure 1 shows the distribution of the numbers of cancers at the 16 anatomical sites, and their relative ranks, in the developed and the developing countries. Overall, the number of cases is quite evenly divided: 49.3% of cases in the developed countries and 50.7% in developing countries, even though the ratio of populations is 1:3. However, the numbers and the rankings of the cancers are quite different. In developed countries, lung cancer is the predominant form of cancer (22.3% of cancers among men) and breast cancer is the most common in women (22.9% of cancers). In the developing countries, cervical cancer poses the major problem, accounting for 24% of cancers among women; in some areas, such as sub-Saharan Africa and Latin America, it accounts for a considerably greater percentage.

Numbers of deaths

A working group on cancer statistics at the World Health Organization (1976) estimated that approximately one death in every five in western countries could be attributed directly to cancer. Estimates of the numbers of deaths due to different causes have also been prepared (Hakulinen *et al.*, 1986a). The basis for these estimates was a simple statistical model, introduced by Preston (1976), which gave a summary of mortality from 17 broad groups of causes (one such group being the neoplasms) in over 200 populations in various stages of development. This study suggested that 4.2 million deaths had been due to cancer in the world in 1980.

Table 3 shows the relative importance of cancer as a cause of death in relation to other causes, in the world as a whole and in several different regions. On a world scale, cancer is third in importance, well behind the infectious diseases and disorders of the circulatory system. However, cancer is relatively much more important in developed countries (19.2% of deaths). It appears to be less important in the developing world (5.5% of deaths) partly because of the younger

Table 2. The most frequent cancers throughout the world, 1980

Ranking	Males			Females		
	Site	No.	%	Site	No.	%
1	Lung	513.6	15.8	Breast	572.1	18.4
2	Stomach	408.8	12.6	Cervix	465.6	15.0
3	Colon/rectum	286.2	8.8	Colon/rectum	285.9	9.2
4	Mouth/pharynx	257.3	7.9	Stomach	260.6	8.4
5	Prostate	235.8	7.3	Corpus uteri	148.8	4.8
6	Oesophagus	202.1	6.2	Lung	146.9	4.7
7	Liver	171.7	5.3	Ovary	137.6	4.4
8	Bladder	167.7	5.2	Mouth/pharynx	121.2	3.9
9	Lymphoma	139.9	4.3	Oesophagus	108.2	3.5
10	Leukaemia	106.9	3.3	Lymphoma	98.0	3.2

Ranking	Both sexes		
	Site	No.	%
1	Stomach	669.4	10.5
2	Lung	660.5	10.4
3	Breast	572.1	9.0
4	Colon/rectum	572.1	9.0
5	Cervix	465.6	7.3
6	Mouth/pharynx	378.5	6.0
7	Oesophagus	310.4	4.9
8	Liver	251.2	4.0
9	Lymphoma	237.9	3.7
10	Prostate	235.8	3.7
11	Bladder	219.4	3.5
12	Leukaemia	188.2	3.0

age of most of these populations, which results in a lower crude mortality rate from cancer, and the higher proportion of deaths from infectious diseases.

An indication of the changes that have occurred over the last 20 years in the proportions of deaths due to different causes for selected regions is given in Table 4. In all the regions listed, and in people of each sex, an increased proportion of deaths has been certified as due to neoplasms, coinciding in some, but not all, with a reduction in the proportion due to disorders of the circulatory system (the most important single cause of death in all regions shown) and in the number of deaths due to infections. However, the increase in the proportion of deaths due to neoplasms has been greatest in those countries in which there were relatively low proportions in 1960. This increase in the importance of cancer as a cause of death might be expected to continue, particularly in the developing world, where infectious diseases are being controlled and the population is living to greater ages.

Figure 1. Numbers of cases of cancer at 16 anatomical sites in developed and in developing countries, with relative ranks[a]

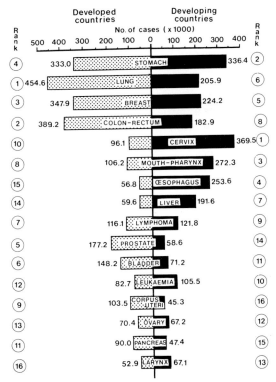

[a] From Parkin *et al.* (1988)

Table 3. Global and regional patterns of annual deaths by cause around 1980 (after Hakulinen *et al.*, 1986b)

Region	All causes (no. of deaths x 1000)	Infections and parasitic diseases (%)	Neo-plasms (%)	Diseases of the circulatory system (%)	Peri-natal condi-tions	Injury and poisoning (%)	Other and unknown (%)
World	50 911	33.1	8.4	26.2	6.4	5.3	20.7
Africa	8 562	48.7	3.1	12.3	8.7	3.8	23.4
Latin America	3 197	31.0	9.0	24.7	8.3	8.3	20.7
North America	2 081	3.6	21.5	54.5	1.2	8.4	10.8
East Asia	8 842	23.0	10.6	33.7	4.3	7.2	21.3
South Asia	20 315	43.8	4.3	15.6	8.4	4.3	23.6
Europe[a]	7 713	8.6	18.1	53.8	1.8	5.8	12.0
Oceania	201	17.7	16.0	42.2	3.2	6.7	14.1
More developed	10 652	7.6	19.2	53.6	1.6	6.4	11.7
Less developed	40 259	39.9	5.5	19.0	7.7	4.9	23.1

[a] Including the USSR

Person-years of life lost due to cancer

In Table 5, the importance of cancer is compared with that of five other broad categories of cause of death – infectious and parasitic diseases, cerebrovascular disorders, other diseases of the circulatory system, respiratory diseases, and injuries and poisoning – in terms of numbers of deaths and of PYLL in people under the age of 70. Data from nine regions in different areas of the world are used. It is clear that, in general, cancer is relatively less important as a cause of death in men under the age of 70 than in women; in women, it is the leading cause of death in eight of these nine countries. For men, circulatory diseases are the leading cause of death in five countries, and cancer the leading cause in three countries. Chile is the only country of the nine in which neither cancer nor circulatory disease, but injury and poisoning, is the most important cause of death in people under the age of 70.

Table 4. Percentages of deaths due to different causes for selected regions, around 1960 and 1980, all ages

Region	Cancer		Infectious/ parasitic diseases		Circulatory diseases		Respiratory diseases		Injury/ poisoning		Other/ unknown	
	1960	1980	1960	1980	1960	1980	1960	1980	1960	1980	1960	1980
Males												
Chile	7	14	9	5	14	24	21	10	10	17	39	30
USA	15	21	2	1	53	48	6	7	9	11	15	12
Japan	14	24	7	2	33	40	7	8	12	9	27	17
Sweden	18	21	1	1	51	55	6	6	8	7	16	10
England and Wales	19	24	1	0[a]	48	49	15	15	5	4	12	8
Portugal	9	14	8	2	25	39	12	9	6	10	40	26
Australia	15	22	1	1	52	48	8	8	9	10	15	11
Females												
Chile	9	18	8	5	16	30	22	10	3	6	42	31
USA	17	21	1	1	56	53	4	6	5	5	17	14
Japan	13	21	5	1	35	46	7	7	6	5	34	20
Sweden	19	22	1	1	54	55	6	6	4	5	16	11
England and Wales	18	21	1	0[a]	55	51	10	14	4	3	12	11
Portugal	9	13	5	2	31	46	10	7	3	4	42	28
Australia	16	21	1	1	55	56	5	5	5	5	18	12

[a] Less than 0.5%

Cancer assumes less importance when examined as a cause of PYLL. The percentage contribution that cancer makes to the total falls in all countries and in people of each sex, and diseases affecting younger persons (infectious diseases, injury and poisoning) assume greater importance.

Most of the variation in the relative importance of cancer as a cause of premature loss of life is due to differences between the countries with regard to other, competing causes of death. This can be seen by comparing *rates* of PYLL per 1000 population. For the regions listed in Table 5, the rate for cancer in males in 1980 varied from 9.4 per 1000 in Chile to 19.3 per 1000 in Hungary, and that in females from 9.5 per 1000 in Spain to 14.3 per 1000 in Hungary. As we saw in the case of deaths (p. 23), the percentage of PYLL due to cancer is increasing in all these areas. Figure 2 shows this percentage at three time periods in six countries. Here, PYLL in a standard population are shown, to illustrate that the rise is independent of the ageing of the population in the 20-year period considered; in fact, if crude rates are used, the increases are only slightly more impressive, so that the ageing of the population has played a relatively small part in increasing the importance of cancer.

Figure 2. Percentage of person-years of life lost due to cancer in persons under 70 years of age, 1960–80

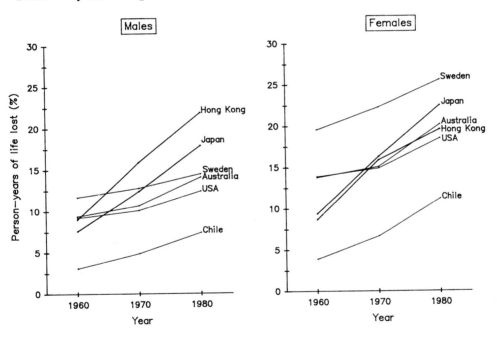

Cancer: Causes, Occurrence and Control

Table 5. Numbers of deaths and person-years of life lost (PYLL) in persons under age 70 for six major groups of causes, 1980; figures are % of total; leading causes of death are in bold type

Region	Cancer	Infectious/ Parasitic diseases	Cardio- vascular disorders	Circulatory diseases	Respiratory diseases	Injury/ poi- soning	Other/ unknown
Deaths							
Males							
Australia	24	1	6	**35**	5	16	13
Chile	13	7	5	10	8	**23**	34
Hong Kong	**31**	4	10	13	13	12	1
Hungary	21	2	10	**29**	6	16	16
Japan	**29**	2	15	15	4	17	18
Kuwait	8	9	3	**21**	8	22	29
Spain	**24**	3	8	22	8	13	22
Sweden	23	1	5	**40**	4	15	12
USA	22	1	4	**34**	5	19	15
Females							
Australia	**32**	1	9	25	5	11	17
Chile	**20**	6	7	11	8	9	39
Hong Kong	**30**	3	12	14	10	10	21
Hungary	**27**	1	13	26	4	9	20
Japan	**35**	2	16	14	4	10	19
Kuwait	10	**14**	3	**14**	10	11	3
Spain	**29**	3	11	20	6	7	24
Sweden	**40**	1	7	2	4	10	16
USA	**32**	1	6	2	5	11	1
PYLL							
Males							
Australia	16	1	3	20	4	**32**	24
Chile	7	9	2	5	10	**28**	39
Hong Kong	**23**	4	5	7	11	21	29
Hungary	15	1	6	20	6	**24**	28
Japan	21	2	10	11	4	**28**	24
Kuwait	5	13	2	11	10	**22**	37
Spain	16	5	4	14	7	**21**	33
Sweden	17	1	4	24	3	**29**	22
USA	13	1	2	19	4	**35**	27
Females							
Australia	**24**	1	5	12	4	20	34
Chile	10	10	3	5	12	**13**	47
Hong Kong	**21**	4	6	8	10	16	35
Hungary	**21**	1	7	15	5	13	38
Japan	**28**	2	9	9	5	17	30
Kuwait	5	**19**	1	8	13	11	43
Spain	**21**	6	5	11	7	11	39
Sweden	**33**	2	5	11	4	19	26
USA	**22**	2	4	14	4	20	34

References

Day, N.E. (1976) A new measure of age-standardized incidence, the cumulative rate. In: Waterhouse, J., Muir, C.S., Correa, P. & Powell, J., eds, *Cancer Incidence in Five Continents*, Vol. III (IARC Scientific Publications No. 15), Lyon, IARC, pp. 443-452

Doll, R. & Cook, P. (1967) Summarising indices for comparison of cancer incidence data. *Int. J. Cancer*, 2, 269-279

Doll, R. & Peto, R. (1981) The causes of cancer: quantitative estimates of avoidable risks of cancer in the United States today. *J. Natl Cancer Inst.*, 66, 1191-1308

Doll, R. & Smith, P.G. (1982) Comparison between registries: age-standardized rates. In: Waterhouse, J., Muir, C.S., Powell, J. & Shanmugaratnam, K., eds, *Cancer Incidence in Five Continents*, Vol. IV (IARC Scientific Publications No. 42), Lyon, IARC, pp. 671-674

Doll, R., Payne, P. & Waterhouse, J., eds (1966) *Cancer Incidence in Five Continents. A Technical Report*, New York, Springer

Doll, R., Muir, C. & Waterhouse, J., eds (1970) *Cancer Incidence in Five Continents*, Vol. II (IARC Scientific Publications No. 15), Lyon, IARC

Haenszel, W. (1950) A standardized rate for mortality defined in units of lost years of life. *Am. J. Public Health*, 40, 17-26

Hakulinen, T., Hansluwka, H., Lopez, A.D. & Nakada, T. (1986a) Global mortality patterns by cause of death in 1980. *Int. J. Epidemiol.*, 15, 226-233

Hakulinen, T., Hansluwka, H., Lopez, A.D. & Nakada, T. (1986b) Estimation of global mortality patterns by cause of death. In: Hansluwka, H., Lopez, A.D., Porapakkham, Y. & Prasartkul, P., eds, *New Developments in the Analysis of Mortality and Causes of Death*, Bangkok, Mahidol University, pp. 177-205

Heasman, M.E. & Lipworth, L. (1966) *Accuracy of Certificates of Cause of Death* (Studies on Medical and Population Subjects No. 20), London, Her Majesty's Stationery Office

Inskip, H., Beral, V., Fraser, P. & Haskey, J. (1983) Methods for age-adjustment of rates. *Stat. Med.*, 2, 455-466

Moriyama, I.M., Baum, W.S., Haenszel, W.M. & Mattison, B.F. (1958) Inquiry into diagnostic evidence supporting medical certificates of death. *Am. J. Public Health*, 48, 1376-1387

Muir, C.S., Waterhouse, J., Mack, T., Powell, J. & Whelan, S., eds (1987) *Cancer Incidence in Five Continents*, Vol. V (IARC Scientific Publications No. 88), Lyon, IARC

Napalkov, N.P. & Eckhardt, S., eds (1982) *Case Control in the Countries of the Council of Mutual Economic Assistance*, Budapest, Akademiai Kiado

Parkin, D.M. (1986) Introduction. In: Parkin, D.M., ed., *Cancer Occurrence in Developing Countries* (IARC Scientific Publications No. 75), Lyon, IARC, pp. 1-23

Parkin, D.M., Läärä, E. & Muir, C.S. (1988) Estimates of the worldwide frequency of sixteen major cancers in 1980. *Int. J. Cancer*, 41, 184-197

Percy, C. & Dolman, A. (1978) Comparison of the coding of death certificates related to cancer in seven countries. *Am. J. Public Health*, 93, 335-350

Preston, S.H. (1976) *Mortality Patterns in National Populations, with Special Reference to Recorded Causes of Death*, New York, Academic Press

Puffer, R.R. & Wynn-Griffith, G. (1967) *Patterns of Urban Mortality* (Scientific Publication No. 151) Washington DC, Pan American Health Organization

Research Group for Population-based Cancer Registration in Japan (1981) Cancer incidence in Japan, 1975 - Cancer registry statistics. In: Segi, M., Tominaga, S., Aoki, K. & Fujimoto, I., eds, *Cancer Mortality Statistics. Japan and the World* (Gann Monograph on Cancer Research No. 26), Tokyo, Japan Scientific Societies Press, pp. 92-116

Rogentine, G.N., Yankee, R.A., Gart, J.J., Nam, J. & Trapani, R.J. (1972) HL-A antigens and disease. Acute lymphocytic leukemia. *J. Clin. Invest.*, 51, 2420-2428

Rogentine, G.N., Trapani, R.J., Yankee, R.A. & Henderson, E.S. (1973) HL-A antigens and acute lymphocytic leukemia: the nature of the HL-A2 association. *Tissue Antigens*, 3, 470-475

Romeder, J.M. & McWhinnie, J.R. (1977) Potential years of life lost between ages 1 and 70: an indicator of premature mortality for health planning. *Int. J. Epidemiol.*, 6, 143-151

Rothman, K.J. (1986) *Modern Epidemiology*, Boston, Little, Brown

Waterhouse, J., Muir, C.S., Correa, P. & Powell, J., eds (1976) *Cancer Incidence in Five Continents*, Vol. III (IARC Scientific Publications No. 15), Lyon, IARC

Waterhouse, J., Muir, C., Shanmugaratnam, K. & Powell, J., eds (1982) *Cancer Incidence in Five Continents*, Vol. IV (IARC Scientific Publications No. 42), Lyon, IARC

West, R.R. (1976) Accuracy of cancer registration. *Br. J. Prev. Soc. Med.*, *30*, 187-192

World Health Organization (1976) *Cancer Statistics* (Tech. Rep. Ser. 632), Geneva

World Health Organization (1977) *ICD-9 International Classification of Diseases, 1975 Revision*, Vol. 1, Geneva

World Health Organization (1978) *ICD-9 International Classification of Diseases, 1975 Revision*, Vol. 2, Geneva

Chapter 2. Objectives and methods of descriptive epidemiology

We pointed out earlier (p. 15) that a major purpose of descriptive epidemiology is to provide information helpful in elucidating the etiology of cancer. Using the measurement tools discussed above, the most basic strategies consist of investigating differences in the risk for cancer according to variables that are conveniently summarized as 'person, place and time', or a combination of these. 'Personal' variables include those details about individuals (sometimes called 'demographic factors') that are generally recorded in routine statistics systems, such as age, sex, race (or nationality), religion, marital status and occupation. 'Place' normally refers to place of residence, and studies of this variable involve geographical comparisons of risk. Studies of risk for cancer rates over 'time' result in trends in risk. Comparative studies involving combinations of these categories are also carried out. Thus, in studies of migrant populations, risks for cancer are usually compared in persons of similar ethnic origin, or at least with similar birthplaces, living in different places or environments, for different periods of time.

The geography of cancer

Geographic epidemiology is the study of the distribution of disease according to the place of residence of those affected. Differences that are observed indicate either that the inhabitants of a particular place have characteristics which are important to their susceptibility to disease, or that the levels of etiological factors in the environment vary. Environmental factors include not only those that can be considered external to the individual – in the biological, chemical or physical environment – but also encompass social and cultural behaviour patterns. The observation of markedly high (or low) rates of particular cancers inevitably provokes the quest for likely explanations in such terms, drawing upon knowledge of the distribution of environmental agents which may be relevant to the cancer.

The units of study in geographical comparisons of disease are generally administrative areas, since information on rates of disease (and on possible etiological agents) are most readily available as by-products of national statistical systems.

Table 6 illustrates the very large range in the incidence rates for individual cancers at the international level – 100–fold for nasopharyngeal cancer in males, for example. International variation is somewhat less marked when comparisons are made between cancer registries in countries with populations of European origin, such as Europe, North America, Australia and New Zealand (Table 7), although large differences remain for some cancers such as those of the lip and oesophagus and melanoma. This suggests the importance of environmental rather than genetic factors in these variations.

Table 6. Worldwide variations in the incidence of cancers at various sites (number of cases per 100 000 population)[a]

Site	ICD-9	Males			Females		
		Highest	Lowest	Ratio	Highest	Lowest	Ratio
Lip	140	Canada, Newfoundland 15.1	Japan, Osaka 0.1	151.0	Australia, South 1.5	UK England and Wales 0.1	16.0
Oral cavity	143–145	France, Bas–Rhin 13.5	Japan, Miyagi 0.5	27.0	India, Bangalore 15.7	Japan, Miyagi 0.2	78.5
Nasopharynx	147	Hong Kong 30.0	UK, South Wales 0.3	100.0	Hong Kong 12.9	USA, Iowa 0.1	129.0
Oesophagus	150	France, Calvados 29.9	Romania, Cluj County 1.2	24.9	India, Poona 12.4	Czechoslovakia, Slovakia 0.3	41.3
Stomach	151	Japan, Nagasaki 82.0	Kuwait: Kuwaitis 3.7	22.2	Japan, Nagasaki 36.1	USA, Iowa 3.0	12.0
Colon	153	USA Connecticut: whites 34.1	India, Madras 1.8	18.9	USA Detroit: blacks 29.0	India, Nagpur 1.8	16.1
Rectum	154	FRG, Saarland 21.5	Kuwait: Kuwaitis 3.0	7.2	FRG; Saarland 13.2	India, Madras 1.3	10.2
Liver	155	China, Shanghai 34.4	Canada, Nova Scotia 0.7	49.1	China, Shanghai 11.6	Australia, New South Wales 0.4	29.0
Pancreas	157	USA Los Angeles: Koreans 16.4	India, Madras 0.9	18.2	USA Alameda: blacks 9.4	India, Bombay 1.3	7.2
Larynx	161	Brazil, São Paulo 17.8	Japan, Miyagi 2.2	8.1	USA, Connecticut: blacks 2.7	Japan, Miyagi 0.2	13.5
Lung	162	USA, New Orleans: blacks 111.0	India, Madras 5.8	19.0	New Zealand: Maoris 68.1	India, Madras 1.2	56.8
Melanoma	172	Australia, Queensland 30.9	Japan, Osaka 0.2	154.5	Australia, Queensland 28.5	India, Bombay 0.2	142.5
Other skin	173	Australia, Tasmania 167.2	India, Madras 0.9	185.8	Australia, Tasmania 89.3	Switzerland, Zurich 0.6	148.8
Breast	175/174	Brazil, Recife 3.4	Finland 0.2	17.0	USA, Hawaii: Hawaiians 93.9	Israel: non-Jews 14.0	6.7

Site	ICD	Highest area	rate	Lowest area	rate	Ratio	Highest area	rate	Lowest area	rate	Ratio
Cervix uteri	180	—		—		—	Brazil, Recife	83.2	Israel: non-Jews	3.0	27.7
Corpus uteri	182	—		—		—	USA, San Francisco Bay Area: whites	25.7	India, Nagpur	1.2	21.4
Ovary, etc	183	—		—		—	New Zealand: Pacific Polynesian Islanders	25.8	Kuwait: Kuwaitis	3.3	7.8
Prostate	185	USA, Atlanta: blacks	91.2	China, Tianjin	1.3	70.2	—		—		—
Testis	186	Switzerland, Basel	8.3	China, Tianjin	0.6	13.8	—		—		—
Penis, etc	187	Brazil, Recife	8.3	Israel: all Jews	0.2	41.5	—		—		—
Bladder	188	Switzerland, Basel	27.8	India, Nagpur	1.7	16.4	Kuwait: non-Kuwaitis	8.5	India, Poona	0.8	10.6
Kidney, etc	189	Canada, Northwest Territories and Yukon	15.0	India, Poona	0.7	21.4	Iceland	10.2	India, Poona	0.8	12.7
Brain	191.2	New Zealand: Pacific Polynesian Islanders	9.7	India, Nagpur	1.1	8.8	Israel: born in Israel	7.6	India, Madras	0.6	13.5
Thyroid	193	USA, Hawaii: Chinese	8.8	Poland, Warsaw City	0.4	22.0	USA, Hawaii: Filipinos	10.8	India, Nagpur	0.6	18.2
Hodgkin's disease	201	Canada, Québec	4.8	Japan, Miyagi	0.5	9.6	Switzerland, Neuchâtel	3.9	Japan, Osaka	0.3	13.0
Non-Hodgkin's lymphoma	200/202	Switzerland, Vaud	11.5	India, Nagpur	1.5	7.7	USA, San Francisco Bay Area: whites	8.7	India, Nagpur	0.7	12.4
Multiple myeloma	203	USA, Alameda: blacks	8.8	Philippines: Rizal	0.4	22.0	USA, Connecticut: blacks	7.4	China, Shanghai	0.4	18.5
Leukaemia	204.8	Canada, Ontario	11.6	India, Nagpur	2.2	5.3	New Zealand: Pacific Polynesian Islanders	10.3	India, Madras	1.1	9.4

*Data from Muir et al. (1987); rates based on fewer than ten cases are excluded.

Table 7. Variations in cancer incidence at various sites in populations of European origin (number of cases per 100 000 population)[a]

Site	ICD-9	Males			Females		
		Highest	Lowest	Ratio	Highest	Lowest	Ratio
Lip	140	Canada, Newfoundland 15.1	UK, Birmingham 0.2	75.5	Australia, South 1.6	UK, England and Wales 0.1	16.0
Oral cavity	143–145	France, Bas–Rhin 13.5	Romania, Cluj County 0.7	19.3	USA, Atlanta: whites 2.4	Yugoslavia, Slovenia 0.3	9.0
Nasopharynx	147	Romania, Cluj County 1.5	UK south-western 0.3	5.0	Romania, Cluj County 0.7	USA, Iowa 0.1	7.0
Oesophagus	150	France, Calvados 29.9	Romania, Cluj County 1.2	24.9	UK, eastern Scotland 5.1	Czechoslovakia, Slovakia 0.3	17.0
Stomach	151	Italy, Parma 44.0	USA, Atlanta: whites 6.1	7.2	Italy, Parma 19.9	USA, Iowa 3.0	6.6
Colon	153	USA, Connecticut: whites 34.1	Romania, Cluj County 4.1	8.3	New Zealand: non-Maoris 28.4	Romania, Cluj County 4.1	6.9
Rectum	154	FRG, Saarland 21.5	Spain, Zaragoza 7.2	3.0	FRG, Saarland 13.2	Poland, Nowy Sacz 4.1	3.2
Liver	155	Switzerland, Geneva 10.2	Canada, Nova Scotia 0.7	14.6	Italy, Ragusa 4.1	Australia, New South Wales 0.4	10.3
Pancreas	157	Switzerland, Neuchâtel 10.4	Spain, Tarragona 3.1	3.4	Denmark 7.0	France, Doubs 1.9	3.7
Larynx	161	Spain, Navarra 17.2	Sweden 2.8	6.1	Switzerland, Neuchâtel 2.3	Sweden 0.3	7.7
Lung	162	UK, western Scotland 100.4	Iceland 24.7	4.1	USA, San Francisco Bay Area: whites 33.3	France, Doubs 2.8	11.9
Melanoma	172	Australia, Queensland 30.9	Poland, Nowy Sacz 1.2	25.8	Australia Queensland 28.5	Spain, Zaragoza 1.4	20.4
Other skin	173	Australia, Tasmania 167.2	FRG, Hamburg 4.9	34.1	Australia, Tasmania 89.3	Switzerland, Zurich 0.6	148.8
Breast	175/174	USA, New York City 0.9	Finland 0.2	4.5	USA, San Francisco Bay Area: whites 87.0	Poland, Nowy Sacz 18.4	4.7

Site	Code	Highest area (rate)	Ratio	Lowest area (rate)	Highest area (rate)	Lowest area (rate)	Ratio
Cervix uteri	180	—	—	—	German Democratic Republic 24.6	Finland 5.5	4.5
Corpus uteri	182	—	—	—	USA, San Francisco Bay Area: whites 25.7	Romania, Cluj County 4.4	5.9
Ovary, etc	183	—	—	—	Norway 15.3	Spain, Zaragoza 5.4	2.8
Prostate	185	USA, Utah 70.2	7.2	Romania, Cluj County 9.8	—	—	—
Testis	186	Switzerland, Basel 8.3	7.5	Spain, Tarragona 1.1	—	—	—
Penis, etc	187	USA, New Mexico: Hispanics 1.7	3.4	Finland 0.5	—	—	—
Bladder	188	Switzerland, Basel 27.8	3.6	Hungary, Vas 7.7	USA, Connecticut: whites 7.4	Hungary, Vas 1.2	6.2
Kidney, etc	189	Iceland 12.2	8.8	Romania, Cluj County 1.7	Iceland 7.6	Romania, Cluj County 1.3	5.8
Brain	191/192	USA, Los Angeles: whites 9.2	3.8	Hungary, Szabolcs 2.4	Iceland 10.0	Hungary, Szabolcs 1.3	7.7
Thyroid	193	Iceland 5.6	14.0	Poland, Warsaw 0.4	Iceland 13.3	Poland, Warsaw City 1.3	10.0
Hodgkin's disease	201	Canada, Québec 4.8	4.8	Hungary, Szabolcs 1.0	Switzerland, Neuchâtel 3.9	Canada, Newfoundland 0.6	6.5
Non-Hodgkin's lymphoma	200/202	Switzerland, Vaud 11.5	4.8	Hungar, Szabolcs 2.4	USA, San Francisco Bay Area: whites 8.7	Hungary, Szabolcs 1.0	8.7
Multiple myeloma	203	Australia, Capital Territory 5.7	5.2	Poland, Warsaw City 1.1	Switzerland, Neuchâtel 3.2	Ireland 0.7	4.6
Leukaemia	204–8	Canada, Ontario 11.6	3.9	Hungary, Szabolcs 3.0	Italy, Varese 8.0	Hungary, Szabolcs 2.7	3.0

[a] Data from Muir et al. (1987); rates based on fewer than ten cases are excluded.

Variations in incidence rates *within* countries may be just as striking as international differences, and these variations can be demonstrated visually by means of atlases of cancer. Very large variations can be seen within the countries of western Europe (Figure 3). The Chinese atlas of cancer mortality (The Editorial Committee for the Atlas of Cancer Mortality in the People's Republic of China, 1979) shows quite clearly enormous variations between counties in mortality rates from several cancers, notably of the oesophagus and nasopharynx.

Findings such as these strongly suggest the action of important environmental factors, and it is often possible to formulate hypotheses on the basis of approximate knowledge of their distribution in the regions concerned. As described above, when quantitative information on the level of potential risk factors is available for the same geographic units for which there are data on cancer incidence (or mortality), geographical correlation studies are possible. Such information may include consumption patterns (intake *per caput*) of foodstuffs, alcohol or tobacco, or levels of pollutants or trace elements in air, soil or water. Many of these ecological studies have been performed. An example of the results of such a study, relating cigarette consumption to rates of mortality from lung cancer, is shown in Figure 4. Geographical correlation studies have the great advantage of being relatively cheap, since the information used has been collected for other purposes; however, they have several drawbacks (see, e.g., Breslow & Enstrom, 1974), the principal one being that cases of disease and levels of exposure to a suspected etiological agent are not being measured in the same individuals.

Localized clusters of cancer cases are frequently reported, which suggest the presence of a similarly localized causative agent. Much interest has been aroused by clusters of Hodgkin's disease (which have provoked speculation about an infectious etiology) and of leukaemia in relation to localized sources of irradiation. The problem with such observations is that the chance occurrence of such groups of cases can be expected even when cases of disease are distributed randomly in space (see Smith, 1982), so that cancer clusters should really excite interest only if they occur more frequently than expected by chance, when they consist of an unusual type of cancer, or when they relate to some localized source of risk identified *a priori* (as in the case of nuclear installations; see p. 161).

It is relatively simple to compare cancer incidence rates between populations living in urban and in rural surroundings, although the exact definitions of 'urban' and 'rural' tend to vary between countries and with time. Urban dwellers show higher risks for cancers at virtually all body sites. The aspects of urban living that are likely to be responsible, such as smoking habits, diet and pollution, are not elucidated by such simple comparisons, however. The difficulties in disentangling the effects of tobacco smoke, indoor and outdoor air pollution and other agents to which city dwellers are exposed are discussed in Part II, Chapter 13.

Variation in risk for cancer related to 'personal' factors

Having demonstrated the degree of variation in the frequency of cancer that exists between areas, a logical sequence is to investigate possible differences in the frequency of cancer among people within the same area but who have some feature that identifies them as different from other residents, such as their sex,

Figure 3. Variations in cancer incidence in the countries of the European Economic Communities[a]

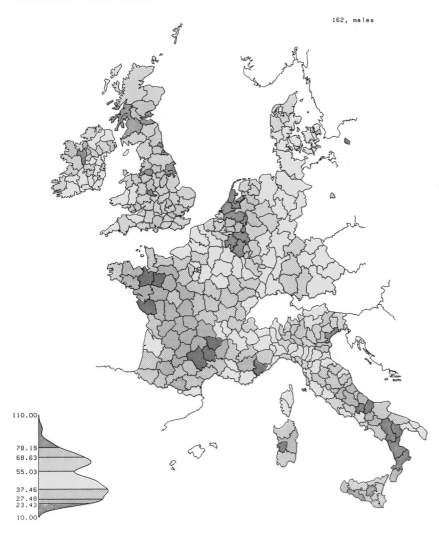

[a] From Smans *et al.* (1990)

age, religion, race or ethnicity. Any differences in cancer frequency would indicate that some aspect of their way of living was associated with the factor under examination and with the etiology of cancer.

Age

Age is the single most important determinant of risk for cancer, and the relationship is so strong that the possible effects of age must be allowed for in every epidemiological study (this is the purpose of carrying out age standardization, discussed above, p. 16).

Figure 4. International correlation between consumption of manufactured cigarettes in 1950 and mortality rates from lung cancer in persons aged 35–44 in the mid-1970s[a]

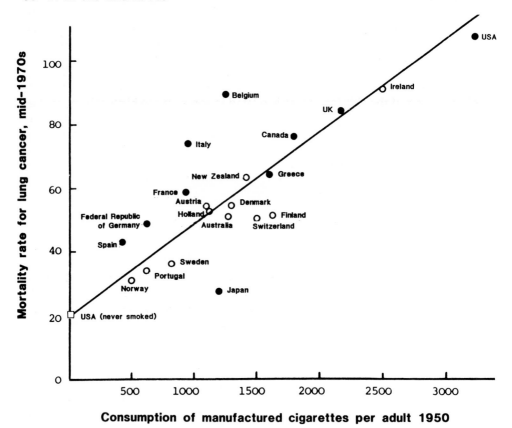

Consumption of manufactured cigarettes per adult 1950

[a] From Doll & Peto (1981). Comparison restricted to developed countries (excluding Africa, all of Asia except Japan, and all except North America) with populations >1 million

For many forms of epithelial cancers that are not hormone-dependent, the relationship between log (age) and log (incidence or mortality) is found to be linear (Cook *et al.*, 1969). In other words, if I_t denotes the incidence at age t, then

$$I_t = b \times t^k,$$

where b and k are constants. This relationship is found to hold over all the age ranges between 30 and 79 years (Doll, 1971).

Doll (1971) noted that, for lung cancer, the value of k in the above relationship differed between smokers and nonsmokers. When, however, age was replaced by duration of smoking, the resulting value of k was the same as that for nonsmokers. It is reasonable to suppose that the same explanation underlies the relationship between age and other cancers, and that the shape of the age-incidence curve relates to the accumulation throughout life of exposure to carcinogenic events.

Although the rates of some cancers do, in fact, fit the relationship described above quite well, this is by no means always so. Rates for older people are often lower than such a curve would imply, either because of poorer ascertainment of cancer in older people or because the pool of individuals who are susceptible to a particular cancer is becoming exhausted. One must also be aware that individuals of different ages in a given population represent different generations (or birth cohorts), and, if the risk for cancer is related in some way to birth cohort, studies of the influence of age should be confined to populations with approximately similar birth dates. Taking such factors into account, the age–mortality curves for three common tumours in England and Wales are as shown in Figure 5 (Osmond & Gardner, 1983). While the relationship between age and mortality is linear for lung cancer, for breast cancer there is a clear inflection at about the age of the menopause, and rates of mortality (and incidence) from cervical cancer cease to increase at all in women over the age of 50. The meaning of such striking patterns is known only in the most general terms; for breast cancer, they are presumed to be related to levels of sex hormones.

Gender

Differences in rates between males and females are often expressed in terms of a 'sex ratio', that is, the ratio of the incidence in people of one sex in relation to that in the other. One of the most striking and consistent features of cancer is that age-specific rates at nearly all body sites are higher in males than in females. Apart from breast cancer, the exceptions to this observation comprise a rather interesting group of cancers: those of the gall-bladder and thyroid, which are generally more common in females, and malignant melanoma of the skin and cancers of the eye, salivary gland and proximal colon, for which the risk is approximately equal in the two sexes. Since few of these differences are explicable in terms of different exposures to carcinogens, we must conclude that they represent differences in susceptibility. What this means in biological terms is still obscure.

Ethnic group

Comparisons between different ethnic groups living in the same country or region demonstrate substantial variations in incidence and mortality. Cancer registries in the USA, in particular, provide data not only on the white and black populations, but also on persons of Japanese, Chinese, Filipino, Hawaiian and Latin American ancestry (Muir *et al.*, 1987). Figure 6 shows the incidence rates for the three major ethnic groups in Singapore. There are very large differences in risk for cancers at several sites.

These remarkable differences in cancer rates between people residing in the same area have two possible explanations: they are due either to differences in genetic susceptibility or to differences in life style. Studies of migrant populations, in which cancer risk is compared in persons of similar ethnic (genetic) backgrounds living in different environments, are particularly useful in investigating this question (see below).

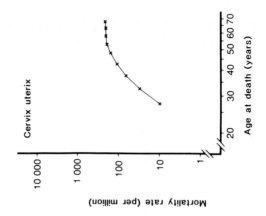

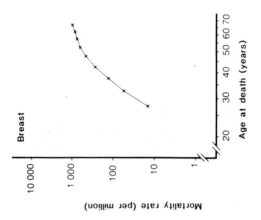

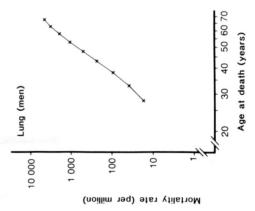

^a From Osmond *et al.* (1983). The mortality rates shown are derived from fitting an age-period-cohort model to data for England and Wales, and represent the values in relation to age that are independent of the effects of the other two factors.

Figure 6. Age-standardized incidence rates for cancers at selected sites in Singapore, by ethnic group and sex, 1978–82[a]

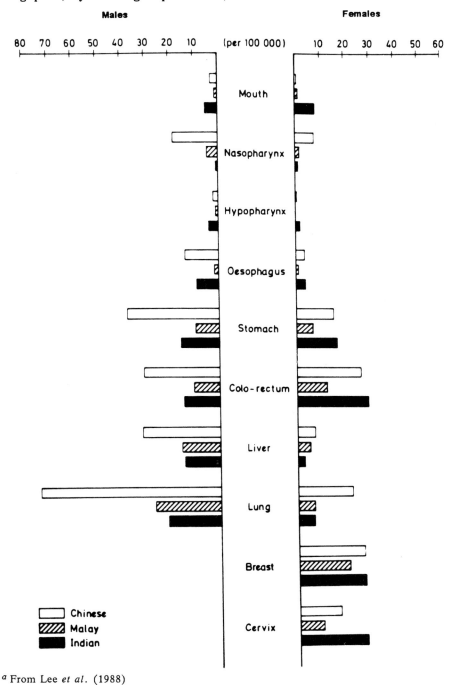

[a] From Lee *et al.* (1988)

Religion

Religious belief may be associated with a set of rules of conduct which help determine a characteristic life style. Members of a particular religious group are therefore worth examining to see whether these differences in life style have produced characteristic patterns of cancer. Ideally, for such comparisons to be valid, the groups being studied should be of the same ethnic stock, adhere to the tenets of their faith, live in the same community and be equally willing and able to seek medical advice; these conditions are not always met. However, there are well substantiated differences in cancer pattern by religion. The longest recognized of these are the virtual absence of penile cancer in Jewish males and the low levels of cancer of the uterine cervix in Jewish women. The contrasting frequencies of cervical and penile cancer in Hindus (high) and Muslims (low) in India are well known (Jussawalla & Jain, 1976).

Members of the Church of Jesus Christ of Latter-day Saints (Mormons) and Seventh-day Adventists living in the USA have been studied extensively. These groups exhibit rates that are substantially lower than national rates for cancers at sites related to use of tobacco and alcohol and for cancers at other sites, such as the large bowel, which are thought to be unrelated to these risk factors.

Occupation

Studies of cancer risk in relation to occupation have been very valuable in identifying carcinogenic hazards. In descriptive epidemiology, details of occupation must be known for cancer patients at the time of their death; in the great majority of such studies, mortality data are used, since occupation is rather poorly recorded by cancer registries. If rates are to be calculated, the numbers of persons at risk (i.e., who may be exposed) in each occupational group must also be known. Although several technical difficulties arise in such studies, mainly relating to the accuracy of statements about 'usual occupation' by relatives of dead patients and the comparability of data from death certificates and the census, significant relationships have been demonstrated between many categories of job and the risks for different cancers. The studies of mortality by occupation that are carried out in England and Wales every ten years have revealed, for example, that electrical workers appear to have a higher than average risk for leukaemia and butchers a higher risk for lung cancer; both of these associations have subsequently been the subject of more detailed studies (Logan, 1986).

The names given to different jobs – 'occupational titles' – are often broad and vague and usually provide little information about exposure to precise agents which may be carcinogenic. This problem has been approached recently by the creation of job-exposure matrices, which define the chemical (or physical) agents likely to be encountered in different occupations, so that risk can be studied in relation to specific exposures, rather than to job title (Hemon & Goldberg, 1989).

Social status

Quite dramatic differences in cancer risk are evident according to some measures of 'social status' (Townsend & Davidson, 1987; Whitehead, 1987). Social status embraces many interrelated variables, including education, income, diet and probable smoking habits, so that the demonstration of apparent differences does little to further etiological insights. The measurement of social status may be based on various sources of information, including an individual's occupation or residential area (as in the UK) or his income or educational level (as in the USA). In studies of occupational mortality, the social class of workers has been taken into consideration to try to separate the effects of the work environment from those of the general way of life of persons pursuing a particular occupation (Fox & Adelstein, 1978). These issues are discussed in detail in Part II, Chapter 16.

Trends of cancer with time

Trends in the risk for cancer with time in defined populations are of particular interest since they imply changes in exposure to environmental factors. Changes due to variation in genetic susceptibility in a population would be seen only if there were fairly widespread migration of individuals in or out of the region; changes that are the result of genetic variation between generations within a stable population would be relatively small and occur very slowly.

Choice of data

Changes in risk can be studied over quite short intervals; however, in order to analyse the likely components of the changes (see below), longer periods are preferable. In general, data on incidence, from cancer registries, cover shorter periods than do data on mortality, which have often been recorded nationally for many years. These two types of data also have other advantages and disadvantages.

Death is a clearly defined event, and its registration is usually a legal requirement. Trends in mortality are, however, influenced not only by changing risk (incidence) but also by changes in survival (see p. 17). The frequent unreliability of statements of 'underlying cause of death' was also discussed earlier (p. 18). Spurious changes in mortality rates may be caused by changes in the registration process, resulting in improvements in the validity of such statements. Thus, fewer deaths would be allocated to vague categories such as 'senility' or just 'cancer', and one would see apparent rises in mortality from better defined categories of cancer.

Neither is cancer registration perfect – there is always the possibility of underregistration (cases being missed) or of the same case being included more than once, and the quality of registration is quite likely to vary over time. In addition, the definition of what exactly constitutes an 'incident cancer' may change – for example, the extension of screening programmes or more intensive use of autopsy may reveal clinically undetected lesions with the cellular appearance of malignancy. If such cases are registered along with clinically diagnosed cases, marked changes in incidence rates can result.

Other factors influence time trends in both incidence and mortality. One is the availability and efficiency of techniques available for diagnosis. These include new X-ray methods and new biochemical tests as well as an increased ability to take tissue samples from the deeper seated organs of the body. These improvements take place over time and frequently occur at different times and to differing degrees in various parts of the world. A further problem relates to changes in the International Classification of Diseases – notable examples are in the categories relating to liver cancer and cancer of the uterus (cervix and corpus), for which mortality rates are very difficult to compare over time owing to differences in the detail provided in the changing codes.

Components of change

Standardized rates, as described above (p. 16), provide a summary index that is independent of age, so that temporal changes in age-standardized incidence (or mortality) rates provide a convenient overview of the magnitude of increase or decrease for the population as a whole. Figure 7 illustrates changes in age-standardized mortality rates in the USA between 1930 and 1985. Such changes can be summarized as annual rates of increase (or decrease) – lung cancer mortality in males, for example, has risen at an average annual rate of 4.6% between 1930 and 1985. Crude rates of incidence or mortality are of little use for studying time trends, since they also reflect any changes in the age structure of the population, as well as the risk for cancer in each age group.

Standardized rates can, however, hide the fact that time trends may be quite different in different age groups. Figure 8 shows the time trends in lung cancer rates in the USA for men of different ages. It is clear that mortality has actually been declining in young men in recent years, starting in the youngest age group (25–34) in about 1960, although the age-standardized mortality (for all ages) was continuing to increase as recently as 1985. Figure 9 shows the same age-specific mortality rates, but the year of *birth* is plotted on the x axis instead of the year of death. When presented in this way, it is clear that the decline in mortality rates among men under the age of 50 began with the generation (or birth cohort) that was born around 1928–32.

Figure 10 shows a different pattern – that of mortality from Hodgkin's disease in the USA between 1950 and 1984. We can see a decline in the rates for men of all age groups in recent years, but the decline began at a fixed period (1965–69) and affected all the age groups (and all birth cohorts) in a similar manner. This decline is associated with improved treatment methods introduced in the late 1960s.

Ideally, one would like to be able to analyse time trends, in order to assess the degree of risk due to age, that due to the year of birth and that associated with the year of diagnosis or death. Age, birth cohort and calendar time period are in practice dependent on each other: when two of these are known, the third is fixed; thus, given a person's age at a particular date, his birth cohort is also known. Various approaches have been made to modelling the effects of age, cohort and period (Osmond & Gardner, 1982; Holford, 1983; Clayton & Schifflers, 1987), but the basic problem remains that the components cannot be identified when there is a uniform trend in all age groups. In general terms, however, when strong environmental factors are responsible for changing risk, they generally affect successive birth cohorts, as in the example of lung cancer given above. Clear 'period' effects are generally the result of improvements in therapy or the introduction of successful screening programmes, as in the case of cervical cancer in the Nordic countries (Hakama, 1980; see p. 72).

An interesting attempt to project cancer incidence in Finland over a long period of time has been made by the Finnish Cancer Registry (Hakulinen *et al.*, 1989).

Figure 7. Age-standardized rates for death from cancers at selected sites in males, USA, 1930–85[a]

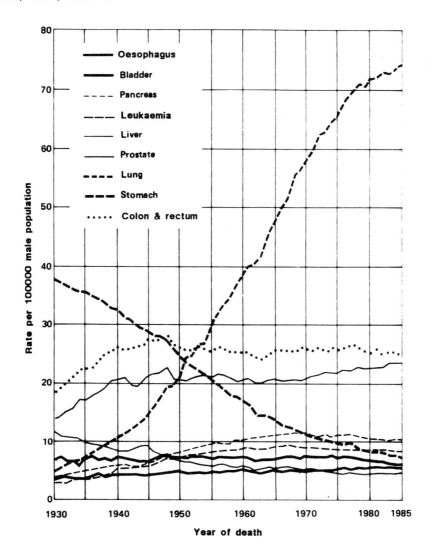

[a] From Silverberg & Lubera (1988); adjusted to the age distribution of the 1970 US census population

Figure 8. Age-specific rates for death from lung cancer among white men in the USA[a]

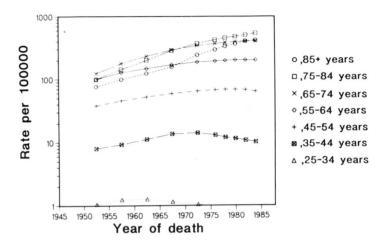

o ,85+ years
□ ,75-84 years
× ,65-74 years
◇ ,55-64 years
+ ,45-54 years
⊠ ,35-44 years
△ ,25-34 years

[a] From Devesa *et al.* (1987)

Studies of migrants

Studies of variations in cancer risk by ethnic origin inevitably raise questions as to whether any differences observed are the result of genetic differences in susceptibility to environmental carcinogens or of differences in life style between the groups. One approach to resolving this problem is to study migrant populations, and to compare their risk of cancer with that of persons of the same genetic background living in the place of origin of the migrants, and with that of persons in the new host country, who share a common external environment. The objective is to see how much the risk for cancer changes from the country of origin to the host country and, if possible, to study how rapidly such changes occur.

Haenszel and Kurihara (1968), studying Japanse migrants to the USA, found that Issei (Japanese born in Japan) had mortality rates from gastric cancer that were much closer to those in Japan than to those in the USA. The rates for Nisei (Japanese born in the USA), although lower than those prevailing in Japan, were still higher than those for whites in the USA. This suggests that some exogenous factor is disappearing gradually from the environment of the migrants and of their descendants. In the same period, mortality rates from intestinal cancer had risen to approach that for white US males, among both Issei and Nisei males, suggesting exposure to a new carcinogen or removal of exposure to some protective factor. By contrast, the same authors found no difference between the rates of mortality from breast cancer in Japanese in Japan and those in the USA. More recently, however, breast cancer mortality rates among Nisei and among third-generation Japanese in the USA were found to be similar to those of whites (Dunn, 1977), suggesting that an environmental factor has now exerted its effect. The two most comprehensive studies of the change in risk in migrant populations in relation to their duration of residence in the new countries are those of migrants to Australia

Figure 9. Mortality rates from malignant neoplasms of the trachea, bronchus and lung among white men in the USA, by birth cohort in five-year intervals during 1947–77[a]

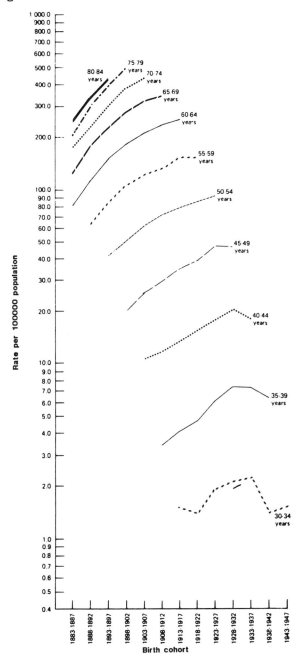

[a] From US Department of Health and Human Services (1982)

Figure 10. Age-specific rates for death from Hodgkin's disease among white men in the USA[a]

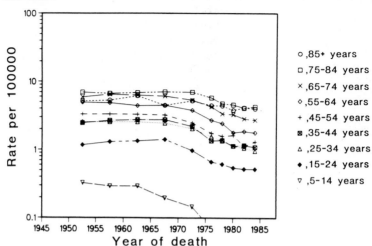

[a] From Devesa *et al.* (1987)

(McMichael *et al.*, 1980; Armstrong *et al.*, 1983) and to Israel (Steinitz *et al.*, 1989). Figure 11 illustrates how the risks for two cancers – breast cancer and malignant melanoma – in migrant populations to Israel change with the length of stay in the new environment. The baseline incidence here is that of Jews born in Israel, and the migrant rates are expressed relative to this. For breast cancer, the risk of Jews born in North Africa is less than half that of Israel-born Jews for recent migrants, but rises very rapidly with duration of stay; this seems not to be the case for Jews born in Asia (predominantly the Middle East). For malignant melanoma, all migrants retain risks much lower than those of Israel-born Jews, but, particularly for European Jews, the risk rises with duration of stay.

The interpretation of the findings outlined above is complex. For one thing, a migrant population is not suddenly plunged into a completely changed environment in the host country. The first generation of migrants often clings to many of the customs of their country of origin; this is particularly true of dietary practices. Hence, changes in risk may not appear for many years. For another, people who migrate are rarely representative of the population of their country of origin as a whole. Migrant populations may be composed of self-selected individuals, often young and healthy, seeking to improve their way of life in another country, or they may comprise persons displaced by war, persecution or famine. Staszewski *et al.* (1970) discussed many of the difficulties associated with studies of migrants.

The most important single conclusion to derive from migrant studies is that, for a group as a whole, it is the new 'environment' that determines cancer risk and not the genetic component associated with the ethnic stock of the migrants. In other words, it is the factors that accompany acculturation to the host country that largely explain international, racial and ethnic variations in cancer rates. Differences in the speed of acculturation, and whether the responsible factors act

Figure 11. Risks for malignant melanoma and for breast cancer among migrants to Israel, by duration of stay, according to region of origin, adjusted for age, sex and period[a]

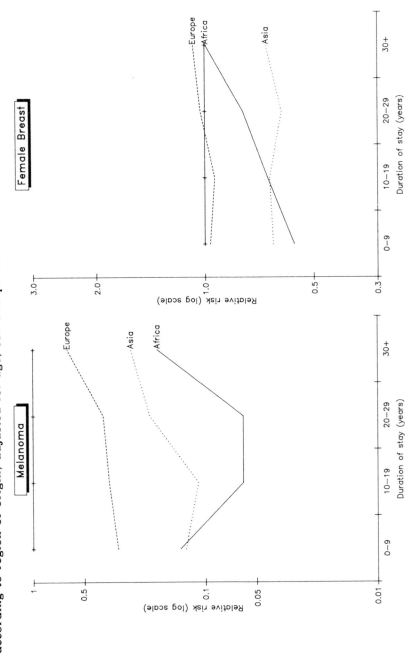

[a] From Steinitz *et al.* (1989)

on early or late stages of carcinogenesis, must be invoked to explain variations in the rapidity with which migrant groups assume the rates of the host country. If acculturation is slow (as it may have been initially with Japanese in North America), or if the factors concerned affect the early stages of carcinogenesis, the change in rates may take place over more than one generation. If, however, acculturation is rapid, and the factors concerned affect the late stages of carcinogenesis, rates may change over a few years. For cancers of relatively obscure etiology, such as breast cancer and large-bowel cancer, insights such as these can be of importance in the formulation of etiological hypotheses.

References

Armstrong, B.K., Woodings, T.L., Stenhouse, N.S. & McCall, M.G. (1983) *Mortality from Cancer in Migrants to Australia - 1962-1971*, Perth, NH & MRC Research Unit in Epidemiology and Preventive Medicine, Raine Medical Statistics Unit, Department of Medicine, University of Western Australia

Breslow, N.E. & Enstrom, J.E. (1974) Geographic correlations between cancer mortality rates and alcohol-tobacco consumption in the United States. *J. Natl Cancer Inst.*, *53*, 631-639

Clayton, D. & Schifflers, E. (1987) Models for temporal variation in cancer rates. I. Age-period and age-cohort models. *Stat. Med.*, *6*, 449-467

Cook, P., Doll, R. & Fellingham, S.A. (1969) A mathematical model for the age distribution of cancer in man. *Int. J. Cancer*, *4*, 93-112

Devesa, S.S., Silverman, D.T., Young, J.L., Pollack, E.S., Brown, C.C., Horm, J.W., Percy, C.L., Myers, M.H., McKay, F.W. & Fraumeni, J.F. (1987) Cancer incidence and mortality trends among whites in the United States, 1947-84. *J. Natl Cancer Inst.*, *79*, 701-770

Doll, R. (1971) The age distribution of cancer: implications for models of carcinogenesis. *J. R. Stat. Soc. Ser. A*, *134*, 133-155

Doll, R. & Peto, R. (1981) The causes of cancer: quantitative estimates of avoidable risks of cancer in the United States today. *J. Natl Cancer Inst.*, *66*, 1191-1308

Dunn, J.E. (1977) Breast cancer among American Japanese in the San Francisco Bay area. *Natl Cancer Inst. Monogr.*, *47*, 157-160

Fox, A.J. & Adelstein, A.M. (1978) Occupational mortality: work or way of life. *J. Epidemiol. Community Health*, *32*, 73-79

Haenszel, W. & Kurihara, M. (1968) Studies of Japanese migrants. I. Mortality from cancer and other diseases among Japanese in the United States. *J. Natl Cancer Inst.*, *40*, 43-68

Hakama, M. (1980) Trends in the incidence of cervical cancer in the Nordic countries. In: Magnus, K., ed., *Trends in Cancer Incidence. Causes and Practical Implications*, Washington DC, Hemisphere Publishing Corp., pp. 279-292

Hakulinen, T., Kenward, M., Luostarinen, T., Oksanen, H., Pukkala, E., Söderman, B. & Teppo, L. (1989) *Cancer in Finland in 1954-2008. Incidence, Mortality and Prevalence by Region*, Helsinki, Finnish Cancer Registry

Hemon, D. & Goldberg, M. (1989) *Methodology of Assessment of Occupational Exposure in the Context of Epidemiological Detection of Cancer Risks* (Series EUR 11810), Luxembourg, Commission of the European Communities

Holford, T.R. (1983) The estimation of age, period and cohort effects for vital rates. *Biometrics*, *39*, 311-324

Jussawalla, D.J. & Jain, D.K. (1976) *Cancer Incidence in Greater Bombay 1970-72*, Bombay, Indian Cancer Society

Lee, H.P., Day, N.E. & Shanmugaratnam, K., eds (1988) *Trends in Cancer Incidence in Singapore, 1968-1982* (IARC Scientific Publications No. 91), Lyon, IARC

Logan, W.P.D., ed. (1986) *Cancer Mortality by Occupation and Social Class 1851-1971* (IARC Scientific Publications No. 36; Studies on Medical and Population Subjects, No. 44), Lyon, IARC

McMichael, A.J., McCall, M.G., Hartshorne, J.M. & Woodings, T.L. (1980) Patterns of gastro-intestinal cancer in European migrants to Australia. The role of dietary change. *Int. J. Cancer*, *25*, 431-437

Muir, C., Waterhouse, J., Mack, T., Powell, J. & Whelan, S., eds(1987) *Cancer Incidence in Five Continents*, Vol. V (IARC Scientific Publications No. 88), Lyon, IARC

Osmond, C. & Gardner, M.J. (1982) Age period and cohort models applied to cancer mortality rates. *Stat. Med.*, *1*, 245-259

Osmond, C. & Gardner, M.J. (1983) Interpretation of disease time trends: is cancer on the increase? A simple cohort technique and its relationship to more advanced models. *J. Epidemiol. Community Health*, *37*, 274-278

Osmond, C., Gardner, M.J., Acheson, E.J. & Adelstein, A.M. (1983) *Trends in Cancer Mortality 1951-1980: Analyses by Period of Birth and Death. England and Wales (Series DH1, No. 11)*, London, Her Majesty's Stationery Office

Silverberg, E. & Luberg, J.A. (1988) Cancer statistics, 1988. *CA Cancer J. Clin.*, *38*, 5-22

Smans, M., Muir, C.S. & Boyle, P., eds (1990) *Atlas of Cancer Mortality in the European Economic Community* (IARC Scientific Publications No. 107), Lyon, IARC

Smith, P.G. (1982) Spatial and temporal clustering. In: Schottenfeld, D. & Fraumeni, J.F., eds, *Cancer Epidemiology and Prevention*, Philadelphia, Saunders, pp. 391-407

Staszewski, J., Slomska, J., Muir, C.S. & Jain, D.K. (1970) Sources of demographic data on migrant groups for epidemiological studies of chronic diseases. *J. Chronic Dis.*, *23*, 351-373

Steinitz, R., Parkin, D.M., Young, J.T., Bieber, C.A. & Katz, L. (1989) *Cancer Incidence in Jewish Migrants to Israel, 1961-1981* (IARC Scientific Publications No. 98), Lyon, IARC

The Editorial Committee for the Atlas of Cancer Mortality in the People's Republic of China (1979) *Atlas of Cancer Mortality in the People's Republic of China*, Shanghai, China Map Press

Townsend, P. & Davidson, N. (1987) *The Black Report*, London, Penguin

US Department of Health and Human Services (1982) *The Health Consequences of Smoking: Cancer. A Report of the Surgeon General*, Washington DC, US Public Health Service

Whitehead, M. (1987) *The Health Divide*, London, Health Education Authority

Chapter 3. Descriptive epidemiology of cancers at specific sites

In this section, we present the descriptive epidemiology of specific cancers in relation to the variables described above. In order to illustrate the level of geographic variation encountered, data on incidence in 20 populations in different areas of the world are presented in the Appendix. Although this part is not directly concerned with risk factors, which are discussed in detail in Part II, the descriptive epidemiology of a cancer is sometimes meaningful only when set in the context of information about possible etiological agents.

Unless otherwise stated, data on the incidence and percentage frequencies of different cancers are taken from *Cancer Incidence in Five Continents, Vol. V* (Muir *et al.*, 1987) or from *Cancer Incidence in Developing Countries* (Parkin, 1985). Data on time trends are those for the USA, 1947–84 (Devesa *et al.*, 1987), the Nordic countries (Hakulinen *et al.*, 1986), England and Wales, 1951–80 (Osmond *et al.*, 1983) and for Singapore, 1968–82 (Lee *et al.*, 1988).

Cancer of the lip

In general, lip cancers are not common, comprising less than 5% of cancers in most populations. Many of the observed variations in incidence may be due to different practices in classifying cancers of the anterior oral cavity to 'lip' or other parts of the mouth.

The highest reported incidence rates for lip cancer are for males in Newfoundland, Canada (15.1), in other Canadian provinces and in Australia; low rates are observed in Japan and India and among US blacks. Rates are normally five to ten times higher in males than in females, and the sex disparity is even greater in countries where the incidence in males is high. A striking racial variation is noted in the USA, where rates in whites are mostly more than five times higher than those in blacks.

In most white populations, lip cancer is the commonest type of oral cancer, accounting for up to half of all cases, and the lower lip is involved much more often than the upper lip. Persons living in rural areas and those employed in outdoor occupations, such as sailors, fishermen and farmers, have high rates of lip cancer, and higher incidences are seen in latitudes near the equator; these findings suggest a relationship with exposure to sunlight. The relationship between latitude and lip cancer risk is not as clear as for skin cancer, however: Finland is at the same latitude as Sweden and has the same amount of solar radiation, yet lip cancer rates in Finland are twice as high as those in Sweden for both men and women (Lindqvist & Teppo, 1978; Smith, 1982).

Cancers of the tongue and mouth

Cancers of the tongue and mouth are most common in Indian populations and have long been associated with the chewing of betel quid (IARC, 1985). Indian migrant populations who retain this habit, such as those in Singapore, also retain their high rates for these cancers, while those who abandon the habit, as in Fiji, do not. Cancers of the tongue and mouth account for up to 50% of all cancers in some parts of India, and for 15–30% in other populations in which chewing habits are widespread, such as in Sri Lanka, Papua New Guinea and Viet Nam. Rates are also notably high among men in Brazil, the Caribbean and France, but very few other populations show rates in excess of 3.0 per 100 000 in people of either sex. The almost universal excess among males is usually between two and ten fold.

Mortality rates from cancers of the tongue and mouth in England and Wales have decreased in successive generations born since the middle of the last century, but they have increased again for cohorts born since 1910 (Osmond *et al.*, 1983); a similar recent increase has been observed in the incidence of these cancers in Scotland for cohorts born since 1920 (MacFarlane *et al.*, 1987). Mortality from cancer of the tongue in young white males aged 10–29 years in the USA doubled between 1950 and 1980 (Depue, 1986). The decline and subsequent increase in mortality rates in successive cohorts in the UK has been interpreted as due to a decrease in pipe smoking and a later increase in cigarette smoking and alcohol consumption: these are all known to be risk factors for this cancer (see Part II, pp. 171, 181).

In contrast, a 31% reduction in incidence was recorded for males in Bombay, India, between 1964 and 1982 (Jayant & Yeole, 1987), due to a steadily accelerating decrease in incidence for successive five-year birth cohorts born between 1913 and 1943. A declining frequency of oral cancer has also been reported from Karachi, Pakistan (Zaidi, 1986), which is ascribed to a switch from betel chewing to cigarette smoking.

Cancer of the salivary glands

Salivary gland tumours are generally uncommon, with incidence rates in people of each sex of below 1.0 per 100 000. About 80% of the malignant tumours involve the parotid glands. The most notable observation has been high rates among females in high-risk populations, such as Eskimos. Rates in Canadian Inuits have been estimated to be 20.3 in males and 34.6 in females (Schaefer & Hildes, 1986); somewhat lower rates, of 3.9 in males and 7.7 in females, were observed in Greenland Eskimos (Nielsen *et al.*, 1978). Aleutian Eskimos in Alaska were found to have rates that were three times greater than those of the US population among males and eight times higher among females (Lanier *et al.*, 1980), but this observation is based on very few cases.

Cancer of the nasopharynx

Nasopharyngeal carcinoma (NPC) is rare in most populations, and age-standardized incidence rates are usually below 1.0 per 100 000. Lymphoma and adenocarcinoma comprise only 5–15% of cancers of the nasopharynx. Areas of high risk for NPC are found in south-east Asia and southern China.

The highest recorded incidence rates in the world are in Hong Kong (30.0 in males and 12.9 in females), where NPC is the second most frequent tumour after lung cancer, accounting for 12% of all cancers. In China, high mortality rates are seen in the south-eastern provinces adjacent to Hong Kong: Guangdong (3.8 times the national mortality rate), Guangxi, Fujian and Hunan. The Chinese migrants to other countries retain the differentials in risk of their regions of origin: thus, Hong Kong Chinese who came originally from Guangdong province have incidence rates that are three to four times higher than Hong Kong Chinese who originated from other provinces (Ho, 1967), and Cantonese-speaking Chinese in Singapore have a risk 1.5–1.8 times higher than those of other dialect groups (Lee *et al.*, 1988). NPC is also frequent elsewhere in south-east Asia, with incidence rates in males of 4.7 in Rizal province in the Philippines and 4.0 in Malays in Singapore; NPC comprises about 15% of cancers in males in case series from Viet Nam and Indonesia, and about 5% in Thailand.

Incidence rates (estimated from case series) are also high in Eskimo populations, e.g., 45.3 in Inuit males in Canada (Schaefer & Hildes, 1986) and 12.3 in Greenland Inuits (Nielsen *et al.*, 1977). An area of intermediate risk for NPC is North Africa, where the relative frequencies for males are 5% in Algeria, 10% in Tunisia and 12% in the Sudan.

The age-incidence rates of NPC are unusual. The rates begin to rise in people who are younger (15–24 years) than those who develop most other epithelial cancers, particularly in high-risk populations. The increase with age is less steep (Hirayama, 1978), and there is little or no increase after the sixth decade of life (Henderson, 1974). In the medium-risk populations of North Africa, there appears to be a first peak in incidence in people 15–19 years of age, followed by a fall, before incidence again rises to a plateau in those over the age of 50 (Ellouz *et al.*, 1978). As a result of these different patterns, NPC is a relatively common tumour among children in North Africa (10–20% of children's tumours), whereas it is rare in childhood elsewhere, even in Chinese populations (Parkin *et al.*, 1988). In most populations, there are two to three times more cases of NPC in males than in females.

The risk for NPC in second- and third-generation Chinese immigrants born in the USA is still much higher than that of US whites, but only half that of first-generation emigrants born in China (Zippin *et al.*, 1962; Buell, 1973a); mortality rates from NPC declined in Chinese Americans during 1950–69 (Fraumeni & Mason, 1974). These aspects of the epidemiology of NPC strongly suggest the influence of environmental factors associated with traditional practices (such as diet and cooking methods) and exposure to a common virus at an early age in the etiology of NPC.

Cancers of the oropharynx and hypopharynx

The descriptive epidemiology of cancers of the oropharynx is similar to that of the tongue and mouth, while that of the hypopharynx has features in common with laryngeal cancer. The highest rates are observed in France, particularly in Calvados (where the incidence in males is 31.3 per 100 000), and rates are high in western Switzerland and northern Italy. High rates are also observed in India, southern Brazil and the Caribbean. In the USA, incidence rates in blacks are more than double those in whites. Rates in females are almost invariably much lower than those in males, and usually less than 1.0 per 100 000; the rare exceptions are found mostly in India, where the female incidence of hypopharyngeal cancer is 1.0–2.5 cases per 100 000, but these are still only about one-fourth of the rates in males.

Time trends in mortality from cancer of the pharynx for males in England and Wales are similar to those for oral cancer, with rising rates in generations born since about 1910; mortality rates for females are declining. In the USA, there have been large increases in mortality rates in black males since 1950, but little change has been seen for black females or for whites.

Cancer of the oesophagus

Oesophageal cancer is characterized by an extreme diversity of rates throughout the world. There are usually more cases among males, but in areas of very high incidence the rates in females may exceed those in males. Incidence rates are estimated to be as high as 195.3 per 100 000 females and 165.5 for males in northern Gonbad in the Caspian region of Iran (Day & Muñoz, 1982), and mortality rates are 211.2 in males and 136.5 in females of Linxian county in China (Lu *et al.*, 1985). These rates are in marked contrast to those in, say, Cluj County in Romania (1.2 per 100 000 males and 0.2 for females).

The high-risk areas of the world include the so-called 'Asian oesophageal cancer belt', which stretches from the Caspian littoral in northern Iran, through the southern republics of the USSR (Turkmenistan, Kazakhstan and Uzbekistan) to western and northern China; south-eastern Africa; parts of eastern South America (southern Brazil, Uruguay, Paraguay, northern Argentina); and certain defined areas of western Europe (particularly France and Switzerland). The high rates in China are reflected in the fact that over half of the annual total of cases of oesophageal cancer in the world occur there. In addition, within small areas of these high-risk areas, striking differences have been demonstrated, as for example within the Transkei (Rose & McGlashan, 1975) and within Brittany in France (Tuyns & Massé, 1973).

There are also quite marked differences between ethnic groups – in the USA, for example, incidence rates in blacks are some four-fold higher than those in whites, and in Singapore rates in Chinese are double those in Indians and ten times those in Malays. Even among the Chinese in Singapore, there are marked variations, of at least six fold, in incidence by dialect group (Lee *et al.*, 1988).

Jews who have migrated to Israel from the high-risk areas of Asia have higher incidence rates of oesophageal cancer than migrants from elsewhere, but the differences decrease with increasing duration of residence in Israel. Second-generation Chinese migrants to Singapore have incidence rates that are two to three times lower than those of first-generation migrants, and US residents of Chinese ancestry now have incidence rates that are little different from those in whites. These changes in risk imply the importance of environmental agents in the etiology of this cancer.

International trends in mortality from oesophageal cancer show quite mixed patterns. Age-standardized rates are declining in the Nordic countries, Switzerland and the Federal Republic of Germany, and increasing in France, in US blacks and in Australia. In France, there are quite distinct cohort patterns among men: the lowest mortality rates are seen in the generation that was born in 1912–16, an effect that can quite plausibly be related to a lower consumption of alcohol in young adulthood than by subsequent cohorts (Tuyns & Audigier, 1976). A similar finding has been noted in Australia (McMichael, 1978) and in England and Wales, where there is a good correlation between per-caput consumption of alcohol (as beer or spirits) and cohort-specific mortality for both men and women (Chilvers *et al.*, 1979).

In South Africa, the rise in frequency of oesophageal cancer appears to be relatively recent, reaching high levels only in the 1960s, and is probably linked to an increased consumption of alcohol; but these conclusions were based only on information about the percentage of hospital admissions attributed to this cancer and on mortality rates in the 'coloured' population (Rose, 1973). This trend seems to be persisting, as there is no suggestion that the incidence among African miners in the Cape area (including the Transkei) and Natal has changed recently (Bradshaw *et al.*, 1982). In the 'Asian oesophageal cancer belt', alcohol consumption cannot explain the extremely high incidence rates observed. Some recent data on time trends from Linxian county (China) suggest that both incidence and mortality rates were relatively constant until about 1970 and have since declined among people of all ages (Lu *et al.*, 1985). The authors propose that the effect is due to improved nutrition.

Cancer of the stomach

In 1980, stomach cancer was estimated to be the single most common form of cancer in the world, accounting for some 670 000 new cases per year, or 10.5% of all cancers (see Table 2). It is probably now the second most common, after lung cancer. The highest recorded incidence rates occur in Japan and probably in other areas of the Far East, including the Republic of Korea and parts of China – particularly the north and centre. High incidence rates have also been reported from the USSR (Napalkov *et al.*, 1983), in eastern Europe and in parts of Latin America, particularly Chile and Costa Rica. In Africa, stomach cancer has generally been considered to be relatively rare, but areas of high frequency have been reported in certain mountainous regions, such as Rwanda, south-west Uganda and around Mount Kilimanjaro. In western Europe, age-standardized incidence rates are generally 15–25 cases per 100 000 population, although higher rates exist in some regions, and particularly in northern Italy.

Incidence and mortality rates in males are approximately double those for females, in both high- and low-risk countries. However, the sex ratio (male:female) is not constant by age group: it is approximately unity in people under age 30 and rises to about 2.2 in persons of about 60 years of age. Rates in whites in the USA are approximately half those in blacks. There are marked variations by socioeconomic status, with a difference of almost three fold in mortality rates between the highest and lowest categories of social class in England and Wales.

Several studies of migrants suggest that the risk for stomach cancer changes rather slowly in populations who move from high-risk to lower-risk countries (the usual pattern). Thus, for Chinese in Singapore, who have much higher risks than

Malays or Indians, there is little difference in incidence between those who were born in China and those who were born locally. The work of Haenszel and Kurihara (1968), showing a rather slow fall in mortality rates between generations of Japanese migrants to the USA, has already been described (p. 46), and incidence rates for Japanese in the USA remain three to four times higher than those for whites. However, for at least some European populations who have migrated to the lower-risk countries of Australia (McMichael *et al.*, 1980) and Israel (Steinitz *et al.*, 1989), risk declines with increasing duration of residence.

The most remarkable feature of the epidemiology of gastric cancer is the virtually universal decline in its incidence (and consequent mortality). The decline is about 2–4% per year, but there is quite a lot of variation between different countries and in the time of its onset. Rates are falling more rapidly for females than for males. Because the decline is present at all age groups, it is impossible to judge whether period or cohort effects (see p. 39) are more important. In Japan, where there is a very high risk for cancer of the stomach, the decline in mortality has been less marked than elsewhere and has been most marked in people in the middle range of ages (Tominaga, 1987). It has been suggested that mass screening programmes have played a part in this decrease (see Part III, p. 272), but this does not explain why the decline has been greater in women, who have profited much less from such programmes.

Data from cancer registries indicate that the temporal changes in the incidence of gastric cancer in Norway (Muñoz & Asvall, 1971) and Japan (Hanai *et al.*, 1982) are due largely to the disappearance of the 'intestinal' type of gastric cancer as opposed to the 'diffuse' type. Studies of migrant populations in Colombia suggest that variations in the incidence of cancer of the stomach are due largely to differences in the intestinal type, while the rates for the diffuse variety are relatively constant (Correa *et al.*, 1970).

Cancer of the colon

Cancer of the colon is a disease of economically 'developed' populations. The highest incidence rate is found in the white male population of Connecticut, USA, with an age-standardized rate of 33.2 per 100 000 population. The highest rate among females is now observed in the black population of the USA (31.0 per 100 000). In the remainder of North America and Oceania, age-standardized rates are generally in the range of 20–30 per 100 000. Incidence and mortality rates for US blacks have been increasing and are now more or less the same as those of whites. Incidence rates in northern and western Europe are generally rather lower than in the other 'developed' areas, at 15–20 per 100 000. In developing countries in Africa, Asia and Latin America, the incidence rates for cancer of the colon are generally low, although in places where rapid urbanization and westernization of life styles have occurred, as in southern Brazil and La Plata, Argentina, Hong Kong and Singapore, age-adjusted rates of 10–15 per 100 000 are seen.

Incidence and mortality rates are about the same in males and females, but cancer of the colon is slightly more common in women under the age of 60 and more frequent in men thereafter.

Ethnic differences in the frequency of this type of cancer, particularly as demonstrated by studies of migrants, suggest that environmental factors play a major role in its etiology. Most studies have involved migrants moving from low-risk to high-risk areas, such as Chinese and Japanese to Hawaii or the rest of the USA, or southern Europeans to North America, Australia or the UK. In general, the risk for cancer of the colon in migrants approximates that of the new country. Migrants to Australia from low-risk countries have increasing rates of colon cancer with increasing duration of stay (McMichael *et al.*, 1980), and persons born in Mexico and living in Los Angeles have higher incidences of colon cancer if they migrated as children than if they moved as adults (Mack *et al.*, 1985). Jewish migrants to Israel, however, show no change in risk with increasing duration of stay, even after more than 30 years in the new environment (Steinitz *et al.*, 1989). Incidence rates for Japanese born in the USA now exceed those of US whites (Shimizu *et al.*, 1987), and the same is true of Japanese living in Hawaii (Kolonel *et al.*, 1980).

In general, incidence and mortality rates for cancer of the colon are rising, particularly in areas where the risk was formerly low (Boyle *et al.*, 1985). These changes have been accompanied by changing ratios between the subsites within the colon at which tumours occur, with left-sided tumours (of the descending and sigmoid colon) becoming more frequent (Haenszel & Correa, 1971; de Jong *et al.*, 1972).

Cancer of the rectum

The geographical distribution of rectal cancer is similar to that of cancer of the colon, but incidence and mortality rates are usually rather lower, although it should be remembered that tumours registered as of the 'large intestine' are coded under the same rubric as cancer of the colon, which may inflate the rates of the latter. Generally, rectal cancer is 1.5–2.0 times more common among males than among females, particularly in countries where the incidence is high.

There is little difference between the incidence rates in North America, Europe and Australia, where the age-standardized rates are mainly in the range 15–20 per 100 000 for males and 8–12 for females. In contrast, mortality rates in the USA are among the lowest in developed countries. This difference between incidence and mortality rates is reflected in time trends for the USA, which show quite large declines in mortality rates for blacks and whites of each sex, with little apparent change in incidence, presumably reflecting improved results of therapy. There is no consistent pattern in the time trends for incidence and mortality elsewhere; rates are rising for people of each sex in Japan, Norway, Finland and Italy, and rates are declining in Denmark and in England and Wales.

Migrant studies give substantially the same results as for cancer of the colon. The early studies of Japanese migrants to the USA showed an increased risk after migration but little change in second-generation migrants (Haenszel & Kurihara, 1968). More recent data suggest that the incidence in US-born Japanese males is considerably higher than that in US whites (Kolonel *et al.*, 1980; Shimizu *et al.*, 1987).

Cancer of the liver

Cancer of the liver ranks eighth in numerical importance on a world-wide basis, with 250 000 new cases per year; it accounts for 5.3% of new cancers in males and 2.6% in females. Three-quarters of these cases occur in developing countries. High-incidence areas for cancer of the liver are sub-Saharan Africa, East and south-east Asia (as far west as Burma) and Melanesia. In North America, only populations of Asian origin and Eskimos have high rates. The incidence is low in South America, Australia and New Zealand (except for the Maori and Polynesian inhabitants) and in Europe, although rates in southern Europe (Spain, Italy and Greece) are moderate.

This cancer occurs more commonly in males than in females: the sex ratio for its incidence is about 3:1 in high-risk areas, but closer to 1.5:1 in areas of lower risk.

The geographic distribution of cancer of the liver shows a relatively close correlation with the prevalence of chronic carriers of hepatitis B surface antigen (HBsAg). Thus, in the high-risk areas of sub-Saharan Africa and eastern Asia, the prevalence of carriers of this antigen is over 10% (Figure 12). There are, however, some interesting exceptions – a high prevalence of carriers of HBsAg but a low incidence of cancer of the liver have been reported in Greenland Eskimos (Melbye *et al.*, 1984). Variations in the incidence of liver cancer within several countries of Africa and Asia have also been shown to be correlated with local levels of aflatoxin contamination of foodstuffs (see p. 126).

The great majority of cancers that occur in this organ in adults are hepatocellular carcinomas; tumours of the intrahepatic bile ducts (cholangiocarcinoma) are by contrast rather rare, representing, for instance, 6.4% of malignant tumours of the liver in the USA. However, in parts of south-east Asia, cholangiocarcinoma is a frequent cancer – it comprises 60% of cancers of the liver in north-eastern Thailand. This distribution coincides with endemic areas for liver flukes, *Clonorchis sinensis* and *Opisthorchis viverrini*, which are presumably important etiological agents (Srivanatakul *et al.*, 1988; see p. 195).

Most cancers of the liver that occur in children are hepatoblastomas. These are rare tumours occurring in the early months of life, and the risk shows little geographic or ethnic variation.

Cancer of the pancreas

Cancer of the pancreas is moderately frequent on a world-wide basis, with 120 000 new cases in 1980. It is more important in developed countries, in which it comprises about 3% of incident cases. However, because it is almost invariably fatal, it is now also a major component of mortality from cancer in western countries; for instance, it is the fourth most common cause of death from cancer in people of each sex in the USA. The highest incidence rates in the world have been recorded in black populations in the USA; New Zealand Maoris also have high rates.

Time trends in the occurrence of pancreatic cancer suggest that the rates of incidence and mortality are increasing practically everywhere. Some caution is

Figure 12. A, Prevalence of carriers of hepatitis B surface antigen (as percentage found to have a positive reaction by radioimmunoassay); and **B,** risk for cancer of the liver (cases/100 000 population) in areas of high risk for this cancer – sub-Saharan Africa and eastern Asia[a]

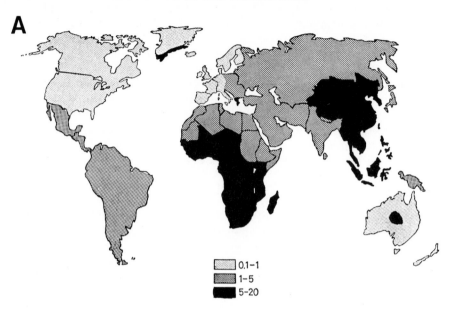

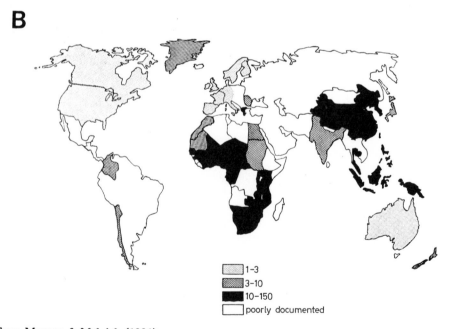

[a] From Maupas & Melnick (1981)

needed in interpreting this observation: pancreatic cancer has been difficult to diagnose, and the increasing availability and sophistication of diagnostic tools might be producing a (spurious) rise in the number of recorded cases; this cancer is recorded particularly inaccurately on death certificates. The increase in mortality rates has generally been greater in males than in females, and has been faster in countries where the rates were low earlier (notably Japan). The increase has levelled off in several countries since about 1970, particularly in the USA where, before that date, mortality rates in black males were rising very rapidly, at 3.9% per year, in comparison with 1.7% in whites.

Moolgavkar and Stevens (1981) drew attention to the similarities in age-specific time trends in mortality from pancreatic cancer and from cancer of the lung in England and Wales and suggested that the cohort-specific changes were related to differences in the prevalence of smoking among males and females in different age groups. These relationships appear to be much less clear elsewhere, for instance, in the USA and Scandinavia.

Cancer of the larynx

Laryngeal cancer is predominantly a cancer of males; the ratio of the numbers of male to female cases in the world in 1980 was estimated to be almost 7:1. The highest incidence rates are reported from southern Brazil, Italy, France and Spain, and high mortality rates are reported from Uruguay, Hungary, Yugoslavia and Cuba. Data on relative frequency suggest that the Middle East and North Africa are also areas of high risk.

The Appendix shows that in several of the areas in which the risk for laryngeal cancer is low, such as the UK, Australia, Pacific populations (Maoris, Hawaiians), USA (whites) and Shanghai, China, the incidence rates for lung cancer are high; in these areas, laryngeal cancers occur mainly in the glottis. However, in populations at high risk – in southern Europe and in US blacks – the incidences of both supraglottic and hypopharyngeal tumours are elevated. These patterns may be related to the effects of alcohol consumption.

Incidence and mortality rates for laryngeal cancer are increasing in males in many countries in southern and eastern Europe, in Scandinavia, in Australia and among US blacks. Examination of the trends in mortality by age group in France and in Australia suggests that these can be related to patterns of alcohol consumption in different generations of males (Tuyns & Audigier, 1976; McMichael, 1978). Ecological studies linking the risk for laryngeal cancer in different populations to per-caput consumption of tobacco and alcohol have generally shown a closer association with the latter factor (Tuyns, 1982).

Cancer of the lung

Lung cancer is almost certainly the commonest cancer in the world today: the annual number of new cases in 1980 was estimated at 660 500 (10.4% of all new cancers), and the number is increasing at a rate of about 0.5% per year. It is most common in the developed regions of the world – in Europe, North America, Australia, the USSR and Japan – and incidence rates are also high in southern South America and the Caribbean. Although the rates are rather lower in South

Africa, south-east Asia and western Asia, and in Micronesia and Polynesia, lung cancer is still the commonest cancer among males in those areas.

The highest incidence rates in the world are found among American blacks (109.0 per 100 000 for males and 28.4 for females), Maoris in New Zealand (101.3 and 68.1 for males and females, respectively) and Scotland (91.1 for males, with a rate of 100.4 for males in the west of Scotland). The lowest are seen in India (5.8 for males and 1.2 for females in Madras) and in African populations (1.1 in males in Dakar). This international variation is well explained by different current and past exposures to the main cause of lung cancer – cigarette smoking. Figure 4 (p. 38) showed the results of one correlation study, in which the risk for lung cancer in young adults was compared with smoking patterns 20 years earlier, as the same generation was entering adult life.

The difference in lung cancer risk for males and females is largely explicable on the basis of smoking habits: rates are lower in females because in almost all countries fewer women smoke, or, when this is no longer the case, they started to smoke at a later period than males, started later in life, smoke less and use brands containing less tar. The risk for lung cancer also tends to be higher in urban than in rural areas. This may be due to the higher prevalence of smoking among city dwellers, but there may also be a contribution of urban air pollution (see Part II, Chapter 13), although comparisons of urban and rural Mormons in Utah, USA, most of whom are nonsmokers, have shown no difference in risk (Lyon *et al.*, 1980a). Studies of lung cancer risk in relation to occupation reveal some interesting discrepancies, suggesting an excess risk due to specific occupational exposures (Table 8). The evidence with regard to single agents that are causally related to lung cancer is described in Part II, Chapter 5.

It is probable that most of the variation in lung cancer risk by ethnic group can be explained by differences in exposure to tobacco smoke. Nevertheless, there are some intriguing exceptions. Chinese women, who are almost all nonsmokers, have much higher rates of lung cancer than might be anticipated (age-standardized rates of 18.5 per 100 000 in Shanghai and 28.8 in Tianjin). A high percentage of such tumours are adenocarcinomas, whereas most of those induced by tobacco smoke are squamous-cell carcinomas. Indoor air pollution has been suspected as a possible etiological factor (Gao *et al.*, 1987).

Time trends in incidence and mortality rates for lung cancer are very striking. This cancer was a relatively rare disease in the early years of this century and has now become the leading cause of death and illness from cancer today. Trends by age group and sex in different countries can be accounted for almost entirely by national tobacco smoking habits, as reflected in the prevalence of smoking in different generations (birth cohorts) and the tar content of the cigarettes they smoked (IARC, 1986). The role of cigarette composition on incidence and mortality rates for lung cancer is discussed on p. 174.

Table 8. Mortality from lung cancer (1970-72) and smoking ratio (1972) by occupation, males, 15–64 years of age, England and Wales[a]

Occupation	Standardized mortality ratio	Smoking ratio[b]
Farmers, foresters, fishermen	84	77
Coal miners (underground)	114	131
Glass and ceramic makers	128	94
Electrical and electronics workers	101	102
Butchers and meat cutters	129	99
Construction workers	144	113
Drivers of buses, coaches	125	128
Clerical workers	79	87
Sales workers	85	91
Administrators and managers	60	76
Medical practitioners	32	33
University teachers	15	52

[a] From Office of Populations and Census Statistics (1978)

[b] $\dfrac{\text{Observed number currently smoking cigarettes}}{\text{Expected number currently smoking cigarettes}} \times 100$

where the expected number is based on age-standardized proportions

The very high rates of lung cancer in industrialized countries reflect the substantial increase in per-caput consumption of cigarettes since the First World War. At present, incidence rates among males in Scandinavia, the UK and North America are rising only in the older generations (e.g., men born before 1925 in Finland, before 1905 in England and before 1930 in the USA), so that in some countries the age-adjusted rates among men are actually falling. Figures 9 and 10 (pp. 47 and 48) showed trends in mortality from lung cancer in US men and, clearly, suggest that the maximal risk is that of the generation born around 1930. This is quite coherent with data on the prevalence of smoking (Figure 13) – which was highest in the generations born 1911–30, of whom, at the age of about 30, some 70% were smokers. Among women, however, smoking is a more recent habit, so that rates are rising in all age groups in most countries, although in the USA there is now a decline in the youngest age groups, and in England there is a fall in generations born since 1925.

In Mediterranean Europe, cigarette smoking is a more recent phenomenon (during the 1930s and 1940s cigarette consumption in the UK was four times that in France), so that lung cancer rates in men are still rising, even though the introduction of low-tar cigarettes has helped to modify the increase. Women in these countries have traditionally been nonsmokers, and their incidence of lung cancer has changed little to date; however, the massive increase in the prevalence of smoking among young females will undoubtedly be reflected in increasing rates quite soon.

The data for developing countries are more sparse. In areas where cigarette smoking is well established among men, such as Singapore, Hong Kong, Israel, Kuwait, Chile and Brazil, the incidence of lung cancer is clearly increasing. With few exceptions, rates for women are now also rising. In other developing countries, such as in Africa, cigarette smoking is too recent a phenomenon to have had much impact.

Figure 13. Changes in the prevalence of cigarette smoking among successive birth cohorts of men, 1900-78[a]

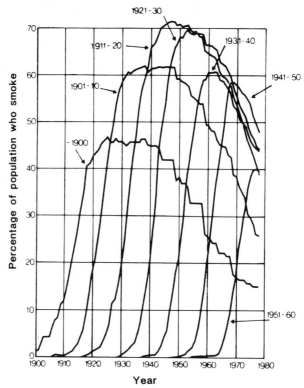

a From US Department of Health and Human Services (1982)

Because the risk for lung cancer in a given generation is closely related to the smoking habits of that generation, and because this habit tends to become established in adolescence and young adult life – long before the occurrence of lung cancer – it is relatively easy to predict the future evolution of the lung cancer epidemic, at least in the medium term. Thus, in the USA, the decline in mortality from lung cancer in men, which has just begun, will continue; however, unless the current prevalence of smoking among females decreases markedly, their rates will continue to rise for another 25 years (Brown & Kessler, 1988). This pattern of increase, in men as well as in women, can be predicted for all of those countries where cigarette smoking is a relatively recent phenomenon.

Mesothelioma

Mesothelioma is defined by its histology; it occurs almost exclusively in the pleura and peritoneum. Although in routine mortality statistics mesothelioma is not usually reported as a separate category, the great majority (70–90%) of deaths classified as cancers of the pleura are probably mesotheliomas (Gardner *et al.*, 1982). In many countries, specialized mesothelioma registers have been set up because mesothelioma is known to be the result of occupational and environmental exposure to asbestos fibres (Wagner *et al.*, 1960; IARC, 1977). There are, however, several difficulties in assessing the available data: information on mortality from mesothelioma may be biased owing to the increased awareness since 1960 of its association with exposure to asbestos, and there is clearly considerable error in attributing it as the cause of death on death certificates (McDonald, 1979).

The annual incidence rates of mesothelioma in the USA in 1973–78 were 0.9 per 100 000 for white males and 0.3 for white females, with lower rates in non-whites. Four times more of these tumours occurred in the pleura in males, while the incidence of peritoneal mesothelioma was similar in people of each sex. More recent data for Australia and the UK suggest crude incidence rates in males of 2.7 and 2.4 per 100 000, respectively (Ferguson *et al.*, 1987), with pleural mesothelioma accounting for about 80% of the tumours.

Localized areas of high incidence have been noted in places where shipbuilding and asbestos insulation are important industries (Tagnon *et al.*, 1980; Enterline & Henderson, 1987). A survey of mortality in 1979–83 in three Turkish villages in which the population is exposed to naturally occurring mineral fibres (erionite) suggested extraordinarily high crude rates for death from malignant mesothelioma – around 800 per 100 000 per year (Baris *et al.*, 1987).

The incidence of mesothelioma is increasing, although part of the observed increase is probably due to better diagnosis and registration. Incidence rates in Connecticut, USA, increased ten times in males and three times in females during the period 1935–78 (Fraumeni & Blot, 1982). In the UK, there was a four-fold increase in the number of deaths certified as being due to mesothelioma between 1968 and 1984; the sex ratio was constant at about 4:1, and there was little change in the age distribution (Jones & Thomas, 1986, 1987). The clearest evidence that the incidence of this cancer is increasing was provided by Spirtas *et al.* (1986), who found that between 1973 and 1980 in the USA, the incidence of pleural mesothelioma among white males increased at an average of 12–13% per year. The increasing trend was confined to older men, and the patterns were considered to be consistent with a cohort effect due to exposure of young men 25–40 years previously.

It seems unlikely that artefacts of diagnosis and death certification can account entirely for these observed trends in mesothelioma incidence, and they are probably the result of patterns of use of asbestos during and shortly after the Second World War (Enterline & Henderson, 1987).

Cancers of the bone

Primary malignant tumours of bone comprise several distinct clinicopathological entities, so that the descriptive epidemiology of this site can be based only on studies in which they can be distinguished. The principal tumours of the bone in the USA are osteosarcomas (36.4%), chondrosarcomas (29.5%) and

Ewing's sarcomas (15.6%) (US Surveillance, Epidemiology and End Results Program, 1973–77). The incidence of osteosarcoma shows two distinct peaks – one in people 15–19 years of age and the other in old people. The adolescent peak appears to be related to bone growth: the bones principally affected are those that grow most rapidly (femur and tibia), and the rates are initially higher in girls (at ages 10–14) but are overtaken by those of boys aged 15–19. Rates in blacks are somewhat higher than those in whites (Parkin *et al.*, 1988). The higher incidence of both osteosarcoma and chondrosarcoma in older people is related to underlying Paget's disease of the bone: people with this condition are estimated to have a risk for developing bone sarcoma that is 13 times higher than that of other people (Price & Jeffree, 1977).

Ewing's sarcoma occurs almost entirely in children and during early adult life, with peak rates of incidence in people in the 15–19 age range. Incidence rates in black children in the USA are only about 10% of those in whites; the risk in sub-Saharan Africa, China, Japan and south-east Asia also appears to be very low.

Soft-tissue sarcomas

Sarcomas are malignant tumours of mesenchymal tissue, such as muscle, fat, fibrous tissue and blood vessels, which can be located in specific organs, in skin or in the connective tissues in between. In routine statistics, these tumours are not reported separately, so that the descriptive epidemiology of soft-tissue sarcomas requires special studies.

Tucker and Fraumeni (1982), reviewing the epidemiology of soft-tissue sarcomas in the USA, found that leiomyosarcoma is the most common form, occurring most commonly in the uterus (with a consequent predominance in females) and the intestinal tract. Liposarcomas are second in frequency, followed by fibrosarcomas and rhabdomyosarcomas; the latter two occur marginally more frequently in blacks. Studies of time trends suggest that incidence and mortality rates for connective tissue tumours are increasing, at least in adults.

Soft-tissue sarcomas comprise 4–8% of all childhood cancers, the main histological types (outside of Africa) being rhabdomyosarcomas and fibrosarcomas, both of which have rather different pathological and clinical characteristics from their adult counterparts.

Kaposi's sarcoma was, until recently, rare in western countries, but in parts of sub-Saharan Africa (particularly central Africa), it occurs at frequencies of 5–10% of all cancers (Hutt, 1981). In its 'endemic' form, the tumour affects predominantly males, and the incidence and sex ratios increase with age. In adults, the tumour progresses slowly and is localized to skin and subcutaneous tissue, particularly of the legs (although autopsy studies show visceral involvement in most cases). In childhood, it takes a more severe course, with lymphatic and visceral involvement. It is this generalized form that has been associated with states of immunosuppression (Penn, 1986) and with infection with human immunodeficiency virus (see p. 192). The latter has resulted in enormous increases in the incidence of this tumour in the population at high risk (Biggar *et al.*, 1987).

Malignant melanoma of the skin

Four types of melanoma are distinguished morphologically. Lentigo maligna melanoma occurs in older individuals with clearly sun-damaged skin; its epidemiological features are very similar to those of non-melanoma skin cancer. Superficial spreading and nodular melanomas occur in younger people and most commonly on body sites that are not continuously exposed to the sun. (The latter may simply be a late stage of the former: Holman *et al.*, 1983.) Finally, acral lentiginous melanomas generally occur on the palms, soles and squamous mucosa and are proportionally infrequent in Europeans. Recent epidemiological studies of the etiology of melanoma have focused mainly on the second and third types.

Cutaneous malignant melanoma remains a relatively infrequent tumour, despite quite marked increases in its incidence in several populations in recent years. Males and females are affected approximately equally. The disease is especially common in fair-skinned populations of European origin living in sunny regions. Thus, the highest reported rates are from Australia and the white populations of Hawaii, California and the southern states of the USA. Incidence rates in Asian populations are low.

The importance of exposure to sunlight might be expected to be reflected by an association between risk for melanoma and latitude of residence. Such a relationship has been proposed for Australia, Canada and the USA (Elwood *et al.*, 1974; Lee, 1982). In Europe, however, the situation is less clear, as incidence rates in the Nordic countries and Switzerland are higher than those in France or Italy. The explanation lies almost certainly in the importance of intermittent (recreational) exposure to sunlight, as well as in differential susceptibility. Thus, there is a strong social class gradient in risk, with higher rates among people of non-manual, professional classes (Lee & Strickland, 1980; Cooke *et al.*, 1984).

In white populations, the sites most often affected are the lower limbs in females and the trunk, head and neck in males. In black populations, malignant melanoma is not particularly rare (representing probably about 2–5% of cancers in Africa), but it occurs mainly on the sole of the foot.

Rapid increases in both incidence and mortality have been observed in people of each sex almost everywhere in the world, even in some countries where the rates are low, such as in Japan (Muir & Nectoux, 1982). The largest average annual increases are about 6% in the Nordic countries, 7% in New Zealand and as much as 11% in the Jewish population of Israel. The increase in risk is evident in people in all age groups, and there is a progressive increase in the risk for successive birth cohorts (Armstrong *et al.*, 1982). Recent data from the USA suggest that the increases in incidence that were evident before 1980 may now have ceased. In any case, it appears that the remarkable changes recorded world-wide are real, and are not due to changes in diagnostic criteria (Van der Esch *et al.*, 1989). In US blacks, there has been almost no change in incidence or in mortality rates.

Data on migrants to Australia and Israel – both sunny environments receiving northern European migrants – show that the risk for melanoma increases with duration of residence in the new environment (see Figure 11, p. 49). In Australia, this change may result in rates that are close to or even higher than those of persons born locally, but it has been suggested that the rise, at least for superficial malignant melanomas, is substantially limited to migrants who arrive in Australia before 15 years of age (Holman & Armstrong, 1984).

Other cancers of the skin

Skin cancers other than malignant melanoma are difficult to study epidemiologically. Most patients with these cancers are treated as hospital out-patients or in general practice; histological examinations are usually not undertaken, since the clinical diagnosis is relatively simple; some persons remain undiagnosed. In many registries, data on these cancers are not collected, and, in those where it is collected, the completeness of registration is usually much less than for other cancers.

About 80% of skin cancers that are not malignant melanoma are basal-cell carcinomas. Most of the remainder are squamous-cell carcinomas, about half of which may arise from malignant transformation of a solar keratosis (Marks *et al.*, 1988). These tumours metastasize infrequently (1–2%), and mortality from such cancers is very low (Scotto *et al.*, 1983; Nixon *et al.*, 1986).

Over 95% of skin cancers other than melanoma are cured by excision, but their importance as a public health problem may be underrated, particularly in areas of high incidence. The highest reported incidence rates are in Australia, where the age-standardized rate was estimated at 555 per 100 000 in a population survey (Giles *et al.*, 1988). The cumulative incidence up to age 74 years was 67%, implying that two out of three persons will have had at least one skin cancer by that age; 10% of affected persons had had two or more skin cancers. In the USA, a one-year survey in eight areas resulted in estimated incidence rates of 233 per 100 000 (standardized to the US 1970 population; Scotto *et al.*, 1983). Incidence rates for skin cancer are not reported in *Cancer Incidence in Five Continents Vol. V* (Muir *et al.*, 1987) from registries in the USA, Israel, Australia (except Tasmania) or New Zealand. In registries that do report these cancers, the rates are highest for males in Tasmania (167) and British Columbia, Canada (109). Incidence rates of 20–60 are typical, and only in Asian populations are the reported rates consistently less than 10 per 100 000.

Susceptibility to skin cancer is inversely related to the degree of melanin pigmentation. Thus, in the USA, whites have about 100 times more skin cancer than blacks. Otherwise, the risk increases steeply with decreasing latitude, and the populations at highest risk live nearest to the equator. Two- to three-fold differences have been demonstrated within Australia and the USA. In the USA and Canada, the gradient is related directly to the amount of 290–320 nm wavelength ultra-violet light (UV-B) reaching the earth's surface, and this relationship is stronger for squamous-cell than for basal-cell tumours (Elwood *et al.*, 1974; Scotto *et al.*, 1983).

Males have about twice as many basal-cell and squamous-cell cancers as females. The anatomical distribution in males and females reflects typical clothing patterns: in males, 60–80% of tumours arise on the face, head and neck, particularly the nose; females have a higher proportion of tumours on the limbs.

In African populations, the great majority (70–85%) of skin cancers are squamous-cell tumours on the lower limbs, arising in association with scar tissue, particularly from tropical ulcers.

A very large American survey in 1977, of almost 30 000 cases (Scotto *et al.*, 1983), showed a 15–20% increase in incidence over that in an earlier survey, in 1971, mainly for basal-cell carcinomas. A recent report on members of a US health plan indicated that the incidence of squamous-cell cancer of the skin increased by about three fold between the 1960s and the 1980s, compared with an approximately four-fold increase for malignant melanoma (Glass & Hoover, 1989).

It has been estimated that the increase in the amount of UV-B radiation that will reach the earth's surface as a result of depletion of stratospheric ozone will be 10–15% or more. Since the large US survey suggested that a 1% increase in UV-B radiation would cause a 1–2% increase in the incidence of skin cancer, and a more recent estimate suggests that the range of increase in incidence may be 1–3% (Jones, 1987), this cancer seems likely to become still more common.

Cancer of the breast

Breast cancer is the third most common tumour in the world (ranked equal with colorectal cancer), after cancers of the lung and stomach (Table 2, p. 24). There were an estimated 572 000 new cases in 1980, or 9% of the global cancer burden. This incidence is particularly striking because breast cancer occurs almost exclusively in women, among whom it ranks first, comprising 18.4% of all cancers. This percentage varies considerably around the world: in high-risk areas, such as North America and western Europe, breast cancer accounts for one in four female cancers, while in low-risk areas such as China and Japan, it accounts for only one in eight to one in 16.

The highest recorded incidence rates are seen in Hawaiian women (93.9 per 100 000) and in US white women (70–90 per 100 000). Incidence rates are high (age-standardized rates of 60–90 per 100 000) in most industrialized countries (with the notable exception of Japan) and in southern Brazil and Argentina; they are intermediate (40–60 per 100 000) elsewhere in South America and in eastern and southern Europe; and low (less than 40) in Central and tropical South America, Africa and Asia. In North America, the cumulative incidence of breast cancer in white women up to age 74 years is 7–9%, which suggests that if current patterns were maintained, one in every 11–14 women would develop breast cancer during her life.

The incidence curve for breast cancer rises with age from 30 to 70 years, but shows a notable inflexion at around 45–54 years, the age of the menopause, after which the risk increases much more slowly with age (see Figure 5). This reduction in the slope of the age-incidence curve is more marked in low-risk areas than in high-risk areas, and in some countries, such as Japan, the incidence actually decreases after 45–54 years of age (Figure 14). There is considerable variation within countries by sociodemographic factors such as race, social class, marital status and region of residence. Three- to four-fold differences in the incidence of breast cancer are observed between Jews (high) and non-Jews (low) in Israel, and between Hawaiians (high) and Filipinos (low) in Hawaii. Breast cancer is more common in single women than in married women: this observation was first made in 1700 by Ramazzini (Petrakis *et al.*, 1982), who noted a high risk among nuns, although mortality in some British nuns is no different from that of the general population (Kinlen, 1982). Widowed and especially divorced women in the USA have even lower rates of breast cancer than married women, among both blacks and whites; rates in single women are almost 50% higher than the rates for widowed women (Swanson *et al.*, 1985). Breast cancer is usually more common in urban than in rural areas and among women of higher rather than lower socioeconomic status; although these factors are interrelated, they appear to have at least partly independent influences on the risk. In England and Wales, for example, breast cancer is slightly more common in rural than in urban areas, but the social class gradient is more marked and women in the highest social class have almost 50% more of this cancer than women in the lowest.

The sex difference in the frequency of breast cancer is perhaps the most obvious feature of its epidemiology. Breast cancer is rare in males, and the incidence is almost invariably less than 1 per 100 000, accounting for less than 0.5% of all cancers in males. The female:male ratio is usually 100 or greater, except in many parts of Africa where it is considerably lower (between 10 and 30), owing, perhaps, to both an elevated incidence of this cancer in men and low rates in women.

Figure 14. Incidence of breast cancer in three areas, with age; U, US whites, 1978–82; Y, Yugoslavia (Slovenia), 1978–81; J, Japan (Miyagi), 1978–82

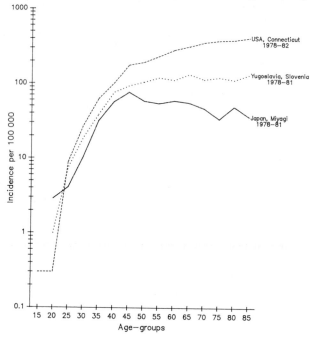

The importance of environmental factors in the etiology of breast cancer is demonstrated by the changes in risk in migrant populations (see p. 46). Rates of breast cancer in European migrants to the USA change relatively rapidly towards those of the US population, but changes in migrant populations from China and Japan are less rapid. This difference may be related to different rates of change in the dietary and reproductive behaviours of these groups (Buell, 1973b; King *et al.*, 1985).

Incidence and mortality rates of breast cancer have been compared in a very large number of studies with average consumption *per caput* of various dietary items (see p. 206). In general, positive correlations have been found with dietary fat, protein (particularly of animal origin) and total calories (Rohan & Bain, 1987). Although these results suggest the importance of diet in the etiology of breast cancer, it is difficult in such ecological studies to allow for the effects of other variables which are themselves associated with dietary habits. Studies of religious groups in the USA, such as Mormons and Seventh-day Adventists, do not provide evidence that diet plays a role: the rates for cancer of the breast among the largely vegetarian Seventh-day Adventists are little different from those of people of similar socioeconomic background who do not belong to this religious group (Lyon *et al.*, 1980b; Phillips *et al.*, 1980a).

Increasing trends in the risk for breast cancer in women have been noted in many countries. There were steady, similar increases in risk (30–50%) in each of the five Nordic countries between 1956 and 1980, which occurred consistently in women aged 30–89 years. The increase was most marked for postmenopausal women, and successive ten-year birth cohorts born 1882–1922 had progressively higher risks; the differences between birth cohorts for premenopausal women were much less marked (Hakulinen *et al.*, 1986). Breast cancer incidence in Singapore increased by an average of 3% per year over the period 1968–82 (Lee *et al.*, 1988); the increase was particularly marked in women of less than 50 years of age and is probably due to an accelerating increase in the risks of successive cohorts, particularly those born 1928–48. Some of the very widespread changes in the incidence of breast cancer may be accounted for by trends in aspects of reproductive behaviour that are known to be associated with the risk for breast cancer, such as progressively smaller family size and later age at first full-term pregnancy (see p. 240). Thus, age-specific trends in mortality from breast cancer in white women in the USA have been shown to be associated with the fertility patterns of the corresponding birth cohorts in early life (Blot *et al.*, 1987). However, the rise in incidence is more marked among US black women than in whites, even though the delay in starting childbearing is more marked in whites than in blacks (White *et al.*, 1987; Krieger, 1988).

Increases in mortality from breast cancer have been less marked than those for incidence. Since survival from breast cancer at different clinical stages has not improved greatly, at least part of the increase in incidence may be due to earlier diagnosis, more complete ascertainment, and perhaps the inclusion in incidence data of cases that would not have become clinically obvious had they not been identified by screening.

Cancer of the uterine cervix

World-wide, cervical cancer is the second most common cancer among women (Table 2). In 1980, there were an estimated 465 600 new cases, accounting for 15% of all cancers diagnosed in women. About 20% of these cases occur in the developed countries and 80% in developing countries, where it is consistently the leading cancer. When all cancer sites for people of each sex are combined, cervical cancer ranks fifth, accounting for 7.3% of all human cancers.

The regions of the world where the risk is highest are sub-Saharan Africa, Central and South America and south-east Asia, where cancer of the cervix constitutes 20–30% of all cancers in women. The highest recorded incidence rates occur in South America and particularly in north-eastern Brazil, with age-standardized rates of 83.2 in Recife and 46.5 in Fortaleza, and in Cali, Colombia, with a rate of 48.2. By contrast, cervical cancer accounts for only 4–6% of all female cancers in North America, Australasia and northern and western Europe; eastern Europe takes an intermediate position.

Low incidence rates are found in middle-eastern populations: in Israel, the rates are 4.0 in Jews and 3.0 in non-Jews, and in Kuwait the rate is 3.9 in Kuwaitis. A zone of relatively low risk, where cervical cancer accounts for less than 10% of female neoplasms, appears to extend from Pakistan to Egypt. Available data suggest, however, considerably higher rates in Morocco, Algeria and Tunisia. Within countries, there are quite large differences between ethnic groups. Among residents in the Los Angeles area of the USA, Latino women have a three-fold greater incidence of cervical cancer than Japanese women. A similar range of incidence rates is observed among the three ethnic groups in Singapore and between the non-Maori and Maori populations of New Zealand.

The rates are generally 1.2–2.3 times higher in urban than in rural populations. Rates are also related to marital status – higher in married women than in single, and higher in widowed or divorced women than in married (Leck *et al.*, 1978). The rates are some four times higher in the wives of unskilled workers than in women married to professional men (Office of Population Censuses and Surveys, 1978), and within these broad groupings there are even more dramatic variations – wives of clergymen have only 12% of the rate of cervical cancer seen in other women of their age, and wives of seamen and fishermen 160% more (Beral, 1974). The degree to which these variations can be explained by different exposures to a sexually transmitted agent has been discussed extensively (Beral, 1974; Skegg *et al.*, 1982).

There have been great declines in incidence and mortality rates for cervical cancer in most countries where organized screening programmes have been introduced (see Part III, p. 278), and the greatest declines are seen in those age groups that are maximally screened (Läärä *et al.*, 1987). However, despite the existence of screening programmes, mortality rates among young women in some countries have been increasing, especially in the generations born since the mid-1930s; this has occurred in the UK (Cook & Draper, 1984), New Zealand (Cox & Skegg, 1986) and Australia (Holman & Armstrong, 1987), although no such increase has occurred in the USA (Chu & White, 1987) or in France among women aged 35 and over (Hill *et al.*, 1989). This increase in mortality from cervical cancer in the UK, New Zealand and Australia has occurred against a steadily decreasing trend observed since the 1950s in most other western countries. Whatever the risk factor(s) involved, it seems that there has been increasing exposure of younger generations of women to varying extents in different countries.

Choriocarcinoma

Choriocarcinoma is a rare tumour which arises from trophoblastic tissue in the placenta. There is a close association with molar pregnancy, in which the parts of the ovum that form the placenta are transformed into grape-like cysts: a woman who has this condition has a 2000 times higher risk of developing choriocarcinoma than women who do not. In 2–20% of cases, a molar pregnancy is followed, usually within one year, by choriocarcinoma.

Mortality data are a poor guide to the occurrence of this tumour because survival rates are high. Incidence should be reported per 100 000 pregnancies, since this is the denominator 'at risk' (see p. 15); however, in most hospital-based series in which choriocarcinoma has been reported, rates are recorded per 100 000 births. As described above (p. 17), hospital series are likely to be subject to varying degrees of selection bias; however, the incidence appears to be high in southern and eastern Asia and in Africa (Bracken *et al.*, 1984). The risk increases steeply with maternal age, and possibly also with the number of pregnancies (Baltazar, 1976).

Cancer of the corpus uteri

With an estimated 149 000 new cases in the world in 1980, the great majority of which are of the endometrium, cancer of the uterine corpus is less than one-third as frequent as cervical cancer in the world as a whole; in developed countries, however, it is now slightly more common. The highest incidence reported (31.1 per 100 000) is in La Plata, Argentina, and high incidence rates are found in US whites, in Canada, in Hawaiians and Maoris and in western Europe. Low rates of incidence (2–4 per 100 000) are seen in Asian populations, except for Jews in Israel and Chinese in Singapore and Hong Kong.

Studies of migrants suggest that the risk increases in populations who move to areas with 'westernized' life styles – for instance, Japanese living in the USA have incidence rates more than six times those in Japan. However, in studies of migrants to Israel and Australia, the risk of first-generation migrants changed hardly at all, in contrast to the situation for cancers of the breast and colon. Similarly, differences in the risks of urban and rural residents and with socioeconomic status are small and inconsistent.

Mortality rates from corpus uterine cancer have declined steeply for women of all age groups. This is probably largely accounted for by high and improving rates of survival. The trends in incidence are more variable: in the USA and to a lesser extent Canada, a substantial increase in the incidence of this cancer among postmenopausal women (most marked at ages 55–64) occurred in the 1970s. The increased risk was ascribed to use of postmenopausal oestrogens; after this was recognized, and use of these drugs fell, incidence rates declined to previous levels, and even below (Austin & Roe, 1982). In addition, 25-35% of postmenopausal women in the USA have had their uterus removed (Lyon & Gardner, 1977). The increase in risk in Europe was much smaller, although small rises have occurred among women over 55 years of age in the Nordic countries.

Cancer of the ovary

Ovarian cancer is an important cause of morbidity and mortality, especially in middle-aged women. It ranks seventh in frequency (4.4%) among all cancers in women, with an estimated 137 600 new cases occurring in the world in 1980. Incidence is high in women in the age range 45–64 years, and survival is poor, partly because the disease has often spread widely when diagnosed. The great majority of ovarian cancers are epithelial carcinomas; germ-cell tumours are uncommon, with a peak in incidence in women aged 15–34 years (as for germ-cell tumours of the testis), and follicular tumours (mainly granulosa-cell) are also rare.

The highest incidence rates of ovarian cancer are reported among white females in northern and western Europe and in North America, where age-standardized rates are 8–15 per 100 000 and cumulative rates up to 74 years of age are 1–2%. In four of the five Nordic countries, incidence rates exceed 14 per 100 000; only in Finland is the rate less than 10. Ovarian cancer is less common in Indian, Chinese and Japanese populations, with rates of 2–5 per 100 000.

Racial differences in the frequency of ovarian cancer are evident in several countries. Blacks and Japanese in the USA have about half the risk for epithelial ovarian tumours seen in whites (Weiss *et al.*, 1977). This difference appears only in women over the age of 40 and is apparent only for epithelial ovarian tumours. Israeli Jews born in Europe have twice the risk of those born in Asia and three times that of Jews from North Africa. Non-Jews in Israel have an even lower risk.

The incidence of ovarian cancer appears to have changed very little over the past 20 or more years in those areas in which adequate data cover the entire period. Recently, however, there has been an increase of 3.4% per year in the incidence of ovarian cancer in Singapore (mainly in women aged 65 and over); in Japan, where ovarian cancer constitutes less than 3% of female cancers, incidence and mortality rates have increased by more than two fold since 1960.

Cancer of the prostate

Prostatic cancer is an important cancer in most developed countries, where the population has a relatively old age structure – particularly in North America, Europe and Australia. It ranks as the fifth most common cancer among males globally, comprising 7.3% of male cancers and 3.7% of all new cancers. More than 90% are adenocarcinomas.

The geographic variation in age-standardized incidence rates is at least 70 fold (see Table 6). The highest incidence rates are found in north-western Europe and in North America; US blacks have a particularly high incidence (see Appendix). High incidence rates are also seen in some Caribbean populations (e.g., 50 per 100 000 in Martinique) and in north-eastern Brazil (44 per 100 000 in Recife), where a large proportion of the population is of African descent. In Africa itself, the rates of prostatic cancer have probably been underestimated. However, despite the fact that the populations contain a large proportion of young people, prostatic cancer is found not infrequently; it comprises 13.2% of male cancers in Gabon, 11.3% in Liberia, 11.2% in the United Republic of Tanzania (Kilimanjaro), 10.7% in Ibadan, Nigeria (estimated minimum age-standardized rate, 22.9) and 5.9% in Bulawayo, Zimbabwe (where the incidence around 1970 was 32.3). Prostatic cancer appears to be uncommon in Indian populations, with rates of less than 10.0, and in China, where rates are less than 2.0 per 100 000. In Japan, rates are less than 10 per 100 000, but Japanese migrants to the USA have a much higher risk, between 20–30 per 100 000, and the rates in Japan itself are increasing. Other migrant groups in the USA also acquire the higher risk of their adopted country.

A difficulty in the epidemiology of prostatic cancer is distinguishing between clinical prostatic cancer and latent carcinoma of the prostate found following operation for prostatic hypertrophy or at autopsy in persons who have died from other causes. The prevalence of latent carcinoma has been studied in autopsy series (Breslow *et al.*, 1977): in men aged 45 and over, the prevalence of small, noninvasive latent carcinoma is about 20%, irrespective of age and regional differences in the incidence of clinical prostatic cancer, while the prevalence of large, invasive latent carcinoma resembles the pattern of incidence of clinical prostatic cancer. For this reason, some of the geographic variation in incidence may be the result of differences in the rate of detection of latent tumours.

In most populations, the incidence of prostatic cancer increases significantly only in men over 50 years of age, but it then increases more rapidly with age than for any other cancer (Cook *et al.*, 1969).

There is considerable variation in risk between different racial and social groups. Blacks in the USA have almost twice the risk of whites at all ages; in 1960, Protestants in New York City had 1.9 times the risk of Jews, while Catholics had an intermediate risk (MacMahon, 1960). In England and Wales, men in the highest social class have about twice the risk of men in the lowest (proportional registration ratios of 140 and 65, respectively, compared with 100 for all men). A similar gradient in incidence, but not in mortality, has been observed in white men in Los Angeles (Ross *et al.*, 1979); however, no socioeconomic gradient was observed in the USA as a whole, among either whites or blacks (Ernster *et al.*, 1978). In the USA, the incidence appeared to be lower in single, separated and divorced men than in married men in all racial groups, but the incidence in widowers was similar to that of married men (Newell *et al.*, 1987a).

Several studies of different populations have shown a positive correlation between average intake of dietary fat and risk for prostatic cancer (e.g., Armstrong & Doll, 1975; Kolonel *et al.*, 1981; see p. 209). The risk for prostatic cancer does not, however, appear to be particularly low among Seventh-day Adventists, a sizable proportion of whom are also vegetarians (Enstrom, 1978; Phillips *et al.*, 1980b).

In most populations, incidence rates are increasing rather rapidly, particularly in those in which incidence has been low (Zaridze *et al.*, 1984). However, the contribution of more frequent diagnosis of latent cancer is probably important.

Mortality rates, too, are generally increasing, although not as rapidly as those for incidence, and in some populations, such as US whites and in the UK and Australia, there has been very little change, which might be related to improvements in survival rates.

Cancer of the testis

Testicular cancers are relatively uncommon, accounting for 1% or less of all male cancers. The highest rates are observed in white populations of northern and western Europe and North America, but age-standardized incidence rates rarely exceed 5 per 100 000. Rates are low in Asia and in black populations.

Age-standardized rates give a misleading picture of testicular cancer, however, since it is primarily a disease of young men: in high-risk populations it is the leading cancer in men aged 20–34 years, accounting for 20% of tumours. Peak incidence rates of up to 10 per 100 000 occur among men aged around 30, with a decline up to the age of 50 years, followed by a small increase after the age of 65. Germ-cell tumours – principally seminoma and teratoma – comprise the great majority of testicular cancers in the age range 15–50 years, and there is also a small early peak in the incidence of germ-cell neoplasms in boys under five years of age.

There are marked differences in the patterns of testicular cancer by race and marital status. The overall incidence of testicular cancer in US whites is four to five times higher than that in blacks, among whom the peak at age 30 is much less marked (Figure 15), while that of other races is intermediate (Spitz *et al.*, 1986). Single men have a higher incidence than married men at all ages, particularly of morphological types other than seminoma; this excess is more marked for blacks than for whites (Newell *et al.*, 1987b).

The incidence of testicular cancer in young white men has increased by two to four times over the last 40 years, while that in men over 60 years of age has remained constant or declined. Similar increases occurred in all five Nordic countries during the same period, although the rates in Denmark have consistently exceeded those in Finland by five fold (Hakulinen *et al.*, 1986). Mortality rates have declined sharply, particularly among younger men, since the introduction of multiple chemotherapy regimes in the 1970s. The widely observed increases in incidence in younger men appear to be due to a cohort effect, with increases in successive US male cohorts born between 1910 and 1959 (Brown *et al.*, 1986; Østerlind, 1986).

Cancer of the penis

Penile cancer is a rare tumour in developed countries, where it comprises less than 1% of male cancers and rates rarely exceed 1.0 per 100 000. The highest recorded incidence rates are seen in Latin America, notably in north-eastern Brazil (Recife and Fortaleza), in the Caribbean and in India. South-east Asia has been reported as an area of high frequency, but recent data suggest that, in the countries where the highest frequencies have been recorded (in Thailand and Viet Nam), penile cancer comprises less than 4% of male cancers. Probably the highest risk is found in certain parts of Africa, particularly in the east in Uganda

Figure 15. Incidence of testicular cancer in US males, 1978–82[a]

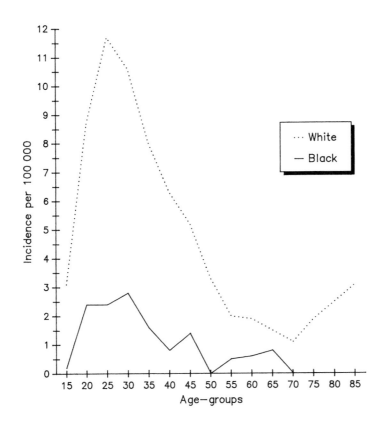

[a] Data from US Surveillance, Epidemiology and End Results Program, 1978-82

and Kenya. In Uganda in the 1960s, penile cancer accounted for 12% of all cancers in males, and very striking differences were noted between different tribal groups; these have been related to variations in the practice of circumcision (Dodge & Linsell, 1963). Schmauz and Jain (1971) noted that the variations in incidence in uncircumcised tribes were related more closely to geographical location than to ethnic origin, and that migrants acquired rates equivalent to those in their new area of residence. The importance of circumcision practices in determining risk for penile cancer is also demonstrated by the very low risk for penile cancer in Jewish populations (this cancer comprising less than 0.1% of all cancers in Israeli Jews) and by the finding that Muslims in Bombay, who are circumcised, have rates considerably lower than Hindus, who are not (Jussawalla & Jain, 1976).

The geographic distribution of penile cancer bears a strong similarity to that of cervical cancer (p. 72), although an examination of published incidence data

(Smith *et al.*, 1980) showed only a weak correlation between them, probably because most of the data were for developed countries. Like cervical cancer, too, penile cancer is reported to occur at increased frequency in people of lower social classes, although this relationship has not been seen in all studies (see Smith *et al.*, 1980).

Cancer of the urinary bladder

An estimated 219 000 new cancers of the urinary bladder occur each year, comprising about 3.5% of all new cancers, and this cancer ranks eleventh on a global basis. More than three-quarters of these tumours occur in men, for whom bladder cancer ranks eighth, representing 5.2% of all new cancers.

The geographic variation in incidence is about ten fold, which is smaller than for many other cancers. This small variation is surprising, because there are well-recognized differences in the classification and registration of bladder papillomas: these are not recorded at all in some registries, so that the comparability of incidence rates is reduced.

The highest recorded incidences of malignant neoplasms of the bladder occur in white male populations in North America and north-western Europe, with age-standardized rates of about 20–25 per 100 000. Bladder cancer is uncommon in eastern Europe and in Indian, Chinese and Japanese populations, with age-standardized rates in males of 2–10 per 100 000. Among females, the age-standardized rates appear not to exceed 10.0 anywhere.

Racial differences within countries are almost as great as the range between countries. Filipinos have at most one-fifth of the risk of whites in the USA (including Hawaii), and blacks consistently about one-half. Males appear universally to have four to ten times higher rates than females. In developed countries, the incidence is up to twice as high in urban and industrialized areas as in rural areas, but this difference is more marked in men than in women.

Transitional-cell tumours typically comprise 90–95% of all bladder cancers, but US blacks have 10% or more squamous-cell cancers, compared to 3% in whites (Schroder *et al.*, 1986). Squamous-cell carcinoma of the bladder is a common tumour in parts of Africa and the Middle East where the bladder parasite *Schistosoma haematobium* is endemic, causing the debilitating disease schistosomiasis (see p. 193). Thus, cancer of the urinary bladder comprises 29% of malignant tumours among men in Cairo, Egypt, and 13% in Baghdad, Iraq. In both areas, it is the most important cancer among males and the second most important among females. High relative frequencies are also found in Malawi, Zambia and Zimbabwe, and in Kuwait and Iran.

Mortality rates for bladder cancer are rising in most countries, with the exception of the USA and Canada; and these changes are more marked in males than in females. Increases in incidence are more marked than those for mortality, and incidence rates in people of each sex are increasing in the USA. The disparity between trends in incidence and mortality probably reflects, in part, improved prognosis; however, it undoubtedly also reflects changes in the definition of bladder carcinoma, which now includes papillomas that would have been excluded in earlier periods. These tumours constitute up to one-third of all urinary bladder cancers.

Cancer of the kidney

In adults, about 75–80% of malignant tumours of the kidney are renal-cell carcinomas, the remainder being cancers of the renal pelvis; other renal-tract cancers, mainly of the ureter, are rare. The range of geographic variation in incidence is rather moderate, and differences in diagnostic ability may account for some of this. The highest incidence rates in the world have been recorded in Eskimo populations and in Scandinavia (Iceland and Sweden). Incidence rates in Asia and Latin America are about one-half to one-third those in European populations.

In western countries, the incidence of renal tumours appears to have increased, at least until recently.

In childhood, the great majority of renal cancers are nephroblastomas (Wilms' tumour), which occur at maximal incidence at between one and three years of age. It used to be thought that the incidence of Wilms' tumour was quite constant throughout the world (Innis, 1972), but there is at least a three- to four-fold range. The highest rates occur in black populations, and the lowest in Chinese, Japanese and Indian populations (Figure 16).

Tumours of the eye

In adults in western countries, the majority of malignant tumours of the eye are malignant melanomas. The estimated rates for these cancers do not show the geographic variations and striking time trends observed for melanoma of the skin (Hakulinen *et al.*, 1978; Strickland & Lee, 1981; see p. 67). The incidence of and mortality from ocular melanoma are very low in black populations (Keller, 1973); however, in Africa, squamous-cell carcinoma of the conjunctival epithelium is relatively frequent.

In children, almost all eye tumours are retinoblastomas. In white populations, these account for 2.5–4% of childhood cancers and occur mainly during the first year of life. In such populations, about 40% of cases are associated with an inherited dominant gene which behaves like a recessive gene (Knudson, 1971). Geographical variations in incidence might arise either from differences in gene frequency (or in the likelihood that those carrying the gene will have children) or from differences in the prevalence of unknown environmental factors responsible for the mutations.

In general, it appears that the risk for retinoblastoma is highest in black populations in North and South America and, probably, Africa. It seems likely that it is the unilateral (mainly nongenetic) form which is responsible for the geographic variation in incidence, implying the presence of environmental factors which enhance the risk.

Cancers of the nervous system

Several factors frustrate systematic study of the epidemiology of tumours of the central nervous system. Firstly, several distinct clinicopathological entities are grouped under this general heading, and, since their etiological factors are probably different, a coherent pattern for the whole group is unlikely to emerge. Secondly, accurate diagnosis of intracerebral and intraspinal lesions is problematic, and it is difficult to distinguish primary from metastatic tumours and to differentiate the many different kinds of primaries. Thirdly, because even benign lesions at these sites may have dramatic consequences for the patient, incidence and mortality rates for these lesions are included, to a variable extent, with those for malignant lesions.

Figure 16. Incidence of malignant kidney tumours in children (aged 0–14) [a]

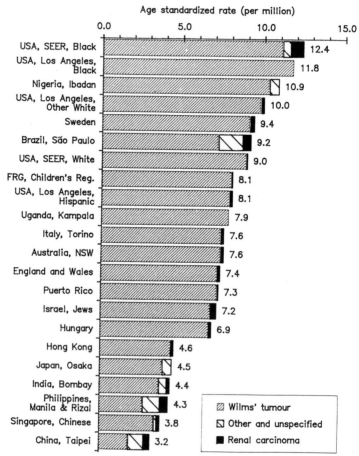

[a] From Parkin *et al.* (1988)

For the group as a whole, age-standardized incidence rates among populations of European origin are usually 5–9 per 100 000 for males and 3–7.5 per 100 000 for females. High rates have been recorded consistently in the Jewish population of Israel, particularly among immigrants of European origin. Incidence rates in Africa and Asia are low, and those in Latin America occupy an intermediate position. These differences also appear to be reflected in the variation in incidence by ethnic group within the USA: age-standardized incidence rates for people of each sex in the US Surveillance, Epidemiology and End Results Program network of registries were 5.9 for whites, 3.6 in Hawaiians, 3.5 for blacks, 2.8 in Puerto Rico, 2.3 for Chinese and Japanese and 1.5 for Filipinos.

Age-specific incidence rates show a bimodal curve, with a small peak in childhood and a second around age 60–70. In adults, the majority of tumours are astrocytomas and undifferentiated glioblastomas. In registration systems in which benign tumours are included, meningiomas form the second most important group, but actual rates depend on the extent of investigation (e.g., by autopsy). Meningiomas are more common in women than in men.

Tumours of the nervous system are the second most important cancer of childhood (except, as in Africa and western Asia, where lymphoma is more common). In children, 30–50% of tumours are astrocytomas, the second most important category being medulloblastoma.

Mortality rates from tumours of the nervous system appear to be increasing in the USA and in several European countries, but since the rise is most marked in older people improved accuracy of certification may be largely responsible.

Cancer of the thyroid

Thyroid cancer is rather rare, generally representing 1–2% of all cancers, although in adolescents and young adults it is one of the most frequent. Incidence rates are about three times higher in females than in males, but the difference depends on age: rates are higher in the young.

The highest rates of thyroid cancer are found in Hawaiian islanders and Polynesian populations, as well as in Filipino migrants to Hawaii and California, but the incidence rate in Rizal province of the Philippines is not high. High rates are also observed in Iceland and in native Alaskan women (Lanier *et al.*, 1976).

Incidence rates for people of each sex appear to be increasing; in US whites and in the Nordic countries, these increases have been greatest in younger age groups. This may be due partly to increased diagnosis of clinically occult lesions, and possibly also to exposure to radiation, particularly in childhood (Ron & Modan, 1982). More people, and especially women, now survive thyroid cancer, and there has thus been a general decline in mortality rates, despite increasing incidence; the sex ratio for mortality from thyroid cancer is also considerably lower than that for incidence.

Various histological types of thyroid cancer exist. Some 3.5% of those in US whites are medullary carcinomas, of which 25% are of genetic origin, constituting part of the multiple endocrine neoplasia type 2 syndrome (see p. 100).

Hodgkin's disease

Hodgkin's disease is distinguishable from the other lymphomas by its histology (by the presence of the so-called Reed-Sternberg giant cell) and its clinical features. It is a relatively uncommon cancer, with age-standardized rates in European populations generally in the range of 2–4 per 100 000 for males and 1.5–3.0 for females. The highest rates have been reported in northern Italy, while rates in Asia, particularly in Japanese and Chinese, are low. The rates appear to be moderate in many parts of Africa.

In western populations, the incidence curve for Hodgkin's disease with age shows a bimodal pattern, initially noted by MacMahon (1957), with a first peak in young adults at about age 25–30, a decline, then a further rise in incidence after age 40–45. In developing countries, however, there is a peak in incidence at age 5–9, with no corresponding peak in young adults. Thus, when incidence is high in childhood it is low in young adults and *vice versa*; and long time series from the same country show changes from the 'childhood' to 'young adult' forms of the disease (Correa & O'Conor, 1971; Gutensohn & Cole, 1977). In the USA, incidence rates among blacks are about 60% those in whites, but the difference is rather greater in young adults than in the elderly. In Japan, Hodgkin's disease shows a unimodal increase with age.

In addition to international variations in incidence, there are also noteworthy variations within countries. Cole *et al.* (1968) reported a north-south gradient within the USA in young adults. Interestingly, in Japan there is also a north-south gradient in mortality, but in the reverse direction: mortality rates are higher in the south.

Migrant studies show that Japanese Americans have mortality rates for Hodgkin's disease that are intermediate between those of white Americans and those of Japanese in Japan, with the shift towards the mortality rates of white Americans for both young and adult forms of the disease (Mason & Fraumeni, 1974).

Many of these epidemiological features of Hodgkin's disease suggest an etiology related to exposure to infectious agents, either in childhood (in developing countries) or delayed until adolescence (in developed countries). Associations of Hodgkin's disease with social class would support this suggestion. Geographic clusters of Hodgkin's disease have been reported in a large number of studies, and cases have been found to occur in individuals with direct or indirect contacts in common; it is doubtful, however, whether these observations are really more frequent than would be expected by chance (Grufferman & Dalzell, 1984).

Non-Hodgkin's lymphoma

Non-Hodgkin's lymphoma is more common than Hodgkin's disease. It is not a single disease entity, and the various subclassifications proposed (mainly on the basis of the morphology of the tumour) probably have little relevance to etiology. For this reason, the descriptive epidemiology of these tumours (with the exception of Burkitt's lymphoma, see below) reveals few distinctive features.

In general, incidence rates are highest in North America and western Europe and lower in eastern Europe and Asia. The rates in Nagasaki, Japan (5.7 in males and 3.4 in females) were much higher than elsewhere in Japan, suggesting the possibility that many of the lymphomas had been induced by exposure to radiation. It has long been known that Africa and the Middle East are apparent high-risk areas for lymphoma, which represent some 7–12% of tumours in males, although such incidence data as are available suggest that the rates may be rather similar to those in European populations. Among children, however, non-Hodgkin's lymphoma is undoubtedly more common in Africa and the Middle East than in Europe or the USA; furthermore, a large proportion of the lymphomas in these populations occur outside the lymph nodes (Salem *et al.*, 1986).

The incidence of these tumours has increased since 1960, especially in western countries (e.g., the Nordic countries and the USA), and, although some of the increase may be due to improved diagnosis and changes in classification, a proportion at least is likely to be real (Barnes *et al.*, 1986).

Mortality rates from non-Hodgkin's lymphoma in the USA are higher among people with higher socioeconomic status and urban residence, and high rates are seen in counties with many residents of Russian (mainly Jewish) or Greek ancestry (Cantor & Fraumeni, 1980).

Burkitt's lymphoma (BL) is a distinct pathological entity arising from B-lymphocytes. First described in Africa, the areas of high risk for BL coincide with those regions affected by holoendemic malaria: sub-Saharan Africa, excepting highland areas, and Papua New Guinea. This environmental link with malaria is supported by studies of migrants; in populations moving from low- to high-incidence areas, the average age of onset of BL is higher than that of people born in endemic areas (Burkitt & Wright, 1966; Morrow *et al.*, 1977). Urban populations in Ghana have lower rates than rural populations (Biggar & Nkrumah, 1979).

The age distribution of BL in endemic areas is highly characteristic, with a peak incidence at five to eight years of age and only rare occurrences before the age of two and after the age of 14. In most series, twice as many boys as girls develop the disease. In the 1970s, the incidence of BL fell in the West Nile district of Uganda and in North Mara district of the United Republic of Tanzania, but, in the latter, this pattern has now been reversed, coinciding with a recrudescence of malaria (Figure 17). There is evidence for seasonal variation in onset of the disease and clustering of cases both geographically and with time.

Awareness of the characteristics of BL has allowed its identification throughout the world, and it is now clear that it comprises a significant percentage (20–30%) of childhood non-Hodgkin's lymphoma in most countries, although incidence rates are much higher in Africa (age-standardized incidence, up to 8 per 100 000 children, compared with 0.2 per 100 000 in whites in the USA). Furthermore, outside the endemic areas, BL is distributed more evenly over different age groups and more frequently involves internal sites, such as the abdominal cavity.

Multiple myeloma

Multiple myeloma is a malignant proliferation of plasma cells originating in the bone marrow, resulting in destruction of bone, especially of the skull. More than any other cancer (except chronic lymphatic leukaemia), it is a disease of old age; it is very rare in people under the age of 35, but rates increase rapidly thereafter to a maximum in people over the age of 75 or 80. More men than women in all age groups have this cancer, and the male:female ratio is highest in countries with the highest rates.

Geographically, the main factors of interest are the high incidence rates in black populations in the USA (age-standardized rates of 9.0 per 100 000 in males and 6.2 per 100 000 in females) and the Caribbean (Martinique and Jamaica), and also in certain Pacific populations, such as Hawaiians in Hawaii and Maoris and Polynesians in New Zealand. Incidence rates in Indians, Chinese, Japanese and Filipinos are low. Migrant populations to the USA appear to retain the risk of their country of origin: age-standardized rates around 1980 were 3.1 for whites, 1.4 for Chinese and 1.0 for Japanese in the USA.

Figure 17. Trends in the incidence of Burkitt's lymphoma in east Africa[a]

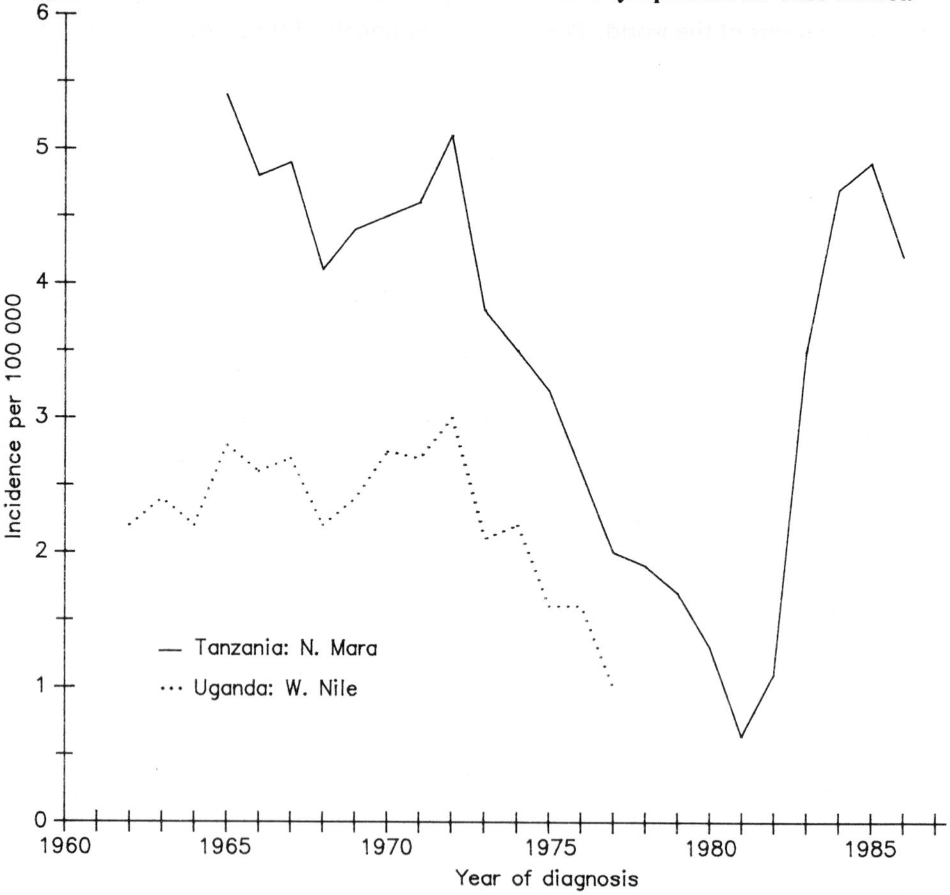

[a] From Geser *et al.* (1989). T, United Republic of Tanzania, North Mara District; U, Uganda, West Nile

As far as can be distinguished from available data, the risk for myeloma in Africa is rather low, although this may be due to the small populations of old people and poor diagnostic methods.

Increases in incidence and mortality rates for myeloma have been observed in most countries, especially in those where the initial rates were low, and these increases are generally greater in older age groups than in the young (Cuzick *et al.*, 1983). A substantial proportion of the increase is probably due to changes in diagnostic methods and in the accuracy of death certification, although it seems unlikely that the rapid increases in mortality rates observed in Japan (4–5% per year) can all be ascribed to these factors.

Leukaemia

The leukaemias are a group of malignancies deriving from the precursor cells of blood and tissue leukocytes. As a group, they represent 3% of the total world cancer incidence, with relatively little variation in this proportion between different regions of the world. They are conventionally distinguished both by the cell type of origin (lymphocytes, myelocytes, monocytes) and by their clinico-pathological behaviour (acute, subacute, chronic). Comparisons of these different subtypes are difficult because the diagnostic accuracy varies, with different proportions remaining unspecified, and because the numbers of cases are small. The descriptive epidemiology of the different varieties is not the same; nevertheless, it is known that different types of leukaemia may share similar etiological factors – as in the case of ionizing radiation (see Part II, Chapter 8), so that considerable overlap might be anticipated.

There is relatively little geographic variation in the incidence of leukaemias as a whole – barely two to three fold, if the figures for Africa are excluded. Table 9 gives data on the frequencies of the different subtypes of leukaemia in 15 populations. The most striking feature is the low risk for chronic lymphatic leukaemia in Chinese, Japanese and Indian populations, which appears to persist when they emigrate to the USA. There is also a suggestion that Pacific populations (Maoris, Hawaiians) have a higher than average risk for acute myeloid leukaemia. Most of the geographical variation is in the risk for acute lymphocytic leukaemia; the incidence in children in Africa appears to be very low. Acute nonlymphocytic leukaemia of childhood shows much less geographic variation in incidence and therefore represents a larger percentage of childhood leukaemia in areas where acute lymphocytic leukaemia is rare.

Leukaemias as a whole show a bimodal curve of incidence, with a first peak in childhood, a trough at ages 15–29, and then a slow rise. The patterns are, however, quite different for the different subtypes (Figure 18): chronic lymphatic leukaemia is a disease of the elderly, the risk for myeloid leukaemias increases slowly with age, while acute lymphocytic leukaemia is essentially a disease of childhood.

Incidence rates are usually higher in males than in females, especially for chronic lymphatic leukaemia, for which the sex ratio is around 2. The sex ratio also varies with age (Figure 18); that for myeloid leukaemias increases progressively with age.

In children (aged under 15), leukaemia is generally the most common cause of cancer, accounting for one-third of all new cases. The commonest subtype is acute lymphocytic leukaemia, which in white populations accounts for 75–80% of cases and shows a distinct peak of incidence in children of two to four years of age. A peak in mortality from leukaemia in children at four years of age was first observed in England and Wales 60 years ago, in white children in the USA 20 years later, and in Japan only in the 1960s (Miller, 1988). The incidence in the black population of the USA is about half that in whites, and the peak at age two to four years is much less marked. In Africa, there is no childhood peak in incidence at all.

Table 9. Age-standardized incidence of leukaemias of different subtypes, around 1980 (per 100 000 population)[a]

Population	Acute lymphocytic		Chronic lymphocytic		Acute myeloid		Chronic myeloid	
	M	F	M	F	M	F	M	F
Puerto Rico[b]	1.3	1.2	0.9	0.4	1.6	1.5	1.1	0.8
USA: whites[b]	1.5	1.2	3.5	1.8	2.7	1.8	1.4	0.9
USA: blacks[b]	0.8	0.6	3.3	1.5	2.1	1.8	1.8	1.0
Canada	1.7	1.4	2.9	1.3	1.9	1.4	1.1	0.7
India, Bombay	0.8	0.5	0.4	0.3	0.9	0.6	0.8	0.6
Israel: Jews	1.3	1.1	2.3	1.5	1.9	1.5	0.9	0.5
Japan, Miyagi	1.2	1.0	*0,1*	*0,1*	1.8	1.5	0.7	0.5
Singapore: Chinese	1.3	1.2	*0,2*	*0,1*	1.5	1.4	0.9	0.6
Czechoslovakia, Slovakia	1.3	1.1	2.8	1.2	1.4	1.3	1.4	0.9
Denmark	1.5	1.1	2.9	1.4	2.6	2.0	0.9	0.7
England and Wales	1.4	1.1	1.6	0.7	1.7	1.3	0.8	0.4
France, Isère	1.9	1.2	2.8	1.0	1.5	0.9	1.5	0.9
Australia, Victoria	1.7	1.7	1.9	1.1	1.9	1.2	1.1	0.9
New Zealand: Maoris	1.9	*1,2*	*0,8*	*1,5*	4.6	2.6	*1,0*	*0,1*
USA, Hawaii: Hawaiians	2.0	*0,6*	*0,0*	*0,0*	4.8	*2,6*	*1,5*	*0,5*

[a] From Muir *et al.* (1987): For rates based on fewer than ten cases among all age groups, the decimal is given by a comma, not a point, and the figure is printed in italics; 0.0/0,0 = a rate greater than 0 but less than 0.05
[b] Data from the US Surveillance, Epidemiology and End Results (SEER) Program

Immunological investigations of acute lymphocytic leukaemia indicate two distinct entities – one derived from T-cells and the other from B-cells. The 'common' form is derived from B-cell precursors, and it is this one which is responsible for the striking peak at age four (Greaves, 1984). In general, there appears to be a lower incidence rate, and less marked age peak, of childhood acute lymphocytic leukaemia in populations with low socioeconomic conditions. It has been suggested (Greaves & Chan, 1986) that this is due to selective underdiagnosis of the 'common' subtype of this disease in such areas, so that the proportion derived from T-cells appears to be correspondingly higher.

The mortality rates for leukaemia as a whole increased up to the 1960s in almost all countries; some of this increase may have been related to improved diagnosis and certification. Since that time, mortality rates have declined, particularly in children and young adults, which is associated with the introduction of effective therapy. Incidence rates, by contrast, show few consistent trends, except for some increases in older age groups, which may be due partly to improved diagnosis.

Figure 18. Incidence of leukaemia of different subtypes with age[a]

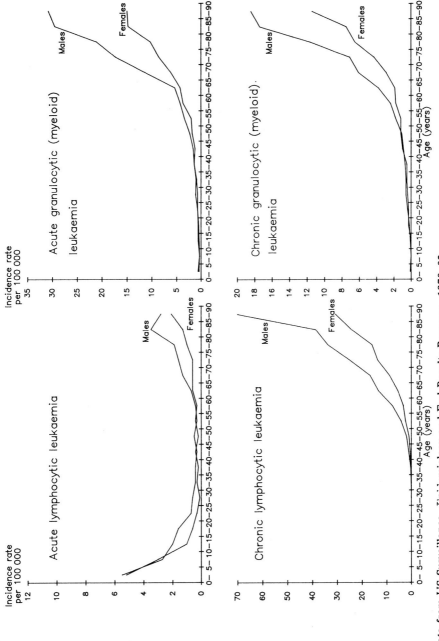

[a] Data from US Surveillance, Epidemiology and End Results Program, 1978–82

References

Armstrong, B. & Doll, R. (1975) Environmental factors and cancer incidence and mortality in different countries, with special reference to dietary practices. *Int. J. Cancer, 15,* 617-631

Armstrong, B.K., Holman, C.D.J., Ford, J.M. & Woodings, T.L. (1982) Trends in melanoma incidence and mortality in Australia. In: Magnus, K., ed., *Trends in Cancer Incidence - Causes and Practical Implications*, Washington DC, Hemisphere Publishing Corp., pp. 399-417

Austin, D.F. & Roe, K.M. (1982) The decreasing incidence of endometrial cancer: public health implications. *Am. J. Public Health, 72,* 65-68

Baltazar, J.C. (1976) Epidemiological features of choriocarcinoma. *Bull. World Health Organ., 54,* 523-532

Barnes, N., Cartwright, R.A., O'Brien, C., Richards, I.D.G., Roberts, B. & Bird, C.C. (1986) Rising incidence of lymphoid malignancies - true or false. *Br. J. Cancer, 53,* 393-398

Baris, I., Simonato, L., Artvinli, M., Pooley, F., Saracci, R., Skidmore, J. & Wagner, C. (1987) Epidemiological and environmental evidence of the health effects of exposure to erionite fibres: a four-year study in the Cappadocian region of Turkey. *Int. J. Cancer, 39,* 10-17

Beral, V. (1974) Cancer of the cervix: a sexually transmitted infection? *Lancet, i,* 1037-1040

Biggar, R.J. & Nkrumah, F.K. (1979) Burkitt's lymphoma in Ghana: urban-rural distribution, time-space clustering and seasonality. *Int. J. Cancer, 23,* 330-336

Biggar, R.J., Herm, J., Goedert, J.K. & Melbye, M. (1987) Cancer in a group at risk of acquired immunodeficiency syndrome (AIDS) through 1984. *Am. J. Epidemiol., 126,* 578-586

Blot, W.J., Devesa, S.S. & Fraumeni, J.F. (1987) Declining breast cancer mortality among young American women. *J. Natl Cancer Inst., 78,* 451-454

Boyle, P., Zaridze, D.G. & Smans, M. (1985) Descriptive epidemiology of colorectal cancer. *Int. J. Cancer, 36,* 9-18

Bracken, M.B., Brinton, L.A. & Hayachi, K. (1984) Epidemiology of hydatidiform mole and choriocarcinoma. *Epidemiol. Rev, 6,* 52-75

Bradshaw, E., McGlashan, N.D., Fitzgerald, D. & Harington, J.S. (1982) Analyses of cancer incidence in black gold miners from southern Africa (1964-79) *Br. J. Cancer, 46,* 737-748

Breslow, N., Chan, C.E., Dhom, G., Drury, R.A.B., Franks, L.M., Gellei, B., Lee, Y.S., Lundberg, S., Sparke, B., Sternby, N.H. & Tulinius, H. (1977) Latent carcinoma of prostate at autopsy in seven areas. *Int. J. Cancer, 20,* 680-688

Brown, C.C. & Kessler, L.G. (1988) Projection of lung cancer mortality in the United States: 1985-2025. *J. Natl Cancer Inst., 80,* 43-51

Brown, L.M., Pottern, L.M., Hoover, R.N., Devesa, S.S., Aselton, P. & Flannery, J.T. (1986) Testicular cancer in the United States: trends in incidence and mortality. *Int. J. Epidemiol., 15,* 164-170

Buell, P. (1973a) Race and place in the etiology of nasopharyngeal cancer: a study based on California death certificates. *Int. J. Cancer, 11,* 268-272

Buell, P. (1973b) Changing incidence of breast cancer in Japanese American women. *J. Natl Cancer Inst., 51,* 1479-1483

Burkitt, D.P. & Wright, D.H. (1966) Geographical and tribal distribution of the African lymphomas in Uganda. *Br. Med. J., i,* 569-573

Cantor, K.P. & Fraumeni, J.F. Jr (1980) Geographic and temporal patterns of non-Hodgkin's lymphoma mortality in US counties, 1950-1975. *Cancer Res., 40,* 2645-2652

Chilvers, C., Fraser, P. & Beral, V. (1979) Alcohol and oesophageal cancer: an assessment of the evidence from routinely collected data. *J. Epidemiol. Community Health, 33,* 127-133

Chu, J. & White, E. (1987) Decreasing incidence of invasive cervical cancer in young women. *Am. J. Obstet. Gynecol., 157,* 1105-1107

Cole, P., MacMahon, B. & Aisenberg, A. (1968) Mortality from Hodgkin's disease in the US. *Lancet, ii,* 1371-1376

Cook, G.H. & Draper, G.J. (1984) Trends in cervical cancer and carcinoma in situ in Great Britain. *Br. J. Cancer, 50,* 367-375

Cook, P.J., Doll, R. & Fellingham, S.A. (1969) A mathematical model for the age distribution of cancer in man. *Int. J. Cancer, 4,* 93-112

Cooke, K.R., Skegg, D.C. & Fraser, J. (1984) Socioeconomic status, indoor and outdoor work, and malignant melanoma. *Int. J. Cancer, 34,* 57-62

Correa, P. & O'Conor, G.T. (1971) Epidemiologic patterns of Hodgkin's disease. *Int. J. Cancer, 8,* 192-201

Correa, P., Cuello, D. & Duque, E. (1970) Carcinoma and intestinal metaplasia of the stomach in Colombian migrants. *J. Natl Cancer Inst., 44,* 297-306

Cox, B. & Skegg, D.C.G. (1986) Trends in cervical cancer in New Zealand. *N.Z. Med. J, 99,* 795-798

Cuzick, J., Velez, R. & Doll, R. (1983) International variations and temporal trends in mortality from multiple myeloma. *Int. J. Cancer, 32,* 13-19

Day, N. & Muñoz, N. (1982) Esophagus. In: Schottenfeld, D. & Fraumeni, J.F., Jr, eds, *Cancer Epidemiology and Prevention,* Philadelphia, Saunders, pp. 596-622

Depue, R.H. (1986) Rising mortality from cancer of the tongue in young white males. *New Engl. J. Med., 315,* 647

Devesa, S.S., Silvermen, D.T., Young, J.L., Pollack, E.S., Brown, C.C., Horm, J.W., Percy, C.L., Myers, M.H., McKay, F.W. & Fraumeni, J.F. (1987) Cancer incidence and mortality trends among whites in the United States, 1947-84. *J. Natl Cancer Inst., 79,* 701-770

Dodge, O.G. & Linsell, C.A. (1963) Carcinoma of the penis in Uganda and Kenya Africans. *Cancer, 16,* 1255-1263

Ellouz, R., Cammoun, M., ben Attia, R. & Bahi, J. (1978) Nasopharyngeal carcinoma in children and adolescents in Tunisia: clinical aspects and paraneoplastic syndrome. In: de-Thé, G. & Ito, Y., eds, *Nasopharyngeal Carcinoma: Etiology and Control* (IARC Scientific Publications No. 20), Lyon, IARC, pp. 115-130

Elwood, J.M., Lee, J.A.H., Walter, S.D., Mo, T. & Green, A.E.S. (1974) Relationship of melanoma and other skin cancer mortality to latitude and ultraviolet radiation in the United States and Canada. *Int. J. Epidemiol., 3,* 325-332

Enstrom, J.E. (1978) Cancer and total mortality among active Mormons. *Cancer, 42,* 1943-1971

Enterline, P.E. & Henderson, V.L. (1987) Geographic patterns for pleural mesothelioma deaths in the United States, 1968-81. *J. Natl Cancer Inst., 79,* 31-37

Ernster, V.L., Selvin, S., Sacks, S.T., Austin, D.F., Brown, S.M. & Winkelstein, W., Jr (1978) Prostatic cancer: mortality and incidence rates by race and social class. *Am. J. Epidemiol., 107,* 311-320

Ferguson, D.A., Berry, G., Jalihovsky, T., Andreas, S.B., Rogers, A.J., Chung Fung, S., Grimwood, A. & Thompson, R. (1987) The Australian Mesothelioma Surveillance Program 1979-1985. *Med. J. Aust., 147,* 166-172

Fraumeni, J.F., Jr & Blot, W.J. (1982) Lung and pleura. In: Schottenfeld, D. & Fraumeni, J.F., Jr, eds, *Cancer Epidemiology and Prevention,* Philadelphia, Saunders, pp. 564-582

Fraumeni, J.F., Jr & Mason, T.J. (1974) Cancer mortality among Chinese Americans, 1950-69. *J. Natl Cancer Inst., 52,* 659-665

Gao, Y.T., Blot, W.J., Zheng, W., Ershow, A.G., Hsu, C.W., Levin, L.I., Zheng, R. & Fraumeni, J.F. (1987) Lung cancer among Chinese women. *Int. J. Cancer, 40,* 604-609

Gardner, M.J., Acheson, E.D. & Winter, P.D. (1982) Mortality from mesothelioma of the pleura during 1968-78 in England and Wales. *Br. J. Cancer, 46,* 81-88

Geser, A., Brubaker, G. & Draper, C.C. (1989) Effect of a malaria suppression program on the incidence of African Burkitt's lymphoma. *Am. J. Epidemiol., 129,* 740-752

Giles, G.G., Marks, R. & Foley, P. (1988) Incidence of non-melanocytic skin cancer treated in Australia. *Br. Med. J., 296,* 13-17

Glass, A.G. & Hoover, R.N. (1989) The emerging epidemic of melanoma and squamous cell skin cancer. *J. Am. Med. Assoc., 262,* 2097-2100

Greaves, M.F. (1984) Subtypes of acute lymphoblastic leukaemia: implications for the pathogenesis and epidemiology of leukaemia. In: Magrath, I., O'Conor, G.T. & Ramot, B., eds, *Pathogenesis of Leukaemias and Lymphomas: Environmental Influences,* New York, Raven Press, pp. 129-139

Greaves, M.F. & Chan, L.C. (1986) Is spontaneous mutation the major 'cause' of childhood acute lymphoblastic leukaemia? *Br. J. Haematol., 64,* 1-13

Grufferman, S. & Dalzell, E. (1984) Epidemiology of Hodgkin's disease. *Epidemiol. Rev.*, *6*, 76-106

Gutensohn, N. & Cole, P. (1977) Epidemiology of Hodgkin's disease in the young. *Int. J. Cancer*, *19*, 595-694

Haenszel, W. & Correa, P. (1971) Cancer of the colon and adenomatous polyps. A review of epidemiologic findings. *Cancer*, *28*, 14-24

Haenszel, W. & Kurihara, M. (1968) Studies of Japanese migrants. I. Mortality from cancer and other diseases among Japanese in the United States. *J. Natl Cancer Inst.*, *40*, 43-68

Hakulinen, T., Teppo, L. & Saxen, E. (1978) Cancer of the eye. A review of trends and differentials. *World Health Stat.*, *31*, 143-158

Hakulinen, T., Andersen, A.A., Malker, B., Pukkala, E., Schon, G. & Tulinius, H. (1986) Trends in cancer incidence in Nordic countries. *Acta Pathol. Microbiol. Immunol. Scand. (Sect. A)*, *94* (Suppl. 288), 62-63

Hanai, A., Fujimoto, I. & Taniguchi, H. (1982) Trends of stomach cancer incidence and histological types in Osaka. In: Magnus, K., ed., *Trends in Cancer Incidence - Causes and Practical Implications*, Washington DC, Hemisphere, pp. 143-154

Henderson, B.E. (1974) Nasopharyngeal carcinoma: present status of knowledge. *Cancer Res.*, *34*, 1187-1188

Hill, C., Benhamou, E., Doyon, F. & Flamant, R. (1989) *Evolution de la mortalité par cancer en France 1950-1985*, Paris, Institut National de Science et de la Recherche Médicale

Hirayama, T. (1978) Descriptive and analytic epidemiology of nasopharyngeal cancer. In: de-Thé, G. & Ito, Y., eds, *Nasopharyngeal Carcinoma: Etiology and Control* (IARC Scientific Publications No. 20), Lyon, IARC, pp. 167-189

Ho, J.H.C. (1967) Nasopharyngeal carcinoma in Hong Kong. In: Muir, C.S. & Shanmugaratnam, K., eds, *Cancer of the Nasopharynx* (UICC Monographs Series 1), Copenhagen, Munksgaard

Holman, C.D.J. & Armstrong, B.K. (1984) Cutaneous malignant melanoma and indicators of total accumulated exposure to the sun: an analysis separating histogenetic types. *J. Natl Cancer Inst.*, *73*, 75-82

Holman, C.D.J. & Armstrong, B.K. (1987) Cervical mortality trends in Australia - an update. *Med. J. Aust.*, *146*, 410-412

Holman, C.D., Armstrong, B.K. & Heenan, R.J. (1983) A theory of the etiology and pathogenesis of human cutaneous malignant melanoma. *J. Natl Cancer Inst.*, *71*, 651-656

Hutt, M.S.R. (1981) The epidemiology of Kaposi's sarcoma. *Antibiotics Chemother.*, *29*, 3-8

IARC (1977) *IARC Monographs on the Evaluation of the Carcinogenic Risk of Chemicals to Humans*, Vol. 14, Asbestos, Lyon, IARC

IARC (1985) *IARC Monographs on the Evaluation of the Carcinogenic Risk of Chemicals to Humans*, Vol. 37, Tobacco Habits Other than Smoking; Betel-quid and Areca-nut Chewing; and Some Related Nitrosamines, Lyon

IARC (1986) *IARC Monographs on the Evaluation of the Carcinogenic Risk of Chemicals to Humans*, (1972) Vol. 38, Tobacco, Lyon, IARC

Innis, M.D. (1972) Nephroblastoma: possible index cancer of childhood. *Med. J. Austr.*, *1*, 18-20

Jayant, K. & Yeole, B.B. (1987) Cancer of the upper alimentary and respiratory tract in Bombay, India: a study of incidence over two decades. *Br. J. Cancer*, *56*, 847-852

Jones, B. & Thomas, P. (1986) Incidence of mesothelioma in Britain. *Lancet*, *i*, 1275

Jones, B. & Thomas, P. (1987) Mesothelioma registry data. *Lancet*, *ii*, 167

Jones, R.R. (1987) Ozone depletion and cancer risk. *Lancet*, *ii*, 167

de Jong, U.W., Day, N.E., Muir, C.S., Barclay, T.H.C., Bras, G., Foster, F.H., Jussawalla, D.J., Kurihara, M., Linden, G., Martinez, I., Payne, P.M., Pedersen, E., Ringertz, N. & Shanmugaratnam, K. (1972) The distribution of cancer within the large bowel. *Int. J. Cancer*, *10*, 463-477

Jussawalla, D.J. & Jain, D.K. (1976) *Cancer Incidence in Greater Bombay 1970-1972*, Bombay, Indian Cancer Society

Keller, A.Z. (1973) Histology, survivorship and related factors in the epidemiology of eye cancers. *Am. J. Epidemiol.*, *97*, 386-393

King, H., Li, J.-Y., Locke, F.B., Pollack, E.S. & Tu, J.-T. (1985) Patterns of site-specific displacement in cancer mortality among migrants: the Chinese in the United States. *Am. J. Public Health*, *75*, 237-242

Kinlen, L.J. (1982) Meat and fat consumption and cancer mortality: a study of strict religious orders in Britain. *Lancet*, *i*, 946-949

Knudson, A.G. (1971) Mutation and cancer: statistical study of retinoblastoma. *Proc. Natl Acad. Sci. USA*, *68*, 820-823

Kolonel, L.N., Hinds, M.W. & Hankin, J.H. (1980) Cancer patterns among migrant and native born Japanese in Hawaii in relation to smoking, drinking and dietary habits. In: Gelboin, H.V., MacMahon, B., Matsushima, T., Sugimura, T., Takayama, S. & Takebe, H., eds, *Genetic and Environmental Factors in Experimental and Human Cancer*, Tokyo, Japan Scientific Societies Press, pp. 327-340

Kolonel, L.N., Harkin, J.H., Lee, J., Chu, S.Y., Nomura, A.M.Y. & Hinds, M.W. (1981) Nutrient intakes in relation to cancer incidence in Hawaii. *Br. J. Cancer*, *44*, 332-339

Krieger, N. (1988) Rising incidence of breast cancer. *J. Natl Cancer Inst.*, *80*, 2

Läärä, E., Day, N.E. & Hakama, M. (1987) Trends in mortality from cervical cancer in the Nordic countries: association with organised screening programmes. *Lancet*, *i*, 1247-1249

Lanier, A.P., Bender, T.R., Blot, W.J., Fraumeni, J.F. Jr & Ward, B. (1976) Cancer incidence in Alaska natives. *Int. J. Cancer*, *18*, 409

Lanier, A.P., Blot, W.J., Bender, T.R. & Fraumeni, J.F. (1980) Cancer in Alaskian Indians, Eskimos and Aleuts. *J. Natl Cancer Inst.*, *65*, 1157-1159

Leck, I., Sibary, K. & Wakefield, J. (1978) Incidence of cervical cancer by marital status. *J. Epidemiol. Community Health*, *32*, 108-110

Lee, H.P., Day, N.E. & Shanmugaratnam, K., eds (1988) *Trends in Cancer Incidence in Singapore 1968-1982* (IARC Scientific Publications No. 91), Lyon, IARC

Lee, J.A.H. (1982) Melanoma. In: Schottenfeld, D. & Fraumeni, J.F., Jr, eds, *Cancer Epidemiology and Prevention*, Philadelphia, Saunders, pp. 984-995

Lee, J.A.H. & Strickland, D. (1980) Malignant melanoma: social status and outdoor work. *Br. J. Cancer*, *41*, 757-763

Lindqvist, C. & Teppo, L. (1978) Epidemiological evaluation of sunlight as a risk factor of lip cancer. *Br. J. Cancer*, *37*, 983-989

Lu, J.-B., Yang, W.-X., Liu, J.-M., Li, Y.-S. & Qin, Y.-M. (1985) Trends in morbidity and mortality for oesophageal cancer in Linxian county, 1959-1983. *Int. J. Cancer*, *36*, 643-645

Lyon, J.L. & Gardner, J.W. (1977) The rising frequency of hysterectomy: its effect on uterine cancer rates. *Am. J. Epidemiol.*, *105*, 439-443

Lyon, J.L., Gardner, J.W. & West, D.W. (1980a) Cancer in Utah: risk by religion and place of residence. *J. Natl Cancer Inst.*, *65*, 1063-1071

Lyon, J.L., Gardner, J.W. & West, D.W. (1980b) Cancer in Mormons and non-Mormons in Utah during 1967-75. *J. Natl Cancer Inst.*, *65*, 1053-1061

MacFarlane, G.J., Boyle, P. & Scully, C. (1987) Rising mortality from cancer of the tongue in young Scottish males. *Lancet*, *ii*, 912

Mack, T.M., Walker, A., Mack, W. & Bernstein, L. (1985) Cancer in Hispanics in Los Angeles County. *Natl Cancer Inst. Monogr.*, *69*, 95-104

MacMahon, B. (1957) Epidemiologic evidence on the nature of Hodgkin's disease. *Cancer*, *10*, 1045-1054

MacMahon, B. (1960) The ethnic distribution of cancer mortality in New York City, 1955. *Acta Unio Int. Cancrum*, *16*, 1716-1724

Marks, R., Rennie, G. & Selwood, T.S. (1988) Malignant transformation of solar keratoses to squamous cell carcinoma. *Lancet*, *i*, 795-797

Mason, T.J. & Fraumeni, J.F., Jr (1974) Hodgkin's disease among Japanese Americans. *Lancet*, *i*, 215

Maupas, P. & Melnick, J.L. (1981) Hepatitis B infection and primary liver cancer. *Prog. Med. Virol.*, *27*, 1-5

McDonald, A.D. (1979) Mesothelioma registries in identifying asbestos hazards. *Ann. N.Y. Acad. Sci.*, *330*, 441-454

McMichael, A.J. (1978) Increases in laryngeal cancer in Britain and Australia in relation to alcohol and tobacco consumption trends. *Lancet*, *i*, 1244-1246

McMichael, A.J., McGall, M.G., Hartshane, J.M. & Woodings, T.L. (1980) Patterns of gastrointestinal cancer in European migrants to Australia: the role of dietary change. *Int. J. Cancer*, *25*, 431-437

Melbye, M., Skirhøj, P., Holgaard Nielsen, N., Vestergaard, B.F., Ebbesen, P., Hart Hansen, J.P. & Bigger, R.J. (1984) Virus-associated cancers in Greenland: frequent hepatitis B virus infection but low primary hepatocellular carcinoma incidence. *J. Natl Cancer Inst.*, *73*, 1267-1272

Miller, R.W. (1988) Geographic and ethnic differences in the occurrence of childhood cancer. In: Parkin, D.M., Stiller, C.A., Bieber, C.A., Draper, G.J., Terracini, B. & Young, J.L., eds, *International Incidence of Childhood Cancer* (IARC Scientific Publications No. 87), Lyon, IARC, pp. 3-7

Moolgavkar, S.H. & Stevens, R.G. (1981) Smoking and cancers of the bladder and pancreas: risks and temporal trends. *J. Natl Cancer Inst.*, *67*, 15-23

Morrow, R.H., Pike, M.C. & Smith, P.G. (1977) Further studies of space-time clustering of Burkitt's lymphoma in Uganda. *Br. J. Cancer*, *35*, 668-673

Muir, C.S. & Nectoux, J. (1982) Malignant melanoma of skin. In: Magnus, K., ed., *Trends in Cancer Incidence - Causes and Practical Implications*, Washington DC, Hemisphere, pp. 365-385

Muir, C., Waterhouse, J., Mack, T., Powell, J. & Whelan, S., eds (1987) *Cancer Incidence in Five Continents, Vol. V* (IARC Scientific Publications No. 88), Lyon, IARC

Muñoz, N. & Asvall, J. (1971) Time trends of intestinal and diffuse types of gastric cancer in Norway. *Int. J. Cancer*, *8*, 144-157

Napalkov, N.P., Tserkovny, G.F. & Merabishvili, V.M., eds (1983) *Cancer Incidence in the USSR* (IARC Scientific Publications No. 48), Lyon, IARC

Newell, G.R., Pollack, E.S., Spitz, M.R., Sider, J.G. & Fueger, J.J. (1987a) Incidence of prostate cancer and marital status. *J. Natl Cancer Inst.*, *79*, 259-262

Newell, G.R., Spitz, M.R., Sider, J.G. & Pollack, E.S. (1987b) Incidence of testicular cancer in the United States related to marital status, histology and ethnicity. *J. Natl Cancer Inst.*, *78*, 881-885

Nielsen, N.H., Mikkelsen, F. & Hansen, J.P.H. (1977) Nasopharyngeal cancer in Greenland: the incidence in an Arctic Eskimo population. *Acta Pathol. Microbiol. Scand. Sect. A*, *85*, 850-858

Nielsen, N.H., Mikkelsen, F. & Hansen, J.P.H. (1978) Incidence of salivary gland neoplasms in Greenland with special reference to anaplastic carcinoma. *Acta Pathol. Microbiol. Scand. Sect. A.*, *86*, 185-193

Nixon, R., Doveistch, A.P. & Marks, R. (1986) Squamous cell carcinoma of the skin: accuracy of clinical diagnosis and outcome of follow-up in Australia. *Med. J. Aust.*, *144*, 235-238

Office of Population Censuses and Surveys (1978) *The Registrar General's Decennial Supplement for England and Wales 1970-72*, London, Her Majesty's Stationery Office

Osmond, C. & Gardner, M.J. (1983) Interpretation of disease time trends: Is cancer on the increase? A simple cohort technique and its relationship to more advanced models. *J. Epidemiol. Community Health*, *34*, 274-278

Osmond, C., Gardner, M.J., Acheson, E.D. & Adelstein, A.M. (1983) *Trends in Cancer Mortality 1951-1980: Analyses by Period of Birth and Death. England and Wales* (Series DHI, No. 11), London, Her Majesty's Stationery Office

Østerlind, A. (1986) Diverging trends in incidence and mortality of testicular cancer in Denmark 1943-1982. *Br. J. Cancer*, *53*, 501-505

Parkin, D.M., ed. (1985) *Cancer Occurrence in Developing Countries* (IARC Scientific Publications No. 75), Lyon, IARC

Parkin, D.M., Stiller, C.A., Draper, G.J. & Bieber, C.A. (1988) The international incidence of childhood cancer. *Int. J. Cancer*, *42*, 511-520

Penn, I. (1986) The occurrence of malignant tumours in immunosuppressed states. *Prog. Allergy*, *37*, 259-300

Petrakis, N.L., Ernster, V.L. & King, M.-C. (1982) Breast. In: Schottenfeld, D. & Fraumeni, J.F., Jr, eds, *Cancer Epidemiology and Prevention*, Philadelphia, Saunders, pp. 855-870

Phillips, R.L., Garfinkel, L., Kuzma, J.W., Beeson, W.L., Lotz, T. & Brin, B. (1980a) Mortality among California Seventh Day Adventists for selected cancer sites. *J. Natl Cancer Inst.*, *65*, 1097-1107

Phillips, R.L., Kuzma, J.W. & Lotz, T.M. (1980b) Cancer mortality among comparable members versus nonmembers of the Seventh-Day Adventist Church. In: Cairns, J., Lyon, J.L. & Skolnick, M., eds, *Cancer Incidence in Defined Populations* (Banbury Report 4), Cold Spring Harbor, NY, CSH Press, pp. 93-108

Price, C.H.G. & Jeffree, G.M. (1977) Incidence of bone sarcoma in SW England 1946-74 in relation to age, sex, tumour site and histology. *Br. J. Cancer, 36*, 511-522

Rohan, T.E. & Bain, C.J. (1987) Diet in the etiology of breast cancer. *Epidemiol. Rev., 9*, 120-145

Ron, E. & Modan, B. (1982) Thyroid. In: Schottenfeld, D. & Fraumeni, J.F., Jr, eds, *Cancer Epidemiology and Prevention*, Philadelphia, Saunders, pp. 837-854

Rose, E. (1973) Esophageal cancer in the Transkei: 1955-69. *J. Natl Cancer Inst., 51*, 7-16

Rose, E.F. & McGlashan, N.D. (1975) The spatial distribution of oesophageal carcinoma in the Transkei, South Africa. *Br. J. Cancer, 31*, 197-206

Ross, R.K., McCurtis, J.W., Henderson, B.E., Menck, H.R., Mack, T.M. & Martin, S.P. (1979) Descriptive epidemiology of testicular and prostatic cancer in Los Angeles. *Br. J. Cancer, 39*, 284-292

Salem, P., Anaissie, E., Allam, C., Geha, S., Hashimi, L., Ibrahim, N., Jabhour, J., Habboubi, N. & Khalyl, M. (1986) Non-Hodgkin's lymphomas in the Middle East. *Cancer, 58*, 1162-1166

Schaefer, O. & Hildes, J.A. (1986) Canada (Eskimos): Inuit Cancer Register 1950-1980. In: Parkin, D.M., ed., *Cancer Occurrence in Developing Countries* (IARC Scientific Publications No. 75), Lyon, IARC, pp. 159-163

Schmauz, R. & Jain, D.K. (1971) Geographical variation of carcinoma of the penis in Uganda. *Br. J. Cancer, 25*, 25-32

Schroder, L.E., Weiss, M.A. & Hughes, C. (1986) Squamous cell carcinoma of bladder: an increased incidence in blacks. *Urology, 28*, 289-291

Scotto, J., Fears, T.R. & Fraumeni, J.F. (1983) *Incidence of Nonmelanoma Skin Cancer in the United States* (NIH Publications No. 83-2433), Bethesda, MD, National Cancer Institute

Shimizu, H., Mack, T., Ross, R.K. & Henderson, B.E. (1987) Cancer of the gastrointestinal tract among Japanese and white immigrants in Los Angeles County. *J. Natl Cancer Inst., 78*, 223-228

Skegg, D.C.G., Corwin, P.A. & Paul, C. (1982) Importance of the male factor in cancer of the cervix. *Lancet, ii*, 581-583

Smith, E.M. (1982) Epidemiology of cancer of the oral cavity and pharynx. In: Correa, P. & Haenszel, W., eds, *Epidemiology of Cancer of the Gastrointestinal Tract* (Developments in Oncology, Vol. 6), The Hague, Martinus Nijhoff, pp. 1-19

Smith, P.G., Kinlen, L.J., White, G.C., Adelstein, A.M. & Fox, A.J. (1980) Mortality of wives of men dying with cancer of the penis. *Br. J. Cancer, 41*, 422-428

Spirtas, R., Beebe, G.W., Connelly, R.R., Wright, W.E., Peters, J.M., Sherwin, R.P., Henderson, B.E., Stark, A., Kovasznay, B.M., Davies, J.N.P., Vianna, J.N., Keehn, R.J., Ortega, L.G., Hochholzer, L. & Wagner, J.C. (1986) Recent trends in mesothelioma incidence in the United States. *Am. J. Ind. Med., 9*, 397-407

Spitz, M.R., Sider, J.G., Pollack, E.S., Lynch, H.K. & Newell, G.R. (1986) Incidence and descriptive features of testicular cancer among United States whites, blacks and Hispanics, 1973-1982. *Cancer, 58*, 1785-1790

Srivanatakul, P., Sontipong, S., Chotiwan, P. & Parkin, D.M. (1988) Liver cancer in Thailand: temporal and geographic variations. *J. Gastroenterol. Hepatol., 3*, 413-420

Steinitz, R., Parkin, D.M., Young, J.L., Bieber, C.A. & Katz, L., eds (1989) *Cancer Incidence in Jewish Migrants to Israel, 1961-1981* (IARC Scientific Publications No. 98), Lyon, IARC

Strickland, D. & Lee, J.A.H. (1981) Malignant melanoma of the eye: stability of rates. *Am. J. Epidemiol., 113*, 700-702

Swanson, G.M., Belle, S.H. & Satariano, W.A. (1985) Marital status and cancer incidence: differences in the black and white populations. *Cancer Res., 45*, 5883-5889

Tagnon, I., Blot, W.J., Stroube, R.B., Day, N.E., Morris, L.E., Peace, B.B. & Fraumeni, J.F., Jr (1980) Mesothelioma associated with the shipbuilding industry in coastal Virginia. *Cancer Res., 40*, 3875-3879

Tominaga, S. (1987) Decreasing trend of stomach cancer in Japan. *Gann, 78*, 1-10

Tucker, M.A. & Fraumeni, J.F., Jr (1982) Soft tissue. In: Schottenfeld, D. & Fraumeni, J.F., Jr, eds, *Cancer Epidemiology and Prevention*, Philadelphia, Saunders, pp. 827-836

Tuyns, A.J. (1982) Incidence trends of laryngeal cancer in relation to national alcohol and tobacco consumption. In: Magnus, K., ed., *Trends in Cancer Incidence - Causes and Practical Implications*, New York, Hemisphere, pp. 199-214

Tuyns, A.J. & Audigier, J.C. (1976) Double wave cohort increase for oesophageal cancer in France in relation to reduced alcohol consumption during the Second World War. *Digestion*, *14*, 197-208

Tuyns, A.J. & Massé, L.M.F. (1973) Mortality from cancer of the oesophagus in Brittany. *Int. J. Epidemiol.*, *2*, 241-245

US Department of Health and Human Services (1982) *The Health Consequences of Smoking: Cancer. A Report of the Surgeon General*, Washington DC, US Public Health Service

Van der Esch, E.P., Muir, C.S., Nectoux, J., MacFarlane, G., Maisonneuve, P., Bharucha, H., Briggs, J., Cooke, R.A., Dempster, A.G., Essex, W.B., Hofer, P.A., Hood, A.F., Ironside, P., Larsen, T.E., Little, J.H., Philipp, R., Pfau, R.S., Prade, M., Pozharisski, K.M., Rilke, F. & Schafler, K. (1990) Temporal change in diagnostic criteria as a cause of the increase of malignant melanoma over time is unlikely. *Int. J. Cancer* (in press)

Wagner, J.C., Skeggs, C.A. & Marchand, P. (1960) Diffuse pleural mesothelioma and asbestos exposure in the north western Cape Province. *Br. J. Ind. Med.*, *17*, 260-271

Waterhouse, J., Muir, C.S., Powell, J. & Shanmugaratnam, K., eds (1982) *Cancer Incidence in Five Continents*, Vol. *IV* (IARC Scientific Publications No. 42), Lyon, IARC

Weiss, N.S., Homonchuche, T. & Young, J.L. (1977) Incidence of histologic types of ovarian cancer: the US Third National Cancer Survey, 1969-71. *Gynecol. Oncol.*, *5*, 161-167

White, E., Daling, J.R., Norsted, T.L. & Chu, J. (1987) Rising incidence of breast cancer among women in Washington State. *J. Natl Cancer Inst.*, *79*, 239-243

Zaidi, S.H.M. (1986) Cancer trends in Pakistan. In: Khogali, M., Omar, Y.T., Gjorgov, A. & Ismail, A.S., eds, *Cancer Prevention in Developing Countries*, Oxford, Pergamon Press, pp. 69-73

Zaridze, D.G., Boyle, P. & Smans, M. (1984) International trends in prostate cancer. *Int. J. Cancer*, *33*, 223-230

Zippin, C., Tekawa, I.S., Bragg, K.U., Watson, D.A. & Linden, G. (1962) Studies on heredity and environment in cancer of the nasopharynx. *J. Natl Cancer Inst.*, *29*, 483-490

PART II

THE CAUSES OF CANCER

Chapter 4. Defining cause

Concepts of causality

Several definitions of disease causality have been proposed over the centuries, and it is not our aim to discuss them all in detail in the context of this book. For practical purposes and for simplification, the theories can be divided into two kinds: those based on mechanistic aspects of causation and those based on the pragmatic, operational consequences of the identification of a given cause.

In *mechanistic interpretations* of causality, a 'cause' may be defined as a factor that is 'necessary' or 'sufficient' for the disease to occur. A well-known example of the mechanistic approach is the Henle–Koch postulates, or criteria, for recognizing bacterial causes of disease: in order to be considered a cause, the suspect agent had (i) to be found in all diseased persons (a necessary cause); (ii) to be absent from the tissues of healthy people (a sufficient cause); and (iii) to be able to induce a similar disease in experimental animals.

For infectious diseases, the requirement of 'sufficiency' had to be modified or abandoned when it became clear that people could be exposed to a pathogen without developing the disease and that, for some infectious agents, 'healthy carriers' actually harboured the pathogen itself. The concept of 'necessary' cause has remained in use: particular lesions that define a disease are obligatorily associated with exposure to the agent. For instance, the microscopic pathological and clinical appearance of tuberculosis is necessarily related to infection with Koch's mycobacterium and theoretically cannot be produced by any other biological agent.

The situation is less clear for cancer. Formulating a mechanistic definition of cancer causation is complicated by the variability that characterizes this biological event. This variability derives from several sources, including interindividual differences in susceptibility to cancer induction and interactions among several causative agents (multifactorial causation). One can say only that certain *events* are necessary for cancer induction, without suggesting that there is anything unique about the factors that are required to produce them.

It is likely that such events involve changes at the level of the DNA of individual cells and that the probability that these changes will take place is influenced in two ways. The first depends on the randomness associated with each event in the multistage sequence that must be activated in order for cancer to be induced. Thus, the probability of the event taking place is dependent on a combination of low-probability biochemical reactions. The second component is the variability in individual responses, due, for instance, to interindividual (constitutional) differences in the ability to inactivate foreign chemicals or to repair damaged DNA. This means that, for the same dose of a carcinogenic agent, the cells of one individual are at higher risk of undergoing these events than those of another. A clear and extreme example is represented by a rare genetic disease – xeroderma pigmentosum – in which repair of DNA is seriously impaired. In these subjects, the frequency of skin cancer induced by ultra-violet light is enormously elevated, although ultra-violet light can also induce skin cancer in individuals who are not affected by this disease.

The induction and development of cancer are a result of genetic and epigenetic changes occurring in a given cell or clone of cells. Although, in some instances, a single event could be sufficient for cancer development, multiple genetic changes (point mutations, chromosomal translocations, amplification and activation of oncogenes, loss of suppressor genes) and the temporal sequence of such changes may vary for each type of tumour (Varmus & Bishop, 1986; Vogelstein *et al.*, 1988; Bos, 1989).

This model of carcinogenesis allows us to define a cause of cancer as a factor that increases the probability that cancer will develop in an individual. Since a value for probability cannot be estimated from the observation of cancer occurrence in one person (apart from probability one or zero), the study of cancer causation has become an epidemiological undertaking: enough people must be studied so that an adequate estimate can be made of whether cancer risk differs among groups of people exposed to different amounts of different agents.

Developments in epidemiology and public health have led to an *operational definition* of cause, according to which a cause is a factor, the elimination of which decreases the occurrence of a disease in a population. Sometimes this type of causal evidence is direct, such as the reduction in the incidence of lung cancer among ex-smokers as compared to current smokers, and the decline in mortality from specific cancers among workers in industries in which exposure to asbestos or aromatic amines was considerably reduced. In most instances, however, causal evidence is not obtained from such unplanned experiments, but from a combination of observations in human populations and the results of tests on experimental animals. The assessment of a causal relationship is based on inductive inference, i.e., a never-ending process of hypothesis formulation, testing and interpretation.

Neoplasms are ultimately the result of an interplay between hereditary and environmental factors. Both the genetic make-up and the environment vary from one human population to another, and it is the joint task of the geneticist and the epidemiologist to interpret these patterns of variation in order to develop meaningful models of cause. As close relatives often share both genes and a common environment, the relative influence of each may be difficult to isolate.

Within populations, cancers at some sites may be largely independent of environmental variation, some may be considered to be purely environmental, and some (perhaps most) may fall somewhere in between. To complicate matters further, a particular cancer may be seen to be the result of inborn susceptibility for some patients, whereas, for others, the same tumour may be seen to be the effect of a harmful exposure.

For most cancers, an individual's risk is at least partially determined at birth. This has been shown both through the study of cancer incidence in different ethnic groups and through the examination of unusual families with multiple affected members. By studying death certificates and cancer registrations, it was found that Ewing's sarcoma of bone is rarely seen among blacks, neither in Africa nor in the USA (Glass & Fraumeni, 1970). Similarly, a peak in the incidence of testicular cancer following adolescence is seen among white males only (Miller, 1977).

Several hereditary conditions are associated with an increased risk of cancer. For some, this susceptibility has been demonstrated by comparing rates among relatives of cancer patients with the rates in the general population. For others, the increase is so dramatic that it is evident after the evaluation of only a few affected families. Syndromes with cancer as the only manifestation are relatively rare. Neurofibromatosis, for example, is characterized by *café-au-lait* spots and neurofibromas as well as a propensity for malignant neural tumours, soft-tissue sarcomas and leukaemia (Hope & Mulvihill, 1981).

Genes associated with elevated cancer risk may either be common variants of several physiological systems, with apparently normal function, or they may be rare mutations which are clearly deleterious to humans. The antigens of the ABO blood group and of the major histocompatibility complex (HLA) are examples of polymorphic genetic systems which contribute to an individual's uniqueness and are passed from parent to child as codominant traits. Cancer of the stomach occurs slightly more often in persons with blood type A (Aird & Bentall, 1953) and is also a complication of a hereditary form of atrophic gastritis (Bonney *et al.*, 1986). Cancers that are believed to be associated with particular antigens of the HLA system include Hodgkin's disease (Dausset *et al.*, 1982), acute leukaemia (Von Fliedner *et al.*, 1983), papillary thyroid carcinoma (Ozaki *et al.*, 1988) and nasopharyngeal cancer (Lu *et al.*, 1990).

The rate at which carcinogens and other chemicals are metabolized varies from individual to individual in Caucasian populations. The metabolism of debrisoquine, for example, an antihypertensive drug, is thought to be controlled by an enzyme present in at least two allelic forms with different levels of activity (Caporaso *et al.*, 1989). After a test dose of debrisoquine, the rate of appearance of urinary metabolites depends on a person's particular set of alleles. Furthermore, this level appears to differ between patients with lung cancer and healthy controls, the rapid metabolizers being overrepresented among the tumour group (Ayesh *et al.*, 1984).

Blood groups, histocompatibility antigens and enzyme variants represent examples of normal differences among human genes that may affect cancer risk. In general, the magnitude of such risks is small; in fact, it would be surprising if a gene that carries a high risk for a (often) fatal condition were found to be common. There are, however, numerous examples of rare genetic mutations that do confer a very high risk for malignant disease upon the bearer.

For several common cancers, notably breast and colon cancer, there is strong evidence of familial predisposition. Cancers occurring within families tend to appear at younger age and are often bilateral (Knudson & Strong, 1973). The risk to sisters of premenopausal, bilateral breast cancer is particularly high (Anderson, 1974); if the mother is affected as well, it approaches 50% (Schwartz *et al.*, 1985). Through the statistical evaluation of several such breast cancer pedigrees (segregation analysis), it is proposed that the excess risk is best explained by a dominant breast cancer susceptibility gene that is active in a minority of affected families (Bishop *et al.*, 1988; Newman *et al.*, 1988). Linkage studies are under way to define the chromosomal location of the responsible gene. In these studies, the pattern of susceptibility is followed in one or more pedigrees with reference to a series of genetic markers of known chromosomal location. When a marker is found which appears to cosegregate with the disease gene through several generations (to an acceptable degree of statistical certainty), it is concluded that the marker and the disease gene are closely linked. It is hoped that this step will lead to the characterization of the gene responsible for breast tumour development in these families and increase our understanding of the mechanisms involved in nonfamilial breast cancer as well.

However, even before the isolation of a cancer-causing mutation, the knowledge of gene location can be applied to the early diagnosis and prevention of an inherited cancer. The application of the techniques of molecular biology to the detection of carriers of predisposing genes is mentioned in Part III, Chapter 18 (thyroid cancer). Hereditary cancer syndromes for which the chromosomal location is now known include familial adenomatous polyposis, multiple endocrine neoplasia type 1 and 2, hereditary retinoblastoma, dysplastic naevus syndrome (familial malignant melanoma), neurofibromatosis (two types) and Von-Hippel–Lindau disease.

Familial cancer of the colon may appear with and without pre-existing multiple adenomatous polyps. Among families with hereditary polyposis, there are several presentations – with osteomas, epidermoid cysts and congenital retinal pigmentation (Gardner syndrome); brain tumours (Turcots syndrome); or papillary carcinoma of the thyroid. In some families, extracolonic manifestations are absent. The susceptibility gene for familial adenomatous polyposis has been localized to chromosome 5 (Bodmer *et al.*, 1987). Early genetic analyses suggest that the variant forms may be the expressions of a single gene, possibly with several different allelic mutations.

Twenty-five percent of all cases of medullary cancer of the thyroid are due to the presence of a highly penetrant, dominant gene. Families with this form of cancer may contain members affected with pheochromocytomas as well – a combination known as the multiple endocrine neoplasia type 2 syndrome (MEN2a). The gene for MEN2a has been mapped to chromosome 10 with several DNA markers (Mathew *et al.*, 1987; Simpson *et al.*, 1987). Polymorphic DNA markers exist in two or more forms, which are distinguishable by size (alleles). A person may carry the same marker on each of his copies of chromosome 10 (homozygote) or he may carry two copies of different size (heterozygote). If an affected parent is heterozygous for markers which are closely linked to the MEN2a gene, and if it can be determined which marker allele shares the chromosome with the MEN2a mutation, then a marker of this size can be looked for in the child. If the child inherits the marker, he will probably inherit the disease as well. This offers the opportunity of screening affected families for individuals at high risk of thyroid cancer (see p. 282).

A second class of cancer susceptibility genes are responsible for a number of rare, recessive conditions characterized either by immunodeficiency or by impaired DNA repair. The tumour type and incidence vary: less than one in ten children with Fanconi's anaemia will develop leukaemia (Schroeder & Kurth, 1971), whereas 60% of carriers of xeroderma pigmentosum will have skin cancer by the age of 15 (Kraemer *et al.*, 1987). Although (homozygous) patients with these conditions are rare, heterozygous carriers are not. A seven-fold increase in risk for breast cancer has been suggested for women carrying a copy of the gene for ataxia telangectasia (Swift *et al.*, 1987). Assuming a carrier rate of 1%, this finding implies that 5% of breast cancer is attributable to the ataxia trait.

Another mechanism leading to increased susceptibility to cancer is the presence of constitutional chromosomal abnormalities. In persons with trisomy 21 (Down's syndrome), the risk for leukaemia increases 18 fold (Miller, 1970); perhaps 2% of childhood leukaemia is thus attributable to the syndrome (Robinson *et al.*, 1984). Males with Klinefelter syndrome harbour an extra copy of the X chromosome and have an excess number of embryonal teratomas (Lee & Stephens, 1987) and breast cancers (Harnden *et al.*, 1971). Individuals with extra chromosomes present as isolated cases due to new mutations, but structural chromosomal abnormalities may be traceable through several members of a pedigree. Families have been reported with Wilms' tumours and inherited deletions and duplications of chromosome 11 (Turleau *et al.*, 1984). In one notable pedigree with an excess of renal cancers, the tendency for cancer was confined to members with a translocation between chromosomes 3 and 8 (Cohen *et al.*, 1979). Gonadoblastomas are very rare ovarian tumours of childhood, but they occur frequently in the streak gonads of females with gonadal dysgenesis and an XY karyotype – the only clear example of a tumour in which an underlying genetic predisposition is the rule rather than the exception (Scully, 1981).

A final group of (possibly) hereditary cancers is perhaps the most puzzling. In children with hemihypertrophy, the two sides of the body develop at different rates. In these children, there is an increased risk for embryonal cancers, including Wilms' tumour, adenocortical carcinoma and hepatoblastoma (Miller, 1968). The genetics of cancers associated with congenital abnormalities are unclear; either the birth defects and the cancers are different expressions of the same gene, or the cancers represent the most extreme outcome of a general pattern of disorganized growth.

For all sites except retinoblastoma, the fraction of cancer attributable to heredity is small; this may be because the relative risk for cancer among gene carriers a small, but more commonly this is a reflection of the rarity of dominant cancer genes. The influences of genetics and environment may be difficult to separate, even in the same patient. Skin tumours in xeroderma pigmentosum patients are a response to damage by ultraviolet light. Because ultraviolet light is ubiquitous and the xeroderma pigmentosum gene is rare, it makes more sense to think of the disease as having a genetic rather than an environmental etiology. But not all examples are as clear-cut. Second primary cancers, notably sarcomas of bone and soft tissue, often complicate radiation treatment for retinoblastoma (Draper *et al.*, 1986). The vast majority of these second tumours arise in patients with the hereditary variant (Abramson *et al.*, 1984), yet hereditary retinoblastoma represents only one-half of the total (Vogel, 1979). A number of patients developed papillary carcinoma of the thyroid after the injudicious use of radiation in the 1950s as a treatment and as a screening tool. Thyroid tumours were also seen more commonly than expected among the relatives of these patients, even though they did not necessarily receive radiation treatment (De Groot & Paloyan, 1973; Fisher & Edmonds, 1980).

These studies illustrate the potential value of looking for genetic factors when studying environmental risks, and *vice versa*. There is currently much interest in developing risk models and analytical tools which permit the joint consideration of hereditary and environmental factors in risk estimation. Identifying individuals who are genetically susceptible to developing cancer is of practical interest because the information can be used in genetic counselling, in advising the avoidance of harmful environmental exposures (in some instances including radiotherapy) and in promoting increased surveillance aimed at early detection.

It must be recognized that, unless a cause produces an effect in all people exposed (and few, if any, such causes are encountered in nature), its effect manifests itself as an increased probability of getting a cancer, which may or may not be due to increased susceptibility. Smokers can be categorized according to gradations of probabilities of getting lung cancer: smokers of more than two packs a day have a higher probability than smokers of five cigarettes per day; smokers exposed to dusty asbestos are also at particularly high risk and so may be particular subgroups of subjects identifiable through biochemical (possibly genetically determined) markers. Within each such subset, chance still decides who will get cancer. The expectation that by progressive and more refined subgrouping it may eventually be possible to separate out those subsets of people in whom the bulk of the cases of a common cancer will be concentrated may never be completely fulfilled. In fact, existing evidence indicates that the majority of cases of common cancers occur among the relatively large sections of the population who are at moderately increased risk rather than among the much smaller sections who are at very high risk.

Identification of the causes of cancer

The role of epidemiology

Direct, rather than indirect, answers to the question 'Is a particular agent carcinogenic for humans?' can be obtained only from studies of human beings, using an epidemiological approach. Epidemiological studies are prompted by different sources of evidence, which include results from the laboratory and two kinds of observations in humans: anecdotal clinical evidence and results of exploratory analyses of cancer mortality and morbidity statistics, described in Part I.

Sir Austin Bradford Hill (Hill, 1965) suggested that nine criteria should be met ideally in order to establish whether an observed relationship is likely to be causal, having ascertained that the exposed persons are at higher risk than the unexposed:

1. Consistency and unbiasedness of the findings
2. Strength of the association
3. Temporal sequence

4. Biological gradient (dose–response relationship)
5. Specificity
6. Coherence with biological background and previous knowledge
7. Biological plausibility
8. Reasoning by analogy
9. Experimental evidence

The discussion which follows explains these criteria.

The history of carcinogenesis bears a strong imprint of clinical observations that led directly to successful identification of etiological factors, at different levels of detail: from the classic description of scrotal cancer in chimney-sweeps and the late nineteenth century account of bladder cancer in workers exposed to aromatic amines, to the quite recent identification of the occurrence of clear-cell adenoma of the vagina in adolescent daughters of mothers who had been treated with the hormone diethylstilboestrol during pregnancy. Astute clinicians are an excellent first line for gathering etiological clues; however, this picture of successful discoveries is one-sided, as many clinical observations have led nowhere.

The finding that exposure to an individual agent, such as a chemical, is followed by the appearance of a cancer can be regarded as no more than suggestive that there is an association. Still, different degrees can be perceived in the strength of such a suggestion. For instance, if two or more cases of a common cancer (say, of the stomach) are reported following the use of a widely used drug (say, aspirin), the most likely explanation is that the association occurred purely by chance. An association is less likely to be due to chance, however, when two or more isolated cases of a cancer are reported in a presumably small group, for instance, in patients treated with melphalan. This holds particularly strongly when the reported cancer is a well specified, uncommon one, like oat-cell carcinoma of the lung, which occurs after exposure to bischloromethyl ether, or liver angiosarcoma, which occurs after exposure to vinyl chloride.

In fact, virtually all causal associations that were brought to light on the basis of clinical observations belong to this group of 'rare cancer–relatively rare exposure'. The strength of the suggestion of a causal association is even greater when a series of consecutive cases is reported from a single centre, so that a rough estimate of the size of the exposed population can be attempted and the number of cancers that would have been expected if exposure to the agent had not occurred can be computed for comparison with the number actually observed. This proved possible, for instance, for some of the early series of cases of leukaemia in benzene-exposed workers in northern Italy.

The other main source of etiological hypotheses is exploratory analyses, as outlined in Part I, of mortality and incidence rates and their variation with space and time and according to demographic characteristics such as sex, age and social class. Of major importance in this respect is the large variation – often ten fold or even a hundred fold – of the incidence rates for most cancers in adults in different populations, defined according to geographical areas of residence or according to other easily measurable variables like ethnic group, religion and social class. Every type of common cancer – that is, common in at least some populations – can be found, albeit rarely, in other populations, whatever the demographic variable used to define the population. This marked variation in rates according to different and partially independent axes of exploration is unlikely to be explained chiefly by concomitant genetic variations and points to the predominant role of environment (broadly defined) in cancer causation.

Exploratory analyses of currently available data are often expanded into correlation studies, in which population characteristics (e.g., population density, salt consumption level, concentration of atmospheric pollutants in the environment) are related to rates of occurrence of a cancer over a series of sampling units, for instance, geographical areas. For correlation analyses of this type, an important requirement is that there be sufficient variation in both rates and levels of environmental indicators between the different geographical units and as little variation as possible within each unit. Although correlation studies may provide very valuable pointers to etiological factors, however, conclusions derived from them must be interpreted with caution. What appears to apply at the level of a population (for example, a correlation between average salt consumption by geographical area and mortality rates for stomach cancer), may not hold at the level of individuals, i.e., subjects who eat more salt may turn out to be at no increased risk for stomach cancer. Such discrepancies, often referred to as the 'ecological fallacy', between findings at two levels is due to the fact that populations differ in many other respects, and one or more other variables which were not taken into account may be responsible for the observed differences.

Thus, studies are required in which exposure of individuals, rather than of populations, can be assessed. These are more adequate tools for testing etiological hypotheses and for estimating the effects of causative agents. In cohort studies, subjects with different degrees of exposure to the main agent of interest are followed up either from the past to the present (historical cohort study) or into the future (prospective cohort study), and their cancer experience, in terms of mortality or morbidity, is analysed as a function of the level of exposure to the agent under study and of other interfering variables. The historical approach has been and remains the main instrument for studies of the occupational environment when past records of exposure, or at least of employment, are available so as to be able to characterize the cohort adequately, and when the exposure is rare in the general population. Details of occupational history and of exposure to agents within the occupational environment and outside it (for instance, smoking habits) can be searched through ad-hoc, usually time-consuming, inquiries in a restricted subsample of the members of the cohort (often numbering several thousands). Different subsampling schemes can be envisaged, all having in common that the ad-hoc information must be acquired both for subjects who have the cancer and for unaffected ones. Such subsampling within a cohort is known as a 'case–control study within the cohort'.

Prospective cohort studies have been conducted less often than historical studies, but they generate essential information. Suffice it to mention the prospective studies on smoking and cancer that were carried out in the UK, the USA and other countries, and the study of atomic bomb survivors in Japan that is still going on. These investigations not only firmly established the causal role of tobacco smoke and ionizing radiation in the occurrence of cancer at several sites, but have provided data on relationships between degree of exposure and cancer outcome, including the temporal aspects of the evolution of risk subsequent to exposure.

Case–control studies represent the other main approach to investigations of etiology. An extension of the clinical method of inquiring into the past of a patient, a case–control study consists in comparing the exposure histories of cancer cases and of controls. The approach is vulnerable to potential distortions deriving from the selection of controls and from the fact that exposure is ascertained after the cancer has occurred. These distortions can be minimized by appropriate design and conduct of the study, notably when the study includes all cases of cancer that occurred in a defined area during a particular period (a 'population-based case–control study') and not just hospitalized cases. Distortions in the ascertainment of exposure can also be reduced by replacing or cross-checking information obtained by interview against past records – for example, to obtain the dose of medical irradiation received by mothers during pregnancy in a study of leukaemia in their children.

However good the methods and however favourable the circumstances, most epidemiological studies (be they cohort or case–control) have certain limitations. The first is the intrinsic limitation that they are not experiments and the conditions cannot therefore be defined at the outset. The researcher must adjust his methods and analyses to the available material. A second aspect of purely observational studies is limitation of the size of available groups, of the length of exposure or of levels of exposure. For instance, only small groups of workers may have been exposed to a suspected carcinogen, and this may have happened only five or ten years previously – probably insufficient time for a usually long-term adverse effect like cancer to occur. Or, dietary variations within a population may be relatively small, so that the chances of detecting an effect of a dietary component are reduced. These considerations should be kept prominently in mind when interpreting the results of a 'negative' study, i.e., one that does not show an increased cancer risk among exposed subjects. The results may reflect the conditions of observations, which cannot be changed by the investigators, rather than a real absence of risk.

A third aspect of epidemiological studies which is often misinterpreted as a limitation, derives from the way in which an agent is defined and measured. An 'agent' is virtually never a pure chemical, as in a laboratory experiment, and is rarely of a technical or even a commercial degree of purity but is present in the particular circumstances of an 'exposure'. This all-embracing term is adopted in epidemiology to designate any agent to which human beings are exposed. Even more frequently, exposures are to mixtures of chemicals (tobacco smoke, alcoholic drinks) or denote circumstances, relatively well defined, in which certain physical, chemical or biological agents are present. Although exposures of greater degrees of complexity inevitably complicate the task of establishing a causal link with a cancer, as more room is left for interference by confounding factors, this should not be seen as an impediment to making inferences of causality. Thus, provided adequate evidence is at hand, it might be stated that 'social class' is the 'cause' of several cancers (see also Chapter 16). An agent defined at the microscopic or submicroscopic level is not more specific a cause than a macroscopic one.

What we define as a cause is a function of the level of observation we choose: at the level of the total population, 'manual occupation' is a cause of bladder cancer; at the level of the population of manual workers, working in a dye plant is a cause; at the level of the individual, β-naphthylamine comes to be regarded as the cause; and at the level of the cells, its hydroxylated metabolite is the cause. The consistency between these different levels of observation greatly reinforces the plausibility of a causal link. In this sense, research into the mechanisms of action of carcinogens – opening the 'black box' of the organism as a whole (usually considered as such in epidemiological studies) – joins with epidemiology in identifying the steps and agents in the causal chain.

One class of epidemiological study avoids some of the problems discussed above. These are usually called randomized intervention studies, and their methodology is close to that of randomized clinical trials on medical treatment. A number of these studies have recently been started or proposed, with the aim of testing the effectiveness of putative anticarcinogenic factors in preventing cancer (or precancerous lesions). Intervention studies are conducted in subjects without cancer, with the goal of preventing the occurrence of cancer (or other diseases) by modifying the subjects' behaviour (e.g., their diet, smoking habits or amount of physical exercise), by providing supplements (e.g., vitamins or fibre) or by vaccination. Such interventions are not intended to be medical treatment for clinical diseases. The random assignment of subjects to the 'exposure' (i.e., treated subjects) guarantees, in principle, that known and unknown sources of noncomparability will operate equally in treated and untreated people and will not bias the results. In all other types of epidemiological investigation, the absence of randomization makes particularly difficult the interpretation of 'small' observed risks, which might reflect simply an unbalanced distribution between exposed and unexposed subjects of some unknown agent rather than the effect of the exposure of interest.

The era is probably ending in which some of the major environmental carcinogens (tobacco smoking, radiation, occupational carcinogens) can be identified by the traditional epidemiological methods of interview and recording of external exposures. When the link between tobacco smoke and cancer was still a subject of hot controversy – notwithstanding the weight of the epidemiological evidence – epidemiologists reinforced and systematized a set of criteria by which causality could be inferred purely on the basis of epidemiology (Hill, 1965; see p. 102), even in the absence of concordant data from tests in experimental animals (this was the case, at that time – in the early 1960s – for tobacco smoke). Biological plausibility was included among the criteria, but it was clearly a relatively weak and dispensable element. The case of tobacco smoke–cancer has been so persuasively influential that the attitude that epidemiology can stand on its own merits, independently of laboratory data, may have gone further than intended. Although the fall-out from molecular biology in terms of concepts and techniques for measuring exposure and targets is still more a prospect than a reality, it can be expected to materialize within the next decade, opening the way for an epidemiological search for the causes of cancer that has a stronger biological basis.

Biological indicators of exposure and of effect

Biochemical (or molecular) epidemiology can entail two different approaches. One is the assessment of exposures for use in prospective studies or in future retrospective studies. The second involves use of end-points other than cancer in studies of the causes of cancer; these end-points are currently undergoing validation.

Exposure and effect indicators that can be used in epidemiological studies include measurement of a putative carcinogen or its breakdown product, the metabolite, in samples obtained from exposed people, measurement of products of reaction of the chemical within the body, such as a DNA or protein adduct, and observation of early biological changes induced by the exposure (such as changes in the genetic material of the cell – cytogenetic changes). The only approach that has been in widespread, routine use until now is measurement of the chemicals, or their metabolites, in body fluids. Thus, individual exposure to, e.g., cadmium, arsenic, nickel, chromium, 4,4'-methylene bis(2-chloroaniline) (MOCA), benzene and polycyclic aromatic hydrocarbons, can be measured in urine and blood (Aitio *et al.*, 1988). Biological monitoring of this kind is performed in order to provide an estimate of the dose absorbed; however, a relationship between risk for lung cancer and urinary excretion of arsenic has been established relatively reliably (Enterline & Marsh, 1982; Enterline *et al.*, 1987). Biological monitoring differs from monitoring of the environment in that variations in the absorption of different individuals is taken into account.

Interindividual differences in the ability to metabolize chemicals into the metabolites that are the ultimate carcinogens cannot be taken into account in current methods for biological monitoring. The two most promising new approaches in biological monitoring – measurement of adducts with proteins and with DNA – may overcome this problem (Müller & Rajewsky, 1981; IARC/IPCS, 1982; Garner, 1985; Bartsch *et al.*, 1988). Chemical and immunological methods to assess adducts between DNA and polycyclic aromatic hydrocarbons, aflatoxins and methylating and ethylating agents have been developed (Autrup *et al.*, 1983; Strickland & Boyle, 1984; Garner, 1985; Hemminki, 1985; Weston *et al.*, 1988; Perera, 1990), and benzo[*a*]pyrene–DNA adducts have been measured in human lymphocytes (Vähäkangas *et al.*, 1985). The measurement of specific DNA adducts has a distinct advantage over any other monitoring method in that one is measuring damage to the target molecules of carcinogenesis. Protein adducts can also serve as markers of exposure to environmental carcinogens, as a surrogate for DNA. With this method, smaller samples are needed, and, since some protein adducts persist for a long time in the body, one can estimate exposure over extended periods of time. An approach that has come into extensive use is a nonspecific analysis of DNA adducts by so-called 'post-labelling' techniques (Randerath *et al.*, 1989). This is probably the most sensitive method for measuring changes in the structure of cellular DNA, but usually information on the causative agent or on the quality of DNA damage present cannot be derived. In order to estimate the extent and type of genetic damage due to a specific chemical, highly sophisticated, specific analytical techniques must be used.

It has been established that agents that alter the genetic apparatus of cells, causing mutations, are potentially carcinogenic. (For a discussion of the relationship between mutagenicity and carcinogenicity, see p. 113). Analysis of the mutagenicity of body fluids, and especially urine, has been widely applied as a means of estimating exposure of people to genotoxic, and thus potentially carcinogenic, chemicals. Tests have therefore been devised in which the capacity of a biological sample, such as urine, to induce mutation in bacteria is measured. Since the methods are completely unspecific and relate only to the capacity of a metabolite to induce mutations in bacteria, the results are sometimes difficult to interpret. Among the major obstacles to drawing definitive conclusions are the other potentially mutagenic exposures of human subjects, as in their diet and due to personal habits, such as smoking.

Structural changes in specific chromosomes have been linked to cancers of several types. In addition, in populations who have been exposed to ionizing radiation, and are thus at elevated risk for developing cancer, structural chromosomal damage has been a consistent finding, to such an extent that chromosomal aberrations have been used as a measure of the dose of exposure to radiation (International Atomic Energy Agency, 1986). Several carcinogenic chemicals have also been shown to produce chromosomal damage in experimental animals and in humans, and, in some studies, analysis of chromosomal aberrations and other cytogenetic changes, such as micronuclei and sister chromatid exchange, has been used to assess human exposure to carcinogenic agents (Sorsa *et al.*, 1988). The drawbacks to use of such analyses include lack of specificity with regard to the causative agent and unresolved questions about the relationship between these changes and carcinogenesis; there are also several practical analytical problems. Other methods that have been studied for use in molecular epidemiology include measurement of urinary cotinine (and nicotine), as an indicator of exposure to tobacco smoke, and measurement of bile acids in faeces. Endogenous formation of *N*-nitroso compounds has been estimated from the urinary excretion of *N*-nitrosoproline (Ohshima & Bartsch, 1981). Several recent studies on the relationship between diet and cancer have involved measurement of lipid-soluble vitamins, such as A and E, and of selenium in samples collected for various purposes several years before the diagnosis of cancer. A number of projects have been proposed for long-term storage of samples obtained during epidemiological studies that are being carried out now, so that, when specific, reliable methods become available, quantitative measurements of exposure will be possible.

The role of the laboratory

The obstacles to the identification of specific causative factors in the origin of human cancers include (i) the long latent period between exposure to causative agents and overt appearance of the disease; (ii) the multistage nature of the carcinogenesis process; and (iii) the likelihood that most human cancers result from a complex interaction between multiple environmental and endogenous (genetic or other host) factors. Although significant progress has been made, several important general questions have still not been completely resolved; these include the extent to which human cancers are due to specific causes, such as chemicals, hormones and physical and viral agents, the relative contributions of carcinogens that act at various stages of the process of carcinogenesis, the role of nutritional factors and the interactions of endogenous and environmental factors.

Laboratory studies for predicting or detecting agents with potential carcinogenic activity have provided approaches to the prevention of human cancer. Short-term tests for the detection of potential carcinogens (see below) are widely used for prescreening chemicals, and, often, when positive results have been obtained, human exposure has been reduced or substitutes have been introduced. The results of laboratory studies have also frequently extended epidemiological findings in making it possible to isolate and identify the individual carcinogenic and cocarcinogenic components of complex mixtures. It is also only by means of laboratory studies that 'new' naturally occurring and man-made carcinogenic agents can be identified.

Long-term bioassays

The principal end-point of bioassays for carcinogenicity is the induction of neoplasms in experimental animals treated and observed for the major part of their life span. The species and strain of test animals, dose and route of administration of the test agent and full pathology of the main organs are the most important considerations in designing such tests.

The species most frequently used in carcinogenicity bioassays are mice, rats and hamsters, because of practical rather than theoretical considerations: their relatively short life span (less than three years) and small size, the large amount of information available about their physiology and biochemistry, and the large data base concerning the incidence of tumours that arise spontaneously in these animals. Although primates are evolutionarily closer to humans, they are not used routinely for practical reasons.

Oral intake, inhalation and application on the skin are the major routes of administration used. Oral intake and inhalation simulate patterns of human exposure the most closely; exposure *via* the skin is not a major route of human exposure for many compounds, but it is often used because it is easy both to apply nonvolatile compounds in this way and to observe the local tumours that are induced.

The doses selected for carcinogenicity testing are often much larger than those to which humans are exposed. Although the metabolic pathways and other pharmacokinetics that operate at higher doses may differ from those which operate at lower doses, high doses are often necessary in order to evaluate carcinogenicity in relatively small numbers of animals. Generally, groups of 50 animals are used per dose tested; these small numbers make it difficult to obtain conclusive negative results. It should be noted that the carcinogenic potency of chemicals varies considerably – by about 10^7: aflatoxin B_1, a mycotoxin occasionally found as a contaminant in food, produces tumours in 50% of rats at daily doses in the order of micrograms, whereas 10–100 mg of benzidine, a known human carcinogen, are required to induce the same incidence in rats.

Interspecies differences in tumour response can also be large; e.g., mice are much less sensitive than rats to the production of tumours by aflatoxin B_1.

While there are therefore good reasons to include a high dose level in testing a substance of unknown carcinogenic activity, the systematic use of the Maximum Tolerated Dose (MTD) has been severely criticized (Ames *et al.*, 1987). There are, however, only a few instances in which a chemical has been shown to be carcinogenic only when given at the MTD, even within the National Toxicology Program where the MTD is systematically included in the testing design.

Target organs often differ according to species, age, sex and other factors. For instance, aromatic amines can induce bladder tumours in humans, but tumours of the liver and other organs in mice and rats (although they induce bladder tumours in hamsters). Thus, although the results obtained in rodents give a qualitative indication of the carcinogenicity of these compounds, they do not necessarily indicate in which organ the effect will appear.

Both the latent period of many human cancers, i.e., the time that elapses between exposure to carcinogens and the appearance of cancer, and the evidence that certain cancers are caused by an interaction of multiple factors indicate that cancers develop as a multistage process. While it is difficult to divide and define these stages clearly, given our still imperfect knowledge about the mechanisms involved in each, studies of experimental model systems have been used to demonstrate and analyse the stages of initiation, promotion (Berenblum & Shubik, 1949) and progression (Foulds, 1969).

Initiating activity reflects the capacity of an agent to produce irreversible cellular changes that give to cells the potential of progressing to tumours. Since cancer is a disease of multicellular organisms, it presumably represents alterations in the functioning of the genes that are concerned with the regulation of cellular interactions. Initiating events are generally recognized to occur by a genetic mechanism, such as an alteration in DNA sequences or chromosome numbers. This event can involve an alteration in primary DNA structures – a gene mutation or chromosomal translocation – or a change in the number of genes or of entire chromosomes – gene amplification of aneuploidy – or the loss of genes that would otherwise prevent neoplastic growth, as in the case of retinoblastoma (Knudson, 1986) and of some colorectal carcinomas (Bodmer *et al.*, 1987; Solomon *et al.*, 1987).

Interspecies differences in susceptibility to chemically induced cancer

Because of the universality of biological processes, one might expect that all mammals, from rodents to humans, would respond similarly to carcinogens. All of the mammals that have been studied, including such diverse species as cows, horses, sheep, dogs, rats and mice, develop cancer spontaneously, although there can be substantial variation in the frequencies with which different organs are affected.

Imposed on the background of general similarities, however, are individual characteristics that might modulate differences in responses between species. One obvious difference is body size. On the one hand, humans, being larger, have more cells than mice and, therefore, more chance of an individual cell becoming malignant. Small animals, on the other hand, tend to have more rapid cell division, which means that the induction periods of manifest tumours are shorter than in larger mammals (see Peto, 1977).

Another set of variables concerns the fate of environmental chemicals in the body. Although absorption after oral exposure tends to be similar among species, the kind of food into which the chemical is mixed, the gastrointestinal transit time and the microbial flora encountered vary considerably among herbivores, omnivores and carnivores. Penetration of the skin by chemicals is partly modified by the thickness of the skin, the density of sweat glands and fur thickness.

Through evolution, various animal species and man have developed essentially the same metabolic systems for detoxifying and eliminating foreign and unnecessary chemical substances, and metabolic pathways tend to be qualitatively similar in different species, although quantitative differences in the rates and directions of metabolisms are not uncommon. Small animals tend to excrete compounds more rapidly. Variation between human individuals in the activities of the enzymes that catalyse activation and deactivation of carcinogens tends to be much greater than that among laboratory animal species; interindividual differences among humans may even exceed those between, e.g., mice and rats. This has important consequences for the extrapolation of data from rodents to humans: when a large number of people are exposed to a carcinogen, it is probable that some of them are as susceptible to the carcinogen as is the most susceptible animal species.

Some qualitative differences also exist. Guinea-pigs are unable to *N*-hydroxylate aromatic amines to the active carcinogen, as humans, dogs and rodents do, and they are therefore resistant to the carcinogenic action of the parent amine. Cats cannot form glucuronic acid conjugates; the same is true for certain genera of rats. Mice of different inbred lines tend genetically to be either susceptible or resistant to induction of the enzymes that are important in the metabolism of aromatic polycyclic hydrocarbon compounds. Thus, different strains or species of animals and, indeed, individual humans, may metabolize carcinogenic compounds differently, resulting in variations in the degree of tumour induction.

One approach to interspecies extrapolation is to compare the results obtained in bioassays in which two species of animals are exposed to the same substance by the same route. In one such series of bioassays, 266 compounds were tested for carcinogenicity in rats and in mice (Haseman & Huff, 1987). The overall concordance between rats and mice exposed to the same chemical was 74% (198/266). Within each species, the results for males and females were also highly correlated (87% for rats and 89% for mice). In an analysis of bioassays of 250 chemicals, Purchase (1980) found that if a chemical was carcinogenic in one species, there was about an 85% chance that it would be carcinogenic in a second species: cancer was produced at at least one common body site in both species by 64% of 109 carcinogens. The high interspecies correlation shown supports the view that carcinogenicity outcomes in one species may predict similar effects in other species (Tomatis *et al.*, 1989).

Use of data from experiments in animals in predicting human risk

The thorny issue of reliable extrapolation of results obtained under the conditions of experiments in animals to the human situation is an enduring one. The characterization of human health risk must often rely solely on data on experimental animals because relevant epidemiological studies are lacking. The ultimate aim of bioassays designed to evaluate the carcinogenic potential of various chemicals in animal species, particularly in rats and mice, is therefore to evaluate the carcinogenic potential of the chemicals to humans. A major premise underlying these activities is that there is a relationship between the carcinogenicity of chemicals in animals and in humans.

A hindrance to comparing data obtained from bioassays with that from studies of humans is that the two types of study are fundamentally different. Animal bioassays are conducted under standardized, controlled laboratory conditions in which the only variable is administration of the test compound. The animals are genetically very similar, fed the same diet, housed in the same environment and not permitted to vary their exercise or to reproduce, and are given the same dose of the test material regularly throughout their lives by the same route. Humans are exposed accidentally or naturally to varying amounts of the substances in question, and to many other substances, for varying durations. They come from various subpopulations (genetic heterogeneity), eat different diets, live in different places, may have intercurrent diseases, and live much longer.

The qualitative relationship between carcinogenicity in animals and humans appears to be good, i.e., all of the chemicals that are known to cause cancer in humans are also carcinogenic to experimental animals, when adequately tested (Wilbourn *et al.*, 1986). Experimental results would be more useful if they could also provide a quantitative prediction of human risk. In a study promoted by the US National Academy of Sciences (NAS Executive Committee, 1975), in which the carcinogenic potency of several human carcinogens was compared in humans and in experimental animals, experimental animals appeared to be more susceptible than humans, but by no more than two orders of magnitude, that is within the range of what could be seen as an acceptable safety factor. In this study, however, the comparison was made between chemicals for which quantitative data on exposure were crude.

In a recent paper, Allen *et al.* (1988) identified 23 substances which are carcinogenic to animals, humans or both and studied the correlation between carcinogenic potency estimates derived from epidemiological and experimental studies. The correlation was impressively high (up to 90%, depending on which means were used to estimate potency); however, the group of agents studied was very heterogeneous and included several complex mixtures.

Kaldor *et al.* (1988) compared the carcinogenicity potency of cytostatic drugs, for which data on human exposure are rather accurate. The results of this survey would indicate that the potency rankings for cyclophosphamide, chlorambucil and melphalan are very similar in rodents and humans. With the caution imposed by the limited number of chemicals considered, one could at least say that in the only case in which the actual exposure levels were measurable in all species with the same accuracy, there was a quantitative correlation in the carcinogenic response in humans and in two rodent species.

Short-term tests

Many natural and synthetic chemicals, as well as ionizing and ultra-violet radiation, can induce permanent genetic alterations (i.e., mutations) in cells and organisms. Different categories of mutation have been recognized in both genes and chromosomes in all organisms, including man. Such changes are deleterious for normal cell function, and, when they occur in the germinal cells of exposed individuals, they may lead to inherited genetic defects in their offspring. Furthermore, a strong association has been found between the mutagenicity and the carcinogenicity of many physical and chemical agents; accordingly, mutations in somatic cells can indicate potential carcinogenicity.

It is generally agreed that during carcinogenesis alterations occur in the genome of malignant cells that are not present in normal cells. Some of the normal genes present in the genome of every individual regulate growth, and their modification (point mutation or amplification) results in a deregulation which may contribute to the unrestricted growth of the cell and therefore to its malignant transformation. Several such genes have been identified, and many others probably exist. They are called 'oncogenes', a term that has been used to indicate their relationship with neoplastic growth; this term has perhaps incited undue expectations, as if these genes were themselves the cause of cancer, while they are in fact part of the ultimate mechanism of cellular growth. It is not known for any given tumour which factors produce such genetic alterations, the molecular nature of the alterations themselves or the mechanisms by which they bring about neoplastic growth. There is evidence, however, that oncogenes found in tumours are activated in this way. Oncogenes have been detected in human and animal tumours, indicating that their activation is one of the mechanisms by which cells become malignant. There is also good evidence that for most, if not all, human tumours this genetic event is not sufficient to produce cancers (Barbacid, 1987). Some cellular oncogenes (notably of the *ras* family) can attain the ability to transform cells by virtue of specific point mutations in critical regions of their coding sequences (Tabin *et al.*, 1982; Seeburg *et al.*, 1984). Studies of cancer in experimental animals have shown that mutations induced in some cellular oncogenes may be highly specific with respect to a carcinogen and, furthermore, that with some experimental designs 100% *ras* activation can occur (Barbacid, 1987).

A wide variety of organisms is used in short-term tests, from bacteriophages and bacteria to mammalian cells and whole mammals *in vivo*. The tests are characterized by end-points which may be related to postulated mechanisms of carcinogenesis and especially to changes at the level of DNA. The end-points vary from DNA damage, gene mutation, sister chromatid exchange, formation of micronuclei, induction of chromosomal aberrations or aneuploidy, to cell transformation. However, it is not known what categories of genetic or related change are most important in neoplastic growth.

The prototype of methods for detecting mutagenicity is the 'Ames test' (although there are now more than 200 such tests), in which the end-point is the induction of mutation at the gene that governs synthesis of histidine in highly mutable strains of the bacterium *Salmonella typhimurium*. Since many carcinogenic chemicals require metabolic activation before they can interact with DNA, a fraction of rodent liver is included in the assay system.

Positive results obtained in tests for genetic and related effects using prokaryotes, lower eukaryotes, plants, insects or mammalian cells in culture imply that similar effects (and therefore, possibly, carcinogenic effects) could occur in mammals. However, the manifestation of these effects may be affected by metabolic processes in the host that lead to inactive or active derivatives. Evidence showing genetic effects in whole experimental animals and in humans is therefore of greater relevance to the prediction of human risk than evidence from other organisms. Studies that show no such effect in whole animals are less relevant. Results from such tests also provide information about the types of genetic effects produced by an agent. Some of the end-points are clearly genetic in nature (e.g., gene mutations and chromosomal aberrations), others are associated with genetic effects to a greater or lesser degree (e.g., those related to DNA repair, such as unscheduled DNA synthesis). In-vitro tests for tumour-promoting activity and for cell transformation may indicate changes that are not necessarily the result of genetic alterations but that may have specific relevance to the process of carcinogenesis.

Several large surveys have shown that most known initiators and 'complete' carcinogens are mutagenic in at least one test system (McCann *et al.*, 1975; Hollstein *et al.*, 1979; De Serres & Ashby, 1981; Bartsch *et al.*, 1982; Ennever & Rosenkranz, 1987; Zeiger, 1987). Correlations between carcinogenicity and positivity in the Ames test range from 60 to 90% (McCann *et al.*, 1975; McCann & Ames, 1976; De Serres & Ashby, 1981). The selection of chemicals for correlation studies is biased, however, since only those compounds that have been tested for carcinogenicity can be chosen, and the number of chemicals for which there is firm evidence of noncarcinogenicity is very small. Of chemicals that have been adequately tested for carcinogenicity in experimental animals and shown to be carcinogenic, about 80% were found to be mutagenic in the Ames test (Bartsch *et al.*, 1982).

Supplements 6 and 7 to the *IARC Monographs on the Evaluation of Carcinogenic Risks to Humans* give an – albeit limited – opportunity to study the capacity of different short-term tests to detect human carcinogens (Table 10). The sensitivity of tests with different end-points (DNA damage, gene mutation, mitotic recombination, induction of sister chromatid exchange, micronuclei or chromosomal aberrations, or induction of morphological transformation) is 67–85%. When tests with end-points of different phylogenetic orders are combined, the sensitivity varies between 54 and 82%.

One crucial problem in establishing a relationship between carcinogenicity and mutagenicity is that mutagenicity is essentially a single-step event and carcinogenicity a multi-step event. This model of carcinogenicity is an operational one, and the sequence of events might be more or less complicated, but it is reasonable to assume that the different steps do not operate by the same mechanisms. As long as at least one step requires a mutational event, however, a

Table 10. Sensitivity of different short–term tests for detecting human carcinogens[a]

Genetic end-point	Test system							Overall sensitivity (%)
	Prokaryotes	Lower eukaryotes	Insects	Mammalian cells in vitro	Human cells in vitro	Mammalian cells in vivo	Human cells in vivo	
DNA damage	10/14			15/17	9/14	9/10		78
Gene mutation	14/20	11/14	8/14	12/19				67
Mitotic recombination		11/13						85
Sister chromatid exchange				13/15	10/15	8/10	5/11	78[b]
Chromosomal aberration				14/16	10/14		8/13	80[b]
Micronuclei						9/13		69
Transformation				14/16		11/14		83
Overall sensitivity (%)	71	81	57	82	67	79	54	

a From IARC (1987a,b). The numerator gives the number of positive tests and the denominator the number of chemicals tested. Only results based on testing of at least ten chemicals in tests of different phylogenetic orders are given.
b Tests with human cells are excluded, since they represent tests of exposure rather than of genotoxicity.

correlation between carcinogenicity and mutagenicity can be expected; but a mixture of genetic and other events obscures correlation of carcinogenic and mutagenic potency. In fact, only a weak correlation has been observed between mutagenic potency (estimated on the basis of results from one short-term test measuring DNA damage) and carcinogenic potency (McCann *et al.*, 1988).

Further, since many chemicals must undergo biotransformation in order to exert their carcinogenic and mutagenic effects, discrepancies between carcinogenic activity and mutagenic activity, as well as between different assays for mutagenicity, are often a consequence of differences in metabolic capacity and pathways rather than differences at the target level. The standard procedure to compensate for metabolic differences in mutagenicity, by which a liver fraction is used to provide the necessary enzymes for bioactivation, is appropriate for a large number of indirectly acting mutagens and carcinogens; however, the activation of carcinogens and mutagens *in vivo* exhibits variations that are not covered by standard assay procedures.

Agents that act in the late stage of the carcinogenesis process, tumour promoters, are among those compounds that do not appear to bind to DNA and are not mutagenic in conventional assay system. Thus, they escape detection by most of the currently used short-term tests. Incomplete knowledge about the mechanisms of tumour promotion means that no validated short-term test has yet been developed to identify these compounds, and their activity can be detected only in two-stage bioassays. Less time is needed to carry out such tests than for long-term tests, because the end-points are usually benign tumours or neoplastic lesions and because the two carcinogenic factors administered ('initiator' and 'promoter') act synergistically to produce tumours. The model used most frequently is mouse skin, but rat liver and rat bladder systems are being used for screening and for studies of mechanisms of carcinogenesis (Peraino *et al.*, 1984; Ito *et al.*, 1989).

At least two in-vitro short-term tests for tumour promoters are currently being evaluated: inhibition of intercellular communication and enhancement of cell transformation. On the assumption that isolation of an 'initiated' cell from surrounding, normal cells is an important factor in tumour promotion, tumour-promoter-mediated inhibition of intercellular communication has attracted much attention (Trosko *et al.*, 1983; Yamasaki & Weinstein, 1985). Many known and suspected tumour-promoting agents inhibit such communication between Chinese hamster V79 cells, as measured by an assay of metabolic cooperation between cells (Trosko *et al.*, 1982). However, not all tumour-promoting agents can be detected by the metabolic cooperation assay, and further validation of the test is necessary.

In view of the limitations of current knowledge about mechanisms of carcinogenesis, caution should be used in interpreting the results of short-term tests. Although they suggest possible cancer hazards, the results cannot be used by themselves to conclude whether or not an agent is carcinogenic, nor can they be used to predict reliably the relative potencies of compounds as carcinogens in intact animals. Since, with the currently available tests, not all classes of agents that are active in the carcinogenesis process, such as hormones, can be detected, the results cannot be used as the sole criterion for setting priorities for carcinogenicity testing. Negative results from short-term tests cannot be considered as evidence to rule out carcinogenicity, nor does lack of demonstrable genetic activity attribute an epigenetic or any other property to an agent.

Given that certain chemicals with carcinogenic properties cannot be identified by any currently available short-term test or combination of tests, carcinogenicity bioassays in experimental animals remain the main basis for assessing the carcinogenicity of chemicals. Results obtained in laboratory animals thus provide important information for evaluating the potential carcinogenic risk to humans from exposures for which epidemiological data do not exist or before they can materialize, since experimental data may be used to prevent human exposure that would have allowed subsequent epidemiological studies.

Environmental determinants of cancer

A number of individual chemicals, groups of chemicals, mixtures, occupational exposures and industries, cultural habits, and physical and biological factors, have been associated with induction of cancers at various body sites. A list of these exposures is given in Table 11, and the evidence for their associations with cancer is discussed in Chapters 5–11.

For the most part, this list is based on deliberations of IARC working groups (IARC, 1987b, 1988a,b, 1989, 1990a,b), which evaluated all available data from studies on cancer in humans and in experimental animals, from studies of the chemistry, metabolism and kinetics of the exposure and from the results of short-term tests for genetic and related effects. They then made overall evaluations of the carcinogenicity of the exposures to humans. These overall evaluations result in categorization of an exposure into one of four categories: *carcinogenic to humans, Group 1* (a causal relationship has been established between the exposure and human cancer); *probably carcinogenic to humans, Group 2A* (a positive association has been observed between the exposure and cancer for which a causal interpretation is credible, but chance, bias or confounding could not be ruled out with reasonable confidence; together with sufficient evidence of carcinogenicity in animals); *possibly carcinogenic to humans, Group 2B* (sufficient evidence of carcinogenicity in animals, but no adequate data on cancer in exposed humans); *probably not carcinogenic to humans, Group 4*, or *not classifiable as to its carcinogenicity to humans, Group 3*. Biological and other factors not yet evaluated for carcinogenicity in the *IARC Monographs* series are also listed in the table. The table first lists exposures classified in groups 1 and 2A, i.e., those considered by working groups to be either carcinogenic or probably carcinogenic to humans; a list of chemicals classified in group 2B, possibly carcinogenic to humans, is given at the end. Some of these may be reclassified as epidemiological data become available.

Table 11. Exposures that are carcinogenic, or probably or possibly carcinogenic, to humans[a]

Industrial processes entailing exposures that are carcinogenic to humans
Aluminium production
Auramine, manufacture of
Boot and shoe manufacture and repair
Coal gasification
Coke production
Furniture and cabinet making
Haematite mining, underground, with exposure to radon
Iron and steel founding
Isopropyl alcohol manufacture (strong-acid process)
Magenta, manufacture of
Painter, occupational exposure as a
Rubber industry

Chemicals and groups of chemicals that are carcinogenic to humans
Aflatoxins
4-Aminobiphenyl
Arsenic and arsenic compounds[b]
Asbestos
Benzene
Benzidine
Bis(chloromethyl)ether and chloromethyl methyl ether (technical-grade)
Chromium compounds, hexavalent[b]
Erionite
Mustard gas (sulfur mustard)
2-Naphthylamine
Nickel compounds[b]
Radon and its decay products
Talc containing asbestiform fibres
Vinyl chloride

Mixtures that are carcinogenic to humans
Alcoholic beverages
Betel quid with tobacco
Coal-tar pitches
Coal-tars
Mineral oils, untreated and mildly treated
Shale-oils
Soots
Tobacco products, smokeless
Tobacco smoke

Drugs that are carcinogenic to humans
Analgesic mixtures containing phenacetin
Azathioprine

N,N-Bis(2-chloroethyl)-2-naphthylamine (Chlornaphazine)
1,4-Butanediol dimethanesulfonate (Myleran)
Chlorambucil
1-(2-Chloroethyl)-3-(4-methylcyclohexyl)-1-nitrosourea (Methyl-CCNU)
Cyclophosphamide
Ciclosporin
Diethylstilboestrol
Melphalan
8-Methoxypsoralen (Methoxsalen) plus ultra-violet radiation
MOPP and other combined chemotherapy including alkylating agents
Oestrogen replacement therapy
Oestrogens, nonsteroidal[b]
Oestrogens, steroidal[b]
Oral contraceptives, combined[c]
Oral contraceptives, sequential
Thiotepa
Treosulphan

Biological and physical factors that are causally related to cancer in humans
Hepatitis B virus[d]
Human T-lymphotropic virus type 1[d]
Ionizing radiation[e]
Ultra-violet radiation[e]

Occupational exposure entailing exposures that are probably carcinogenic to humans
Petroleum refining

Chemicals and groups of chemicals that are probably carcinogenic to humans
Acrylonitrile
Benz[a]anthracene
Benzidine-based dyes
Benzo[a]pyrene
Beryllium and beryllium compounds
Cadmium and cadmium compounds
p-Chloro-o-toluidine and its strong-acid salts
Dibenz[a,h]anthracene
Diethyl sulfate
Dimethylcarbamoyl chloride
Dimethyl sulfate
Epichlorohydrin
Ethylene dibromide
Ethylene oxide
N-Ethyl-N-nitrosourea

Table 11 (contd)

Formaldehyde
4,4'-Methylene bis(2-chloroaniline) (MOCA)
N-Methyl-N'-nitro-N-nitrosoguanidine (MNNG)
N-Methyl-N'-nitrosourea
N-Nitrosodiethylamine
N-Nitrosodimethylamine
Propylene oxide
Silica, crystalline
Styrene oxide
Tris(2,3-dibromopropyl)phosphate
Vinyl bromide

Mixtures that are probably carcinogenic to humans

Creosotes
Diesel engine exhaust
Polychlorinated biphenyls

Drugs that are probably carcinogenic to humans

Adriamycin
Androgenic (anabolic) steroids
Azacitidine
Bischloroethyl nitrosourea (BCNU)
Chloramphenicol
1-(2-Chloroethyl)-3-cyclohexyl-1-nitrosourea (CCNU)
Chlorozotocin
Cisplatin
5-Methoxypsoralen
Nitrogen mustard
Phenacetin
Procarbazine hydrochloride
Tris(1-aziridinyl)phosphine sulfide (Thiotepa)

Biological factors for which an association with the occurrence of human cancer has been observed but a causal relationship has not been established

Clonorchis sinensis
Epstein-Barr virus
Herpes simplex virus type 2
Human immunodeficiency viruses
Human papilloma virus
Opisthorchis viverrini
Schistosoma haematobium

Exposures that are possibly carcinogenic to humans

Agents and groups of agents:

A-α-C (2-Amino-9H-pyrido[2,3-b]indole)
Acetaldehyde
Acetamide

Acrylamide
AF-2 [2-(2-Furyl)-3-(5-nitro-2-furyl)-acrylamide]
para-Aminoazobenzene
ortho-Aminoazotoluene
2-Amino-5-(5-nitro-2-furyl)-1,3,4-thiadiazole
Amitrole
ortho-Anisidine
Antimony trioxide
Aramite®
Auramine (technical-grade)
Azaserine
Benzo[*b*]fluoranthene
Benzo[*j*]fluoranthene
Benzo[*k*]fluoranthene
Benzyl violet 4B
Bleomycins
Bracken fern
1,3-Butadiene
Butylated hydroxyanisole (BHA)
γ-Butyrolactone
Carbon-black extracts
Carbon tetrachloride
Ceramic fibres
Chloramphenicol
Chlordecone (Kepone)
Chlorendic acid
α-Chlorinated toluenes
Chloroform
Chlorophenols
Chlorophenoxy herbicides
4-Chloro-*ortho*-phenylenediamine
Citrus Red No. 2
para-Cresidine
Cycasin
Dacarbazine
Dantron
Daunomycin
DDT
N,N'-Diacetylbenzidine
2,4-Diaminoanisole
4,4'-Diaminodiphenyl ether
2,4-Diaminotoluene
Dibenz[*a,h*]acridine
Dibenz[*a,j*]acridine
7H-Dibenzo[*c,g*]carbazole
Dibenzo[*a,e*]pyrene
Dibenzo[*a,h*]pyrene
Dibenzo[*a,i*]pyrene
Dibenzo[*a,l*]pyrene

Table 11 (contd)

1,2-Dibromo-3-chloropropane
para-Dichlorobenzene
3,3'-Dichlorobenzidine
3,3'-Dichloro-4,4'-diaminodiphenyl ether
1,2-Dichloroethane
Dichloromethane
1,3-Dichloropropene
Diepoxybutane
Di(2-ethylhexyl)phthalate
1,2-Diethylhydrazine
Diglycidyl resorcinol ether
Dihydrosafrole
3,3'-Dimethoxybenzidine (*ortho*-Dianisidine)
para-Dimethylaminoazobenzene
trans-2-[(Dimethylamino)methylamino]-5-
  [2-(5-nitro-2-furyl)vinyl]-1,3,4-oxadiazole
3,3'-Dimethylbenzidine (*ortho*-Tolidine)
Dimethylformamide
1,1-Dimethylhydrazine
1,2-Dimethylhydrazine
1,6-Dinitropyrene
1,8-Dinitropyrene
1,4-Dioxane
Disperse Blue 1
Ethyl acrylate
Ethylene thiourea
Ethyl methanesulfonate
2-(2-Formylhydrazino)-4-(5-nitro-2-furyl)thia-
  zole
Glasswool
Glu-P-1 (2-Amino-6-methyldipyridol-[1,2-*a*:
  3',2'-*d*imidazole
Glu-P-2 (2-Aminodipyrido[1,2,a:3',2'-*d*]-
  imidazole
Glycidaldehyde
Hexachlorobenzene
Hexachlorocyclohexanes
Hexamethylphosphoramide
Hydrazine
Indeno[1,2,3-*cd*]pyrene
IQ (2-Amino-3-methylimidazo[4,5-*f*]-
  quinoline)
Iron-dextran complex
Lasiocarpine
Lead compounds, inorganic
MeA-α-C (2-Amino-3-methyl-9*H*-pyrido-
  [2,3-*b*]indole)
Medroxyprogesterone acetate
Merphalan
2-Methylaziridine

Methylazoxymethanol and its acetate
5-Methylchrysene
4,4'-Methylene bis(2-methylaniline)
4,4'-Methylenedianiline
Methyl methanesulfonate
2-Methyl-1-nitroanthraquinone (uncertain
  purity)
N-Methyl-*N*-nitrosourethane
Methylthiouracil
Metronidazole
Mirex
Mitomycin C
Monocrotaline
5-(Morpholinomethyl)-3-[(5-nitrofurfuryli-
  dene)amino]-2-oxazolidinone
Nafenopin
Niridazole
Nitrilotriacetic acid and its salts
5-Nitroacenaphthene
6-Nitrochrysene
Nitrofen (technical-grade)
2-Nitrofluorene
1-[(5-Nitrofurfurylidene)amino]-2-
  imidazolidinone
N-[4-(5-Nitro-2-furyl)-2-thiazolyl]acetamide
Nitrogen mustard *N*-oxide
2-Nitropropane
1-Nitropyrene
4-Nitropyrene
N-Nitrosodi-*n*-butylamine
N-Nitrosodiethanolamine
N-Nitrosodi-*n*-propylamine
3-(*N*-Nitrosomethylamino)propionitrile
4-(*N*-Nitrosomethylamino)-1-(3-pyridyl)-
  1-butanone (NNK)
N-Nitrosomethylethylamine
N-Nitrosomethylvinylamine
N-Nitrosomorpholine
N'-Nitrosonornicotine
N-Nitrosopiperidine
N-Nitrosopyrrolidine
N-Nitrososarcosine
Oil Orange SS
Panfuran S (containing dihydroxymethyl-
  furatrizine)
Phenazopyridine hydrochloride
Phenobarbital
Phenoxybenzamine hydrochloride
Phenyl glycidyl ether
Phenytoin

Table 11 (contd)

Ponceau MX	Trichlormethine
Ponceau 3R	Trp-P-1 (3-Amino-1,4-dimethyl-5*H*-pyrido-
Potassium bromate	[4,3-*b*]indole)
Progestins	Trp-P-2 (3-Amino-1-methyl-5*H*-pyrido-
1,3-Propane sultone	[4,3-*b*]indole)
β-Propiolactone	Trypan blue
Propylthiouracil	Uracil mustard
Rockwool	Urethane
Saccharin	Mixtures:
Safrole	Bitumens, extracts of steam-refined and
Slagwool	air-refined
Sodium *ortho*-phenylphenate	Carrageenan, degraded
Sterigmatocystin	Chlorinated paraffins of average carbon
Streptozotocin	chain length C_{12} and average degree of
Styrene	chlorination approximately 60%
Sulfallate	Diesel fuel, marine
2,3,7,8-Tetrachlorodibenzo-*para*-dioxin	Fuel oils, residual (heavy)
(TCDD)	Gasoline
Tetrachloroethylene	Gasoline engine exhaust
Thioacetamide	Polybrominated biphenyls
4,4'-Thiodianiline	Toxaphene (Polychlorinated camphenes)
Thiourea	Exposure circumstances:
Toluene diisocyanates	Carpentry and joinery
ortho-Toluidine	Textile manufacturing industry

[a] From IARC (1987b, 1988a,b, 1989, 1990a,b), unless otherwise specified

[b] The evaluation of carcinogenicity to humans applies to the group of chemicals as a whole and not necessarily to all individual chemicals within the group.

[c] There is also conclusive evidence that these agents protect against cancer of the ovary and endometrium.

[d] See Chapter 11

[e] See Chapter 8

References

Abramson, D.H., Ellsworth, R.M., Kitchin, D. & Tung, G. (1984) Second nonocular tumors in retinoblastoma survivors. Are they radiation induced? *Ophthalmology*, *91*, 1351-1355

Aird, I. & Bentall, H.H. (1953) A relationship between cancer of stomach and the ABO blood group. *Br. Med. J.*, *i*, 799-801

Aitio, A., Järvisalo, J., Riihimäki, V. & Hernberg, S. (1988) Biologic monitoring. In: Zenz, C., ed., *Occupational Medicine. Principles and Practical Applications*, 2nd ed., Chicago, Yearbook Medical Publishers, pp. 178-197

Allen, B.C., Crump, K.S. & Shipp, A.M. (1988) Correlation between carcinogenic potency of chemicals in animals and humans. *Risk Anal.*, *8*, 531-544

Ames, B.N., Magaw, R. & Gold, L.S. (1978) Ranking possible carcinogenic hazards. *Science*, *236*, 271-280

Anderson, D.E. (1974) Genetic study of breast cancer: identification of a high risk group. *Cancer*, *34*, 1090-1097

Autrup, H., Bradley, K.A., Shamsuddin, A.K.M., Wakhisi, J. & Wasunna, A. (1983) Detection of putative adduct with fluorescence characteristics identical to 2,3-dihydro-2-(7'-guanyl)-3-hydroxyaflatoxin B₁ in human urine collected in Murang'a District, Kenya. *Carcinogenesis*, *4*, 1193-1195

Ayesh, R., Idle, J.R., Ritchie, J.C., Chrothers, M.J. & Hetzel, M.R. (1984) Metabolic oxidation phenotypes as markers for susceptibility to lung cancer. *Nature*, *312*, 169-170

Barbacid, M. (1987) Ras genes. *Ann. Rev. Biochem.*, *56*, 779-827

Bartsch, H., Tomatis, L. & Malaveille, C. (1982) Mutagenicity and carcinogenicity of environmental chemicals. *Regul. Toxicol. Pharmacol.*, *2*, 94-105

Bartsch, H., Hemminki, K. & O'Neill, I.K., eds (1988) *Methods for Detecting DNA Damaging Agents in Humans: Applications in Cancer Epidemiology and Prevention* (IARC Scientific Publications No. 89), Lyon, IARC

Berenblum, I. & Shubik, P. (1949) An experimental study of the initiating stage of carcinogenesis and a re-examination of the somatic mutation theory of cancer. *Br. J. Cancer*, *3*, 109-118

Bodmer, W.F., Bailey, C.J., Bodmer, J., Bussey, H.J., Ellis, A., Gorman, P., Lucibello, F.C., Murday, V.A., Rider, S.H., Scambler, P., Sheer, D., Solomon, E. & Spurr, N.K. (1987) Localization of the gene for familial adenomatous polyposis on chromosome 5. *Nature*, *328*, 614-616

Bonney, G.E., Elston, R.C., Correa, P., Haenszel, W., Zavala, D.E., Zarama, G., Collazos, T. & Cuello, C. (1986) Genetic etiology of gastric carcinoma: I. Chronic atrophic gastritis. *Genet. Epidemiol.*, *3*, 213-224

Bos, J.L. (1989) *Ras* oncogenes in human cancer: a review: *Cancer Res.*, *49*, 4682-4689

Caporaso, N., Pickle, L.W., Bale, S., Ayesh, R., Hetzel, M. & Idle, J. (1989) The distribution of debrisoquine metabolic phenotypes and implications for the suggested association with lung cancer risk. *Genet. Epidemiol.*, *6*, 517-524

Cohen, A.J., Li, F.P., Berg, S., Marchetto, D.J., Tsai, S., Jacobs, S.C. & Brown, R.S. (1979) Hereditary renal-cell carcinoma associated with a chromosomal translocation. *New Engl. J. Med.*, *310*, 592-595

Dausset, J., Colombani, J. & Hors, J. (1982) Major histocompatibility complex and cancer, with special reference to human familial tumours (Hodgkin's disease and other malignancies). *Cancer Surv.*, *1*, 119-147

De Serres, F.J. & Ashby, J., eds (1981) *Evaluation of Short-term Tests for Carcinogens* (Progress in Mutation Research, Vol. 1), Amsterdam, Elsevier/North Holland

Draper, G.J., Sanders, B.M. & Kingston, J.E. (1986) Second primary neoplasms in patients with retinoblastoma. *Br. J. Cancer*, *53*, 661-671

Ennever, F.K. & Rosenkranz, H.S. (1987) Prediction of carcinogenic potency by short-term genotoxicity tests. *Mutagenesis*, *2*, 39-44

Enterline, P.E. & Marsh, G.M. (1982) Cancer among workers exposed to arsenic and other substances in a copper smelter. *Am. J. Epidemiol.*, *116*, 895-911

Enterline, P.E., Henderson, V.L. & Marsh, G.M. (1987) Exposure to arsenic and respiratory cancer. A reanalysis. *Am. J. Epidemiol.*, *125*, 929-938

Fisher, C. & Edmonds, C.J. (1980) Papillary carcinoma of the thyroid in two brothers after chest fluoroscopy in childhood. *Br. Med. J.*, *281*, 1600-1601

Foulds, L. (1969) *Neoplastic Development*, Vol. 1, London, Academic Press

Garner, R.C. (1985) Assessment of carcinogen exposure in man. *Carcinogenesis*, *6*, 1071-1078

Glass, A.G. & Fraumeni, J.F. (1970) Epidemiology of bone cancer in children. *J. Natl Cancer Inst.*, *44*, 187-199

de Groot, L. & Paloyan, E. (1973) Thyroid carcinoma and radiation. A genetic endemic. *J. Am. Med. Assoc.*, *225*, 487-491

Harnden, D.G., Maclean, N. & Langlands, A.O. (1971) Carcinoma of the breast and Klinefelter's syndrome. *J. Med. Genet.*, *8*, 460-461

Haseman, J.K. & Huff, J.E. (1987) Species correlation in long-term carcinogenicity studies. *Cancer Lett.*, *37*, 125-132

Hemminki, K. (1985) Nucleic acid adducts of chemical carcinogens and mutagens. *Arch. Toxicol.*, *52*, 249-285

Hill, A.B. (1965) The environment and disease: association or causation? *Proc. R. Soc. Med.*, *58*, 295-300

Hollstein, M., McCann, J., Angelosanto, F.A. & Nichols, W.W. (1979) Short-term tests for carcinogens and mutagens. *Mutat. Res.*, *65*, 133-226

Hope, D.G. & Mulvihill, J.J. (1981) Malignancy in neurofibromatosis. *Adv. Neurol.*, *29*, 33-55

IARC (1987a) *IARC Monographs on the Evaluation of Carcinogenic Risks to Humans*, Suppl. 6, *Genetic and Related Effects: An Updating of Selected IARC Monographs from Volumes 1 to 42*, Lyon

IARC (1987b) *IARC Monographs on the Evaluation of Carcinogenic Risks to Humans*, Suppl. 7, *Overall Evaluations of Carcinogenicity: An Updating of IARC Monographs, Volumes 1 to 42*, Lyon

IARC (1988a) *IARC Monographs on the Evaluation of Carcinogenic Risks to Humans*, Vol. 43, *Man-made Mineral Fibres and Radon*, Lyon

IARC (1988b) *IARC Monographs on the Evaluation of Carcinogenic Risks to Humans*, Vol. 44, *Alcohol Drinking*, Lyon

IARC (1989) *IARC Monographs on the Evaluation of Carcinogenic Risks to Humans*, Vol. 45, *Occupational Exposures in Petroleum Refining; Crude Oil and Major Petroleum Fuels*, Lyon

IARC (1990a) *IARC Monographs on the Evaluation of Carcinogenic Risks to Humans*, Vol. 46, *Diesel and Gasoline Engine Exhausts and Some Nitroarenes*, Lyon

IARC (1990b) *IARC Monographs on the Evaluation of Carcinogenic Risks to Humans*, Vol. 47, *Some Organic Solvents, Resin Monomers and Related Compounds, Pigments and Occupational Exposures in Paint Manufacture and Painting*, Lyon

IARC/IPCS (1982) Development and possible use of immunological techniques to detect individual exposures to carcinogens. *Cancer Res.*, 42, 5236-5239

International Atomic Energy Agency (1986) *Biological Dosimetry: Chromosomal Aberration Analysis for Dose Assessment* (Tech. Rep. Ser. No. 260), Vienna

Ito, N., Imaida, K., Hasegawa, R. & Tsuda, H. (1989) Rapid bioassay methods for carcinogens and modifiers of hepatocarcinogenesis. *C.R.C. Crit. Rev. Toxicol.*, 19, 385-415

Kaldor, J.M., Day, N.E. & Hemminki, K. (1988) Quantifying the carcinogenicity of antineoplastic drugs. *Eur. J. Cancer Clin. Oncol.*, 24, 703-711

Knudson, A.G., Jr (1986) Genetics of human cancer. *J. Cell Physiol. (Suppl.)*, 4, 7-11

Knudson, A., Strong, L.C. & Anderson, D.E. (1973) Heredity and cancer in man. *Prog. Med. Genet.*, 9, 113-158

Kraemer, K.H., Lee, M.M. & Scotto, J. (1987) Xeroderma pigmentosum. *Arch. Dermatol.*, 123, 241-250

Lee, M.W. & Stephens, R.L. (1987) Klinefelter's syndrome and extragonadal germ cell tumours. *Cancer*, 60, 1053-1057

Lu, S., Day, N., Degos, L., Lepage, V., Huang, P., Chan, S., Simons, M., MacKnight, B., Easton, D., Zeng, Y. & de-Thé, G. (1990) The genetic basis for carcinoma of the nasopharynx (NPC): evidence of linkage to the HLA locus *Nature*, (in press)

Mathew, C.G.P., Chin, K.S., Easton, D., Thorpe, K., Carter, C., Liou, G.I., Fong, S.L., Bridges, C.D.B., Haak, H., Nieuwenhuijszen Kruseman, A.C., Schifter, S., Hansen, H.H., Telenius, H., Telenius-Berg, M. & Ponder, B.A.J. (1987) A linked genetic marker for multiple endocrine neoplasia, type 2A on chromosome 10. *Nature*, 328, 527-528

McCann, J. & Ames, B.N. (1976) A simple method for detecting environmental carcinogens as mutagens. *Ann. N.Y. Acad. Sci.*, 271, 5-13

McCann, J., Choi, E., Yamasaki, E. & Ames, B.N. (1975) Detection of carcinogens as mutagens in the *Salmonella*/microsome test: assay of 300 chemicals. *Proc. Natl Acad. Sci. USA*, 72, 5135-5139

McCann, J., Gold, L.S., Horn, L., McGill, R., Graedel, T.E. & Kaldor, J. (1988) Statistical analysis of Salmonella test data and comparison to results of animal cancer tests. *Mutat. Res.*, 205, 183-195

Miller, R.W. (1968) Relation between cancer and congenital defects: an epidemiologic evaluation. *J. Natl Cancer Inst.*, 40, 1079-1085

Miller, R.W. (1970) Neoplasia and Down syndrome. *Ann. N.Y. Acad. Sci.*, 171, 637-644

Miller, R.W. (1977) Ethnic differences in cancer occurrence: genetic and environmental influences with particular reference to neuroblastoma. In: Mulvihill, J.J., Miller, R.W. & Fraumeni, J.F., eds, *Genetics and Human Cancer*, New York, Raven Press, pp. 1-14

Müller, R. & Rajewsky, M.F. (1981) Antibodies specific for DNA components structurally modified by chemical carcinogens. *J. Cancer Res. Clin. Oncol.*, 102, 99-113

NAS Executive Committee (1975) *Pest Control. An Assessment of Present and Alternative Technologies*, Vol. 1, Washington DC

Newman, B., Austin, M.A., Lee, M. & King, M.C. (1988) Inheritance of human breast cancer: evidence for autosomal dominant transmission in high-risk families. *Proc. Natl Acad. Sci. USA*, *85*, 3044-3048

Ohshima, H. & Bartsch, H. (1981) Quantitative estimation of endogenous nitrosation in humans by monitoring *N*-nitrosoproline excreted in the urine. *Cancer Res.*, *41*, 3658-3662

Ozaki, O., Ito, K., Kobayashi, K., Suzuki, A., Manabe, Y. & Hosado, Y. (1988) Familial occurrence of differentiated, nonmedullary thyroid carcinoma. *World J. Surg.*, *12*, 565-571

Peraino, C., Staffeldt, E.F., Carnes, B.A., Ledeman, V.A., Blomquist, J.A. & Vesselinovitch, S.D. (1984) Relationship of histochemically detectable altered heptocyte foci to hepatic tumorigenesis. In: Börzsönyi, M., Lapis, K., Day, N.E. & Yamasaki, H., eds, *Models, Mechanisms and Etiology of Tumour Promotion* (IARC Scientific Publications No. 56), Lyon, IARC, pp. 37-55

Perera, F., Jeffrey, A., Santella, R.M., Brenner, D., Mayer, J., Latriano, L., Smith, S., Young, T.-L., Tsai, W.Y., Hemminki, K. & Brandt-Rauf, P. (1990) Macromolecular adducts and related biomarkers in biomonitoring and epidemiology of complex exposures. In: Vainio, H., Sorsa, M. & McMichael, A.J., eds, *Complex Mixtures and Cancer Risk* (IARC Scientific Publications No. 104), Lyon, IARC (in press)

Peto, R. (1977) Epidemiology, multistage models, and short-term mutagenicity tests. In: Hiatt, H.H., Watson, J.D. & Winston, J.A., eds, *Origins of Human Cancer*, Book C, *Human Risk Assessment*, Cold Spring Harbor, NY, CSH Press, pp. 1403-1428

Purchase, H.G. (1980) Validation of tests for carcinogenicity. In: Montesano, R., Bartsch, H. & Tomatis, L., eds, *Molecular and Cellular Aspects of Carcinogen Screening Tests* (IARC Scientific Publications No. 27), Lyon, IARC, pp. 343-349

Randerath, K., Liehr, J.G., Gladek, A. & Randerath, E. (1989) Use of the ^{32}P-postlabelling assay to study transplacental carcinogens and transplacental carcinogenesis. In: Napalkov, N.P., Rice, J.M., Tomatis, L. & Yamasaki, H., eds, *Perinatal and Multigeneration Carcinogenesis* (IARC Scientific Publications No. 96), Lyon, IARC, pp. 189-205

Robison, L.L., Nesbit, M.E., Sather, H.N., Level, C., Shahidi, N., Kennedy, A. & Hammond, D. (1984) Down syndrome and acute leukemia in children: a 10 year retrospective survey from Children's Cancer Study Group. *J. Pediatr.*, *105*, 235-242

Scully, R.E. (1981) Neoplasia associated with anomalous sexual development and abnormal sex chromosomes. *Pediatr. Adolesc. Endocr.*, *8*, 203-217

Schroeder, T.M. & Kurth, R. (1971) Spontaneous chromosomal breakage and high incidence of leukemia in inherited disease. *Blood*, *37*, 96-112

Schwartz, A.G., King, M.C., Belle, S.H. & Satariano, W.A. (1985) Risk of breast cancer to relatives of young breast cancer patients. *J. Natl Cancer Inst.*, *75*, 665-668

Seeburg, P.H., Colby, W.W., Capon, D.J., Goeddel, D.V. & Levinson, A.D. (1984) Biological properties of human C-Ha-ras 1 genes mutated at codon 12. *Nature*, *312*, 71-75

Simpson, N.E., Kidd, K.K., Goodfellow, P.J., McDermid, H., Myers, S., Kidd, J.J., Jackson, C.E.M., Duncan, A.M.V., Farer, L.A., Brasch, K., Castiglione, C., Genel, M., Gertner, J., Greenberg, C.R., Gusella, J.F., Holden, J.J.A. & White, B.N. (1987) Assignment of multiple endocrine neoplasia type 2a to chromosome 10 by linkage. *Nature*, *328*, 528-530

Solomon, E., Voss, R., Hall, V., Bodmer, W.F., Jass, J.R., Jeffreys, A.J., Lucibello, F.C., Patel, I. & Rider, S.H. (1987) Chromosome 5 allele loss in human colorectal carcinomas. *Nature*, *328*, 616-619

Sorsa, M., Pyy, L., Salomaa, S., Nylund, L. & Yager, J.W. (1988) Biological and environmental monitoring of occupational exposure to cyclophosphamide in industry and hospitals. *Mutat. Res.*, *204*, 465-479

Strickland, P.Y. & Boyle, J.M. (1984) Immunoassay of carcinogen modified DNA. *Prog. Nucleic Acids Res.*, *31*, 1-58

Swift, M., Reitnauer, P.J. & Morrell, D. (1987) Breast and other cancers in families with ataxia-telangiectasia. *New Engl. J. Med.*, *316*, 1290-1294

Tabin, C.J., Bradley, S.M., Bargmann, C.I., Weinberg, R.A., Papageorge, A.G., Scolnick, E.M., Dhar, R., Lowy, D.R. & Chang, E.H. (1982) Mechanism of activation of a human oncogene. *Nature*, *300*, 143-149

Tomatis, L., Aitio, A., Wilbourn, J. & Shuker, L. (1989) Human carcinogens so far identified. *Jpn. J. Cancer Res.*, *80*, 795-807

Trosko, J.E., Yotti, L.P., Warren, S.T., Tsushimoto, G. & Chang, C.C. (1982) Inhibition of cell-cell communication by tumor promoters. In: Hecker, E., Fusenig, N.E., Kunz, W., Marks, F. & Thielmann, H.W., eds, *Cocarcinogenesis and Biological Effects of Tumour Promoters*, New York, Raven, pp. 565-585

Trosko, J.E., Chang, C.C. & Metcalf, A. (1983) Mechanisms of tumour promotion: potential role of intercellular communication. *Cancer Invest.*, *1*, 511-526

Turleau, C., de Grouchy, J., Tournade, M.F., Gagnadoux, M.F. & Junien, C. (1984) Del 11p/aniridia complex: report of three patients and a review of 37 observations from the literature. *Clin. Genet.*, *26*, 356-362

Vähäkangas, K., Newman, M.J., Shamsuddin, A., Sinopoli, N., Mann, D.L., Wright, W.E. & Harris, C.C. (1985) Detection of benzo[*a*]pyrene diol epoxide-DNA adducts in peripheral blood lymphocytes and antibodies to the adducts in sera from coke oven workers. *Proc. Am. Assoc. Cancer Res.*, *26*, 88

Varmus, H. & Bishop, J. (1986) Biochemical mechanisms of oncogene activity: proteins encoded by oncogenes. Introduction. *Cancer Surv.*, *5*, 153-158

Vogel, F. (1979) Genetics of retinoblastoma. *Human Genet.*, *52*, 1-54

Vogelstein, B., Fearon, E.R., Hamilton, S.R., Kern, S.E., Preisinger, A.C., Leppert, M., Nakamura, Y., White, R., Smits, A.M.M. & Bos, J.L. (1988) Genetic alterations during colorectal-tumour development. *New Engl. J. Med.*, *319*, 525-532

Von Fliedner, V.E., Mercia, H., Jeannet, M., Barras, C., Feldge, A., Imbach, P. & Wyss, M. (1983) Evidence for HLA-linked susceptibility factors in childhood leukemia. *Human Immunol.*, *8*, 183-193

Weston, A., Willey, J.C., Manchester, D.K., Wilson, V.L., Brooks, B.R., Choi, J.S., Poirier, M.C., Trivers, G.E., Newman, M.J., Mann, D.L. & Harris, C.C. (1988) Dosimeters of human exposure to carcinogens: polycyclic aromatic hydrocarbon-macromolecular adducts. In: Bartsch, H., Hemminki, K. & O'Neill, I.K., eds, *Methods for Detecting DNA Damaging Agents in Humans: Applications in Cancer Epidemiology and Prevention* (IARC Scientific Publications No. 89), Lyon, IARC, pp. 181-189

Wilbourn, J.D., Haroun, L., Heseltine, E., Kaldor, J., Partensky, C. & Vainio, H. (1986) Response of experimental animals to human carcinogens: an analysis based upon the IARC Monographs programme. *Carcinogenesis*, *6*, 1853-1863

Yamasaki, H. & Weinstein, I.B. (1985) Cellular and molecular mechanisms of tumour promotion and their implications for risk assessment. In: Vouk, V.B., Butler, G.C., Hoel, D.G. & Peakall, D.B., eds, *Methods for Estimating Risk of Chemical Injury: Human and Non-human Biota and Ecosystems*, New York, John Wiley, pp. 155-180

Zeiger, E. (1987) Carcinogenicity of mutagens. Predictive capability of the Salmonella mutagenesis assay for rodent carcinogenicity. *Cancer Res.*, *47*, 1287-1296

Chapter 5. Single environmental agents

Acrylonitrile

Acrylonitrile, used in the synthesis of synthetic fibres and resins, has been shown to increase the incidences of respiratory cancers and of cancers at other sites in some studies, but not in others. These conflicting results are offset, however, by the findings of experimental studies, which show that it induces tumours at a variety of sites in rats. Acrylonitrile is therefore probably carcinogenic to humans (IARC, 1979a, 1987a).

Aflatoxins

Aflatoxins are compounds produced by fungal strains that are distributed ubiquitously, except in colder climatic areas such as northern Europe and Canada. Virtually all foods are potentially susceptible to contamination with these compounds, and samples of nearly every major dietary staple have been found to contain some level of aflatoxin at one time or another. Although it has been known for over 25 years that aflatoxins are highly carcinogenic to experimental animals, producing liver tumours in mice, rats, fish, ducks, marmosets, tree shrews and monkeys, clear evidence for a causal association with cancer in humans has been difficult to obtain. The major problem is the difficulty in assessing past exposure to aflatoxin at the individual level. There is, however, suggestive evidence that aflatoxins are carcinogenic to humans. A positive correlation between estimated aflatoxin intake or level·of aflatoxin contamination of market food samples and cooked food and incidence of or mortality from hepatocellular cancer was observed in early studies in Uganda, Swaziland, Thailand and Kenya. Similar correlations have been reported from China, Mozambique, the Philippines and the USA, where there is considerable geographical variation in the occurrence of this cancer. A highly significant correlation was found between hepatocellular cancer incidence or mortality and aflatoxin intake in summary analyses of data obtained from studies conducted in different regions of Africa and Asia. The results of a case-control study in the Philippines support this conclusion (IARC, 1976a, 1987a). One major difficulty in interpreting previous studies had been potential confounding due to infection with hepatitis B virus, which is endemic in many areas where the relationship between aflatoxin intake and hepatocellular carcinoma has been examined; however, in three recent studies, both factors were taken into account, and the association was still evident (Bosch & Muñoz, 1989). Additional suggestive evidence for an association between exposure to aflatoxins and liver cancer comes from two studies of workers in grain processing in Sweden and Denmark, among whom a 2.5-fold increase in risk for cancers of the liver and biliary tract was reported (Alavanja et al., 1987; Olsen et al., 1988).

Alkene oxides

This group includes highly reactive compounds which are directly acting alkylating agents and are thus capable of reacting with genetic material without transformation in the body. Several such agents have been found to be carcinogenic in experimental animals. Epoxides, as these compounds are also known, are widely used industrially, and large numbers of people are exposed – for instance, to ethylene oxide and propylene oxide, which are produced in huge volumes. Another source of exposure is the use of these compounds as sterilizing agents for a wide variety of products, including medical supplies and food.

Ethylene oxide has been the object of a number of small studies, but, although these indicate that a causal relationship between exposure to ethylene oxide and leukaemia is possible, they suffer from various disadvantages, especially confounding exposures to other chemicals, which make their interpretation difficult (IARC, 1985a, 1987a). Although the epidemiological data on **epichlorohydrin** (IARC, 1976b, 1987a), **propylene oxide** (IARC, 1985b, 1987a) and **styrene oxide** (IARC, 1985c, 1987a) are inadequate, the experimental data indicate that these compounds are carcinogenic to animals. These findings, in conjunction with the known activity of all three chemicals as alkylating agents and their activity in a number of short-term tests for genetic and related activity, lead to the conclusion that the three compounds are, like ethylene oxide, probably carcinogenic to humans.

The experimental data that demonstrate the carcinogenicity of **diepoxybutane** (IARC, 1976c, 1987a), **diglycidyl resorcinol ether** (IARC, 1985d, 1987a; used as an epoxy resin) and **glycidaldehyde** (IARC, 1976d, 1987a; used in wool and leather preparation) are also compelling, and these compounds are considered to be possibly carcinogenic to humans.

Alkyl esters, lactones and sultones

This group, which includes many important chemical intermediates, has again been little studied epidemiologically, for the same reasons as mentioned above. They, too, are alkylating agents. Thus, despite the inadequacy of the studies that have been carried out in humans, the results of experimental tests indicate that **diethyl sulfate** (IARC, 1974a, 1987a) and **dimethyl sulfate** (IARC, 1974b, 1987a) are probably carcinogenic to humans. **Ethyl methane sulfonate** (IARC, 1974c, 1987d) and **methyl methane sulfonate** (IARC, 1974d, 1987d), which have been tested for use as male contraceptives, are clearly carcinogenic in experimental animals, and they, along with the related compounds **1,3-propane sultone** (IARC, 1974e, 1987a), **β-butyrolactone** (IARC, 1976e, 1987a) and **β-propiolactone** (IARC, 1974f, 1987a), must be considered possibly carcinogenic to humans.

Alkyl halides

Compounds in this group of somewhat heterogeneous chemistry are widely used. They are found in industry and agriculture, as, for example, fumigants, solvents, degreasing agents, cutting fluids, propellants and refrigerants, as raw materials for plastics and textiles and as anaesthetics.

The most notorious member of this group is **vinyl chloride** (IARC, 1979b, 1987a), used as the basis for polyvinyl chloride (PVC). This chemical is carcinogenic to humans, inducing a rare tumour of the liver, angiosarcoma. The first angiosarcoma of the liver in a polymerization worker was detected in 1961, but the relationship between the development of this tumour and exposure to vinyl chloride was described only in 1974. Subsequently, a large number of epidemiological studies have substantiated the causal association. Several studies also confirm that exposure to vinyl chloride causes other forms of cancer – hepatocellular carcinoma, brain tumours, lung tumours and malignancies of the lymphatic and haematopoietic system.

Vinyl bromide (IARC, 1986a, 1987a), which is closely related to vinyl chloride, has not been the subject of epidemiological studies, but the finding that it also induces a dose-related incidence of angiosarcoma of the liver in rats exposed by inhalation indicates that it is probably carcinogenic to humans.

Information on the cancer risk of people exposed to two further chemical intermediates of this class of compounds, **1,2-dichloroethane** (IARC, 1979c, 1987a) and **1,3-dichloropropene** (IARC, 1986b, 1987a), is lacking, but both are highly carcinogenic to experimental animals, indicating that they are possibly carcinogenic to humans as well.

This group of compounds also includes a number of well-known solvents – **carbon tetrachloride** (IARC, 1979d, 1987a), **dichloromethane** (IARC, 1986c, 1987a), **chloroform** (IARC, 1979e, 1987a; previously used as an anaesthetic) and **tetrachloroethylene** (IARC, 1979f; 1987a; used widely in dry-cleaning). The available epidemiological data on these four compounds are too sparse to draw conclusions; but, again, all four are carcinogenic in animals and must therefore be considered to be possibly carcinogenic to humans.

The group also comprises agents used as fumigants in foods destined for human consumption or in the soil in which they are grown. One, **ethylene dibromide** (IARC, 1977a, 1987a), is also used as a lead scavenger in gasoline. Several epidemiological studies have been carried out on people exposed to this compound, but the possibility of deriving meaningful conclusions from them is limited by several factors, including the mixed exposures of the subjects. Experiments in animals, however, have demonstrated its carcinogenicity, and tests carried out *in vitro* show that it induces DNA damage and chromosomal effects in human and other mammalian cells. This combination of evidence indicates that ethylene dibromide is probably carcinogenic to humans. For another fumigant, **1,2-dibromo-3-chloropropane** (IARC, 1979g, 1987a), the available epidemiological data are again uninformative, but experiments in animals exposed by inhalation, the route of human exposure, indicate a clear carcinogenic response.

The two halogenated ethers, **bis(chloromethyl)ether** (BCME; IARC, 1974g, 1987a) and **chloromethyl methyl ether** (CMME, **technical-grade**; IARC, 1974h, 1987a), which formerly occurred as chemical intermediates, are indisputably carcinogenic to humans. Numerous epidemiological studies and case reports have demonstrated that workers exposed to CMME and/or BCME have an increased risk for a specific form of lung cancer, with risks rising to ten fold or more in heavily exposed workers.

Dimethylcarbamoyl chloride (IARC, 1976f, 1987a), produced from phosgene (a chemical warfare agent), is used as an intermediate in the production of certain drugs, for the treatment of myasthenia gravis, and of pesticides. No epidemiological study has been carried out on this compound, but its clear carcinogenicity in experimental animals and its activity in a wide range of tests for genetic and related effects indicate that it is probably carcinogenic to humans.

Aromatic amines

The group of aromatic amines includes some very important industrial chemicals used as intermediates in the manufacture of dyes and pigments for textiles, paints, plastics, paper and hair dyes, in drugs, in pesticides, and as antioxidants in the preparation of rubber for the manufacture of tyres and cables.

Studies of bladder cancer among workers in the dyestuffs industry, and later among rubber workers, hold an important place in the history of occupationally related cancers. A series of case reports, the first of which appeared at the end of the last century, indicated that workers exposed to 'aniline' dyes were at increased risk for bladder cancer. This evidence led the International Labour Organization (International Labour Office, 1921) to declare certain aromatic amines as human carcinogens. The epidemiological study of Case *et al.* (1954), on hazards for workers in the chemical industry, established that **benzidine** (IARC, 1982a, 1987a) and **2-naphthylamine** (IARC, 1974i, 1987a) were carcinogenic to humans. In another study carried out at about the same time, it was shown that rubber workers had also had an increased risk for bladder cancer, attributed largely to exposure to aromatic amines. **4-Aminobiphenyl** (IARC, 1972a, 1987a) was widely used in the industry at that time, and it was shown shortly afterwards that it caused bladder cancer in humans. The first law banning the use of a carcinogen was passed in the UK in 1969 with respect to 4-aminobiphenyl. The epidemiological findings subsequently prompted discontinuation of production and prevented widespread use of 4-aminobiphenyl in other countries.

Epidemiological studies of cancer in relation to other specific aromatic amines have either been inadequate or nonexistent or have been confounded by concomitant exposures to other chemicals, and it has not been possible to establish clear causal relationships with individual exposures. Thus, **benzidine-based dyes** (IARC, 1987a) and **4,4′-methylenebis(2-chloroaniline)** (MOCA, a curing agent for plastics, which is structurally related to benzidine; IARC, 1974j, 1987a) are probably carcinogenic to humans, but the epidemiological data are inadequate. Both MOCA and the three benzidine-based dyes for which experimental data were available have been demonstrated to be carcinogenic to animals, producing tumours at various sites. Oral administration of MOCA to dogs induced tumours of the urinary bladder.

The **manufacture of auramine** (IARC, 1987a; which also involves exposure to other chemicals) is causally associated with an increased incidence of bladder cancer; however, it has been impossible to distinguish the causative agent.

Technical-grade auramine (IARC, 1972b, 1987a) nevertheless induces tumours at various sites in experimental animals and is thus considered to be possibly carcinogenic to humans. The **manufacture of magenta** (IARC, 1987a) was the process first associated with bladder cancer, in 1895, and Case's survey of workers in the chemical industry also showed an association between magenta production and an increased incidence of bladder cancer. A study in Italy corroborated this finding. The identity of the actual causative agent has, however, remained unknown, and experiments in animals with magenta and *para*-magenta revealed little evidence of a carcinogenic effect. Other suspects include the precursor compounds *ortho*-**toluidine** (IARC, 1982b, 1987a) and **4,4'-methylene bis(2-methylaniline)**, which are possibly carcinogenic to humans, and *ortho*-nitrotoluene.

3,3'-Dichlorobenzidine (IARC, 1982c, 1987a) and **3,3'-dimethoxybenzidine** (*ortho*-dianisidine; IARC, 1974k, 1987a) are also possibly carcinogenic to humans, although no adequate epidemiological study is available. These compounds have been made in the same factories as benzidine, however, and may therefore have contributed to the increased risk for bladder cancer associated with exposure to benzidine. In addition, tests in a wide variety of animal species have shown the carcinogenicity of these two compounds beyond doubt; both produce tumours of the urinary bladder in various species as well as tumours at many other sites.

For a number of other aromatic amines (see Table 11), no epidemiological study is available; however, experimental studies have again clearly demonstrated their carcinogenicity, and they are thus considered possibly to be carcinogenic to humans.

Benzene

Benzene (IARC, 1982d, 1987a), which is carcinogenic to humans, occurs as a natural constituent of crude petroleum oil and is produced in large quantities by a synthetic process. It was used for many years as a solvent, and this use continues in many countries. Elsewhere, it is now used mainly as a chemical intermediate, but it also occurs in gasoline fumes and as an emission from the burning of fossil fuels. Numerous case reports first demonstrated a relationship between exposure to benzene and the occurrence of various types of leukaemia. These reports were recently corroborated by the results of four epidemiological studies on workers exposed to benzene in three countries, in which levels of exposure to benzene were measured. Three independent studies have demonstrated an increased incidence of acute nonlymphocytic leukaemia in such workers, and one showed an increased risk for myelogenous leukaemia in refinery workers exposed to benzene. In a Chinese cohort study of more than 28 000 workers exposed to benzene, a six-fold increase in risk for leukaemia was seen. Mortality was especially high for workers engaged in organic synthesis, painting and rubber production.

Fibres and crystals

Asbestos (IARC, 1977b, 1987a), a naturally occurring rock, is one of the best known causes of human cancer; the carcinogenic hazard associated with the inhalation of asbestos dust has been recognized since at least the 1950s. Occupational exposure to most forms of asbestos results in an increased risk for lung cancer, and mesothelioma. Mesothelioma, a rare tumour derived from the cells lining the peritoneum, pericardium or pleura, occurs at a high rate in workers exposed to asbestos, such as shipyard workers, construction workers and asbestos miners. Several studies have also shown increased risks for cancer of the larynx; some indicate a risk for cancer of the gastrointestinal tract.

It has not been possible to establish a threshold dose below which no pathogenic effect will be seen. No clear excess of cancer has been associated with the presence of asbestos fibres in drinking-water (see also p. 233), but mesotheliomas have been observed in individuals living in the neighbourhood of asbestos factories and mines and in people living with asbestos workers.

Studies of talc miners and millers have also shown an increased risk for lung cancer, but only in those exposed to **talc containing asbestiform fibres** (IARC, 1987a,b). Mesotheliomas have been reported in these workers.

Fibre size is a crucial factor in determining the carcinogenicity of asbestos, and this led to the hypothesis that other fibres of similar size to asbestos could also induce tumours. Evidence for the application of this hypothesis came initially from experimental studies, but it was confirmed for humans by a series of studies of villagers in Turkey exposed to **erionite** (IARC, 1987a,c), a zeolite mineral from which many houses in that areas are built. The studies demonstrated very high mortality from malignant mesothelioma, mainly of the pleura, in three Turkish villages where there was erionite contamination and where exposure had occurred ever since birth. In corroboration of this finding, high incidences of mesotheliomas were induced in experimental animals exposed to erionite by inhalation and by intrapleural and intraperitoneal administration.

Since the demonstration that asbestos fibres are carcinogenic to humans, a search has been undertaken for a 'safe' mineral fibre that could be used to replace asbestos in the many applications in which it has been found to be invaluable. The so-called 'man-made mineral fibres' (IARC, 1987a, 1988) would seem to be a suitable group substitute, since it should be feasible to regulate the dimensions of the fibres to specific sizes, different from those which are hazardous. However, **glass-wool, rockwool** and **slagwool** and **ceramic fibres**, which are used as replacements for asbestos in some applications, are also possibly carcinogenic to humans.

The mineral dust **crystalline silica** (IARC, 1987a,d) is probably carcinogenic to humans. Exposure to silica occurs during mining and quarrying of coal and other minerals (metal and nonmetal), during stone cutting and construction, during production of glass and ceramics, in foundries and in other occupations such as sandblasting, polishing and grinding. Epidemiological studies of both exposed populations and of silicotics (persons diagnosed as having silicosis after occupational exposure to silica) indicate the carcinogenicity to the lung of a working environment contaminated with crystalline silica, particularly in combination with other exposures. There is not yet enough evidence to establish the association as causal, however, because, in most of the industries studied, except the granite and stone industry, the effect of silica cannot be separated from those of other carcinogenic exposures, such as tobacco smoking.

Fluorides used in drinking-water

A larger number of ecological epidemiological studies have been performed to compare cancer incidence or mortality in groups of people who consume water with high and low natural concentrations of fluoride, and in people using artificially fluoridated and nonfluoridated water; other studies have followed time trends of different cancers before and after the fluoridation of drinking-water. These studies, which cover the range of doses of fluoride in drinking-water to which humans are exposed, are mutually consistent in that their results do not show a positive association between exposure to fluoride and overall cancer rates or rates of different cancers (IARC, 1982e, 1987a).

Formaldehyde

Exposure to formaldehyde is widespread, resulting mainly from its employment in the production of plastics and resins, including urea-formaldehyde resins used as adhesives in the manufacture of particle-board and plywood, and in cosmetic and laboratory products. A number of epidemiological studies, using different designs, have been completed on persons in a variety of occupations with exposure to formaldehyde. Although excess occurrence of cancers at a number of sites has been reported, the evidence for the possible involvement of formaldehyde is strongest for cancers of the nose and of the nasopharynx, which could come into direct contact with formaldehyde through inhalation. Living in 'mobile homes', which contain particle-board, was reported to be a risk factor for nasopharyngeal cancer. Sinonasal cancer was associated with employment in jobs in which there is potential contact with formaldehyde in studies in Denmark and in the Netherlands. In the latter, the histological type of sinonasal cancer was found to be different from that associated with exposure to wood dust, which is an established risk factor for this cancer (see p. 143). No other cancer occurred in excess consistently across the various studies. Studies in rats have shown that exposure to formaldehyde by inhalation results in an increased incidence of tumours of the nasal cavity, at a very specific site. The two sets of evidence taken together indicate that formaldehyde is probably carcinogenic to humans (IARC, 1982f, 1987a).

Metals

Arsenic and arsenic compounds are carcinogenic to humans. A large number of case reports have appeared in the medical literature of skin and other cancers in people exposed to arsenic compounds medicinally, environmentally (in drinking-water) and occupationally, but it is primarily studies of occupational exposure to inorganic arsenic, especially in mining and copper smelting, that demonstrated an increased risk for cancer of the lung. In one study, an almost ten-fold increase in the incidence of lung cancer was found in smelter workers who were most heavily exposed to arsenic, and a relatively clear dose-response relationship was seen with cumulative exposure. This finding is corroborated by a number of other studies in different countries (IARC, 1980a, 1987a).

An increased incidence of lung cancer was also observed among workers in chromate-producing industries and among chromium platers and chromium alloy workers. However, a clear distinction between the relative carcinogenicity of chromium compounds of different oxidation states or solubilities was difficult to achieve. More recent studies have shed some light on this problem: the increased incidence of respiratory cancer has now been shown to occur predominantly among people who work with **hexavalent chromium compounds**. These include producers and users of chromate pigment, chrome platers, stainless-steel welders and foundry workers handling chromium–nickel alloy (IARC, 1987a, 1990).

Both of the latter two groups of workers are also exposed to **nickel compounds**. However, the studies that have most clearly demonstrated the association between exposure to nickel compounds and risk for cancer, particularly of the lung and nasal sinuses, concern workers in nickel refineries. The early studies in Wales (UK) and Norway were confirmed by later reports from Canada, the USA, New Caledonia, Slovakia and the USSR. It is still not possible to state with certainty which nickel compounds are human carcinogens. A large amount of evidence has accrued, however, that nickel refining carries a carcinogenic risk particularly to workers in processes that entail exposure to nickel (sub)sulfides, oxides or soluble nickel salts and mixed copper–nickel oxide (IARC, 1990).

The evidence for an association between **beryllium and beryllium compounds** and cancer in humans is confined to studies on two groups of workers at beryllium extraction, production and fabrication facilities in the USA, who were found to have a greater incidence of lung cancer than comparison populations, and to data from the US Beryllium Case Registry, in which subjects who had suffered from acute berylliosis (which usually follows heavy exposure to beryllium) were found to have an elevated risk for dying from lung cancer. This evidence is supported by the results of a large number of tests in experimental animals in which beryllium and many of its compounds produced lung tumours after exposure by inhalation or intratracheally (IARC, 1980b, 1987a).

Some early, small studies suggested that exposure to **cadmium** may be associated with increased incidences of respiratory and prostatic cancers. Cadmium salts cause both local tumours at the sites of their injection and testicular tumours in experimental animals, and recent studies showed that exposure by inhalation to cadmium chloride causes pulmonary tumours in rats (IARC, 1976g, 1987a). Recent epidemiological studies (Ades & Kazantzis, 1988; Kazantzis *et al.*, 1988) have not confirmed the early findings on prostatic cancer but have consistently shown a small excess of lung cancer in cadmium production workers and in nonferrous smelters exposed to cadmium.

Inorganic lead compounds also produce tumours at various sites when given to experimental animals. Small increases in risk for respiratory cancer were observed in smelter and battery plant workers, but these studies showed no clear trend with length or degree of exposure and could have been confounded by factors such as smoking and exposure to arsenic. Due to the inconsistency of the epidemiological studies, these compounds were evaluated as being possibly carcinogenic to humans (IARC, 1980c, 1987a).

Mustard gas

Mustard gas (sulfur mustard) was used in large quantities as a chemical warfare agent during the First World War; by 1919, US production had risen to approximately 18 000 kg per day, and, for some time after July 1917, large areas of soil in the region of battle lines in France were contaminated with mustard gas. It was used in Ethiopia in 1936, and production and stockpiling of this chemical have continued. It is used as a model compound in biological studies on alkylating agents. Clear evidence that mustard gas is carcinogenic to humans comes primarily from studies of workers who produced mustard gas in Japan and the UK during the Second World War, who experienced an increased risk for cancer of the respiratory tract (IARC, 1975, 1987a)

N-*Nitroso compounds*

N-Nitroso compounds occur ubiquitously in the human environment but cannot be studied for carcinogenicity in humans as individual compounds. We are exposed to *N*-nitroso compounds after their formation in the environment and subsequent absorption from food, water, air, and industrial and consumer products; after their formation within the body from precursors absorbed separately from food, water and air; due to the consumption or smoking of tobacco; and from naturally occurring compounds.

A causal relationship between exposure to *N*-nitroso compounds and carcinogenic risk to humans has yet to be established; however, many animal species and organs are susceptible to the carcinogenic action of the majority of such compounds, and it has been shown that alkylating metabolites are formed from them within the body. Because of these alkylating properties, several members of this group are used as chemotherapeutic agents in the treatment of cancer. For these compounds, therefore, it has been possible to carry out studies on their effects in humans. The evidence that **1-(2-chloroethyl)-3-(4-methylcyclohexyl)-1-nitrosourea** (methyl-CCNU; IARC, 1987a), **bischloroethyl nitrosourea** (BCNU; IARC, 1981a, 1987a) and **1-(2-chloroethyl)-3-cyclohexyl-1-nitrosourea** (CCNU; IARC, 1981b, 1987a) induce second primary cancers in treated patients is discussed below, in Chapter 7.

Even in the absence of epidemiological data, the evidence for the carcinogenicity in experimental systems of several other *N*-nitroso compounds is so compelling that it is reasonable to state that they are probably carcinogenic to humans (see Table 11). Certain other *N*-nitroso compounds are possibly carcinogenic to humans, although the experimental data are not extensive enough to make a more definitive statement. These include the tobacco-specific nitrosamines **4-(*N*-nitrosomethylamino)-1-(3-pyridyl)-1-butanone**, **N-nitrosomethylaminopropionitrile** and **N'-nitrosonornicotine** (IARC, 1985e, 1987a) and others (see Table 11).

Polyhalogenated aromatic and alicyclic compounds

Compounds of this group are very stable in the environment and are used widely in numerous industrial and agricultural applications. Because of these two factors, they are found in almost every corner of the globe, and particularly in the food chain. Further, at least two of them – polybrominated biphenyls and hexachlorobenzene – have been released accidentally into the environment in large quantities, resulting in the exposure of large numbers of the general population to high doses.

Polychlorinated biphenyls (PCBs), because of their physicochemical characteristics and high stability, have been used for a wide variety of industrial purposes. They have also been found in human and animal tissues and in the environment, from Greenland to Antarctica. In 1968, after accidental contamination of rice oil with PCBs, thousands of people in Japan were intoxicated and developed 'Yusho' disease. Occupational exposure to PCBs has been most marked among groups of workers in capacitor manufacturing plants. Epidemiological studies of these two types of population suggest an association between exposure to PCBs and an increased risk for cancer, especially of the liver and biliary tract, indicating that PCBs are probably carcinogenic to humans; however, the numbers of subjects were small, dose–response relationships could not be evaluated, and the role of compounds other than PCBs could not be evaluated. The results of experiments in animals corroborate the findings of the epidemiological studies: tumours of the liver were induced; in addition, PCBs enhanced the effects of other liver carcinogens (IARC, 1978, 1987a).

Polybrominated biphenyls, used as flame retardants in textiles and plastic products such as polyurethane foam, were the centre of an incident in the USA, in which animal feed was contaminated. The available epidemiological data are inadequate for an evaluation of carcinogenicity to humans to be made; however, the finding that these compounds induce malignant liver tumours in experimental animals, as do PCBs, indicates that they are possibly carcinogenic to humans (IARC, 1986d, 1987a).

Hexachlorobenzene, used as a fungicide on seed grain and occurring in industrial wastes from the manufacture of chlorinated compounds, was also the cause of a large accidental poisoning episode, in Turkey. In experimental studies in which hexachlorobenzene was administered orally to mice, rats and hamsters, tumours were induced in the liver and biliary system and at other sites; further, neoplastic liver nodules were induced in offspring of treated animals. These results would indicate that hexachlorobenzene should be considered to be possibly carcinogenic to humans (IARC, 1979h, 1987a).

A number of other compounds in this group are pesticides, also widely used and equally persistent in the environment. The best known is DDT. In spite of the enormously widespread, long-term use of this compound, adequate epidemiological studies on DDT have not been carried out. Thus, although increased risks for certain cancers were noted in some studies, the data are inadequate on which to base an evaluation of carcinogenicity to humans. Nevertheless, oral administration of DDT to mice and rats has been shown to induce tumours at a number of sites, including the liver, and DDT enhances the incidence of liver tumours induced by known carcinogens. The possibility of its carcinogenicity to humans must therefore be envisaged (IARC, 1974l, 1987a).

Hexachlorocyclohexanes, the γ isomer of which is the insecticide lindane, have also been studied inadequately epidemiologically, but the technical grade and the α isomer are carcinogenic to experimental animals, causing liver and lymphoreticular neoplasms (IARC, 1979i, 1987a). *para*-**Dichlorobenzene** is used mainly in the form of solid blocks as a space deodorant and as a moth repellant. No epidemiological study is available, although one report of a series of five cases has suggested an association between leukaemia and exposure to dichlorobenzenes. The compound is carcinogenic to experimental animals (IARC, 1982g, 1987a). **Chlordecone** (IARC, 1979j, 1987a), **mirex** (IARC, 1979k, 1987a) and **toxaphene** (IARC, 1979l, 1987a), all used as insecticides, have not been the object of epidemiological studies or case reports; all, however, are carcinogenic to experimental animals, producing tumours of the liver. All five compounds are thus possibly carcinogenic to humans.

Tris(2,3-dibromopropyl)phosphate

The evidence that tris(2,3-dibromopropyl)phosphate, 'Tris', is probably carcinogenic to humans derives from several sources. The only epidemiological study reported concerned workers with exposure to a wide range of other chemicals and cannot be used to judge the carcinogenicity of this compound. However, Tris, used mainly as a flame retardant in children's clothing, induced tumours at many sites in experimental animals and gave positive results in every short-term test to which it was submitted (IARC, 1979m, 1987a).

Polycyclic aromatic hydrocarbons

Largely as a result of the burning of wood and the more recent utilization of fossil fuels, polycyclic aromatic hydrocarbons are distributed widely in the human environment, albeit at low concentrations. In industrial situations and in the case of exposures to the mixtures described in the next section, the levels of these compounds may often be much higher. Because they almost always occur as mixtures, epidemiological studies have not been able to demonstrate the carcinogenicity to humans of individual compounds. Information from experiments in animals has therefore been essential in establishing their carcinogenicity.

Benzo[a]pyrene (IARC, 1983a, 1987a) is used as the indicator compound for the presence of polycyclic aromatic hydrocarbons in environmental material, since it has been found consistently in mixtures of such compounds. Benzo[a]pyrene and two others, **benz[a]anthracene** (IARC, 1983b, 1987a) and **dibenz[a,h]anthracene** (IARC, 1983c, 1987a), are considered to be probably carcinogenic to humans on the basis of experimental data obtained from both whole animals and in-vitro test systems. Experimental data indicate that other such compounds are possibly carcinogenic to humans (Table 11).

References

Ades, A.E. & Kazantzis, G. (1988) Lung cancer in a nonferrous smelter: the role of cadmium. *Br. J. Ind. Med.*, *45*, 435-442

Alavanja, M.C.R., Malker, H. & Hayes, R.B. (1987) Occupational cancer risk associated with the storage and bulk handling of agricultural foodstuff. *J. Toxicol. Environ. Health*, 22, 247-254

Bosch, F.X. & Muñoz, N. (1989) Epidemiology of hepatocellular carcinoma. In: Bannasch, P., Keppler, D. & Weber, G., eds, *Liver Cell Carcinoma* (Falk Symposium No. 51), Dordrecht, Kluwer Academic Publishers, pp. 3-14

Case, R.A.M., Hosker, M.E., McDonald, D.B. & Pearson, J.T. (1954) Tumours of the urinary bladder in workmen engaged in the manufacture and use of certain dyestuff intermediates in the British chemical industry. Part. I. The role of aniline, benzidine, alpha-naphthylamine and beta-naphthylamine. *Br. J. Ind. Med.*, *11*, 75-104

IARC (1972a) *IARC Monographs on the Evaluation of Carcinogenic Risk of Chemicals to Man*, Vol. 1, *Some Inorganic Substances, Chlorinated Hydrocarbons, Aromatic Amines, N-Nitroso Compounds and Natural Products*, Lyon, pp. 74-79

IARC (1972b) *IARC Monographs on the Evaluation of Carcinogenic Risk of Chemicals to Man*, Vol. 1, *Some Inorganic Substances, Chlorinated Hydrocarbons, Aromatic Amines, N-Nitroso Compounds and Natural Products*, Lyon, pp. 69-73

IARC (1974a) *IARC Monographs on the Evaluation of Carcinogenic Risk of Chemicals to Man*, Vol. 4, *Some Aromatic Amines, Hydrazine and Related Substances, N-Nitroso Compounds and Miscellaneous Alkylating Agents*, Lyon, pp. 277-281

IARC (1974b) *IARC Monographs on the Evaluation of Carcinogenic Risk of Chemicals to Man*, Vol. 4, *Some Aromatic Amines, Hydrazine and Related Substances, N-Nitroso Compounds and Miscellaneous Alkylating Agents*, Lyon, pp. 271-276

IARC (1974c) *IARC Monographs on the Evaluation of Carcinogenic Risk of Chemicals to Man*, Vol. 7, *Some Anti-thyroid and Related Substances, Nitrofurans and Industrial Chemicals*, Lyon, pp. 245-251

IARC (1974d) *IARC Monographs on the Evaluation of Carcinogenic Risk of Chemicals to Man*, Vol. 7, *Some Anti-thyroid and Related Substances, Nitrofurans and Industrial Chemicals*, Lyon, pp. 253-260

IARC (1974e) *IARC Monographs on the Evaluation of Carcinogenic Risk of Chemicals to Man*, Vol. 4, *Some Aromatic Amines, Hydrazine and Related Substances, N-Nitroso Compounds and Miscellaneous Alkylating Agents*, Lyon, pp. 253-258

IARC (1974f) *IARC Monographs on the Evaluation of Carcinogenic Risk of Chemicals to Man*, Vol. 4, *Some Aromatic Amines, Hydrazine and Related Substances, N-Nitroso Compounds and Miscellaneous Alkylating Agents*, Lyon, pp. 259-269

IARC (1974g) *IARC Monographs on the Evaluation of Carcinogenic Risk of Chemicals to Man*, Vol. 4, *Some Aromatic Amines, Hydrazine and Related Substances, N-Nitroso Compounds and Miscellaneous Alkylating Agents*, Lyon, pp. 231-238

IARC (1974h) *IARC Monographs on the Evaluation of Carcinogenic Risk of Chemicals to Man*, Vol. 4, *Some Aromatic Amines, Hydrazine and Related Substances, N-Nitroso Compounds and Miscellaneous Alkylating Agents*, Lyon, pp. 239-245

IARC (1974i) *IARC Monographs on the Evaluation of Carcinogenic Risk of Chemicals to Man*, Vol. 4, *Some Aromatic Amines, Hydrazine and Related Substances, N-Nitroso Compounds and Miscellaneous Alkylating Agents*, Lyon, pp. 97-111

IARC (1974j) *IARC Monographs on the Evaluation of Carcinogenic Risk of Chemicals to Man*, Vol. 4, *Some Aromatic Amines, Hydrazine and Related Substances, N-Nitroso Compounds and Miscellaneous Alkylating Agents*, Lyon, pp. 65-71

IARC (1974k) *IARC Monographs on the Evaluation of Carcinogenic Risk of Chemicals to Man*, Vol. 4, *Some Aromatic Amines, Hydrazine and Related Substances, N-Nitroso Compounds and Miscellaneous Alkylating Agents*, Lyon, pp. 41-47

IARC (1974l) *IARC Monographs on the Evaluation of Carcinogenic Risk of Chemicals to Man*, Vol. 5, *Some Organochlorine Pesticides*, Lyon, pp. 83-124

IARC (1975) *IARC Monographs on the Evaluation of Carcinogenic Risk of Chemicals to Man*, Vol. 9, *Some Aziridines, N-, S- and O-Mustards and Selenium*, Lyon, pp. 181-192

IARC (1976a) *IARC Monographs on the Evaluation of Carcinogenic Risk of Chemicals to Man*, Vol. 10, *Some Naturally Occurring Substances*, Lyon, pp. 51-72

IARC (1976b) *IARC Monographs on the Evaluation of Carcinogenic Risk of Chemicals to Man*, Vol. 11, *Cadmium, Nickel, Some Epoxides, Miscellaneous Industrial Chemicals and General Considerations on Volatile Anaesthetics*, Lyon, pp. 131-139

IARC (1976c) *IARC Monographs on the Evaluation of Carcinogenic Risk of Chemicals to Man*, Vol. 11, *Cadmium, Nickel, Some Epoxides, Miscellaneous Industrial Chemicals and General Considerations on Volatile Anaesthetics*, Lyon, pp. 115-123

IARC (1976d) *IARC Monographs on the Evaluation of Carcinogenic Risk of Chemicals to Man*, Vol. 11, *Cadmium, Nickel, Some Epoxides, Miscellaneous Industrial Chemicals and General Considerations on Volatile Anaesthetics*, Lyon, pp. 175-181

IARC (1976e) *IARC Monographs on the Evaluation of Carcinogenic Risk of Chemicals to Man*, Vol. 11, *Cadmium, Nickel, Some Epoxides, Miscellaneous Industrial Chemicals and General Considerations on Volatile Anaesthetics*, Lyon, pp. 225-229

IARC (1976f) *IARC Monographs on the Evaluation of Carcinogenic Risk of Chemicals to Man*, Vol. 12, *Some Carbamates, Thiocarbamates and Carbazides*, Lyon, pp. 77-84

IARC (1976g) *IARC Monographs on the Evaluation of Carcinogenic Risk of Chemicals to Man*, Vol. 11, *Cadmium, Nickel, Some Epoxides, Miscellaneous Industrial Chemicals and General Considerations on Volatile Anaesthetics*, Lyon, pp. 39-74

IARC (1977a) *IARC Monographs on the Evaluation of Carcinogenic Risk of Chemicals to Man*, Vol. 15, *Some Fumigants, the Herbicides 2,4-D and 2,4,5-T, Chlorinated Dibenzdioxins and Miscellaneous Industrial Chemicals*, Lyon, pp. 195-209

IARC (1977b) *IARC Monographs on the Evaluation of Carcinogenic Risk of Chemicals to Man*, Vol. 14, *Asbestos*, Lyon

IARC (1978) *IARC Monographs on the Evaluation of the Carcinogenic Risk of Chemicals to Humans*, Vol. 18, *Polychlorinated Biphenyls and Polybrominated Biphenyls*, Lyon, pp. 43-103

IARC (1979a) *IARC Monographs on the Evaluation of the Carcinogenic Risk of Chemicals to Humans*, Vol. 19, *Some Monomers, Plastics and Synthetic Elastomers, and Acrolein*, Lyon, pp. 73-113

IARC (1979b) *IARC Monographs on the Evaluation of the Carcinogenic Risk of Chemicals to Humans*, Vol. 19, *Some Monomers, Plastics and Synthetic Elastomers, and Acrolein*, Lyon, pp. 377-438

IARC (1979c) *IARC Monographs on the Evaluation of the Carcinogenic Risk of Chemicals to Humans*, Vol. 20, *Some Halogenated Hydrocarbons*, Lyon, pp. 429-448

IARC (1979d) *IARC Monographs on the Evaluation of the Carcinogenic Risk of Chemicals to Humans*, Vol. 20, *Some Halogenated Hydrocarbons*, Lyon, pp. 371-399

IARC (1979e) *IARC Monographs on the Evaluation of the Carcinogenic Risk of Chemicals to Humans*, Vol. 20, *Some Halogenated Hydrocarbons*, Lyon, pp. 401-427

IARC (1979f) *IARC Monographs on the Evaluation of the Carcinogenic Risk of Chemicals to Humans*, Vol. 20, *Some Halogenated Hydrocarbons*, Lyon, pp. 491-514

IARC (1979g) *IARC Monographs on the Evaluation of the Carcinogenic Risk of Chemicals to Humans*, Vol. 20, *Some Halogenated Hydrocarbons*, Lyon, pp. 83-96

IARC (1979h) *IARC Monographs on the Evaluation of the Carcinogenic Risk of Chemicals to Humans*, Vol. 20, *Some Halogenated Hydrocarbons*, Lyon, pp. 155-178

IARC (1979i) *IARC Monographs on the Evaluation of the Carcinogenic Risk of Chemicals to Humans*, Vol. 20, *Some Halogenated Hydrocarbons*, Lyon, pp. 195-239

IARC (1979j) *IARC Monographs on the Evaluation of the Carcinogenic Risk of Chemicals to Humans*, Vol. 20, *Some Halogenated Hydrocarbons*, Lyon, pp. 67-81

IARC (1979k) *IARC Monographs on the Evaluation of the Carcinogenic Risk of Chemicals to Humans*, Vol. 20, *Some Halogenated Hydrocarbons*, Lyon, pp. 283-301

IARC (1979l) *IARC Monographs on the Evaluation of the Carcinogenic Risk of Chemicals to Humans*, Vol. 20, *Some Halogenated Hydrocarbons*, Lyon, pp. 327-348

IARC (1979m) *IARC Monographs on the Evaluation of the Carcinogenic Risk of Chemicals to Humans*, Vol. 20, *Some Halogenated Hydrocarbons*, Lyon, pp. 575-588

IARC (1980a) *IARC Monographs on the Evaluation of the Carcinogenic Risk of Chemicals to Humans*, Vol. 23, *Some Metals and Metallic Compounds*, Lyon, pp. 39-141

IARC (1980b) *IARC Monographs on the Evaluation of the Carcinogenic Risk of Chemicals to Humans*, Vol. 23, *Some Metals and Metallic Compounds*, Lyon, pp. 143-204

IARC (1980c) *IARC Monographs on the Evaluation of the Carcinogenic Risk of Chemicals to Humans*, Vol. 23, *Some Metals and Metallic Compounds*, Lyon, pp. 40, 208, 209, 325-415

IARC (1981a) *IARC Monographs on the Evaluation of the Carcinogenic Risk of Chemicals to Humans*, Vol. 26, *Some Antineoplastic and Immunosuppressive Agents*, Lyon, pp. 79-95

IARC (1981b) *IARC Monographs on the Evaluation of the Carcinogenic Risk of Chemicals to Humans*, Vol. 26, *Some Antineoplastic and Immunosuppressive Agents*, Lyon, pp. 173-202

IARC (1982a) *IARC Monographs on the Evaluation of the Carcinogenic Risk of Chemicals to Humans*, Vol. 29, *Some Industrial Chemicals and Dyestuffs*, Lyon, pp. 149-183, 391-398

IARC (1982b) *IARC Monographs on the Evaluation of the Carcinogenic Risk of Chemicals to Humans*, Vol. 27, *Some Aromatic Amines, Anthraquinones and Nitroso Compounds, and Inorganic Fluorides Used in Drinking-water and Dental Preparations*, Lyon, pp. 155-175

IARC (1982c) *IARC Monographs on the Evaluation of the Carcinogenic Risk of Chemicals to Humans*, Vol. 29, *Some Industrial Chemicals and Dyestuffs*, Lyon, pp. 239-256

IARC (1982d) *IARC Monographs on the Evaluation of the Carcinogenic Risk of Chemicals to Humans*, Vol. 29, *Some Industrial Chemicals and Dyestuffs*, Lyon, pp. 93-148, 391-398

IARC (1982e) *IARC Monographs on the Evaluation of the Carcinogenic Risk of Chemicals to Humans*, Vol. 27, *Some Aromatic Amines, Anthraquinones and Nitroso Compounds, and Inorganic Fluorides Used in Drinking-water and Dental Preparations*, Lyon, pp. 237-303

IARC (1982f) *IARC Monographs on the Evaluation of the Carcinogenic Risk of Chemicals to Humans*, Vol. 29, *Some Industrial Chemicals and Dyestuffs*, Lyon, pp. 345-389

IARC (1982g) *IARC Monographs on the Evaluation of the Carcinogenic Risk of Chemicals to Humans*, Vol. 29, *Some Industrial Chemicals and Dyestuffs*, Lyon, pp. 215-238

IARC (1983a) *IARC Monographs on the Evaluation of the Carcinogenic Risk of Chemicals to Humans*, Vol. 32, *Polynuclear Aromatic Compounds, Part 1, Chemical, Environmental and Experimental Data*, Lyon, pp. 211-224

IARC (1983b) *IARC Monographs on the Evaluation of the Carcinogenic Risk of Chemicals to Humans*, Vol. 32, *Polynuclear Aromatic Compounds, Part 1, Chemical, Environmental and Experimental Data*, Lyon, pp. 135-145

IARC (1983c) *IARC Monographs on the Evaluation of the Carcinogenic Risk of Chemicals to Humans*, Vol. 32, *Polynuclear Aromatic Compounds, Part 1, Chemical, Environmental and Experimental Data*, Lyon, pp. 299-308

IARC (1985a) *IARC Monographs on the Evaluation of the Carcinogenic Risk of Chemicals to Humans*, Vol. 36, *Allyl Compounds, Aldehydes, Epoxides and Peroxides*, Lyon, pp. 189-226

IARC (1985b) *IARC Monographs on the Evaluation of the Carcinogenic Risk of Chemicals to Humans*, Vol. 36, *Allyl Compounds, Aldehydes, Epoxides and Peroxides*, Lyon, pp. 227-243

IARC (1985c) *IARC Monographs on the Evaluation of the Carcinogenic Risk of Chemicals to Humans*, Vol. 36, *Allyl Compounds, Aldehydes, Epoxides and Peroxides*, Lyon, pp. 245-263

IARC (1985d) *IARC Monographs on the Evaluation of the Carcinogenic Risk of Chemicals to Humans*, Vol. 36, *Allyl Compounds, Aldehydes, Epoxides and Peroxides*, Lyon, pp. 181-188

IARC (1985e) *IARC Monographs on the Evaluation of the Carcinogenic Risk of Chemicals to Humans*, Vol. 37, *Tobacco Habits Other than Smoking: Betel-quid and Areca-nut Chewing; and Some Related Nitrosamines*, Lyon, pp. 209-223, 241-261, 263-268

IARC (1986a) *IARC Monographs on the Evaluation of the Carcinogenic Risk of Chemicals to Humans*, Vol. 39, *Some Chemicals Used in Plastics and Elastomers*, Lyon, pp. 133-145

IARC (1986b) *IARC Monographs on the Evaluation of the Carcinogenic Risk of Chemicals to Humans*, Vol. 41, *Some Halogenated Hydrocarbons and Pesticide Exposures*, Lyon, pp. 113-130

IARC (1986c) *IARC Monographs on the Evaluation of the Carcinogenic Risk of Chemicals to Humans*, Vol. 41, *Some Halogenated Hydrocarbons and Pesticide Exposures*, Lyon, pp. 43-85

IARC (1986d) *IARC Monographs on the Evaluation of the Carcinogenic Risk of Chemicals to Humans*, Vol. 41, *Some Halogenated Hydrocarbons and Pesticide Exposures*, Lyon, pp. 261-292

IARC (1987a) *IARC Monographs on the Evaluation of Carcinogenic Risks to Humans*, Suppl. 7, *Overall Evaluations of Carcinogenicity: Updating of IARC Monographs Volumes 1-42*, Lyon

IARC (1987b) *IARC Monographs on the Evaluation of the Carcinogenic Risk of Chemicals to Humans*, Vol. 42, *Silica and Some Silicates*, Lyon, pp. 185-224

IARC (1987c) *IARC Monographs on the Evaluation of the Carcinogenic Risk of Chemicals to Humans*, Vol. 42, *Silica and Some Silicates*, Lyon, pp. 225-239

IARC (1987d) *IARC Monographs on the Evaluation of the Carcinogenic Risk of Chemicals to Humans*, Vol. 42, *Silica and Some Silicates*, Lyon, pp. 39-143

IARC (1988) *IARC Monographs on the Evaluation of Carcinogenic Risks to Humans*, Vol. 43, *Man-made Mineral Fibres and Radon*, Lyon, pp. 39-171

IARC (1990) *IARC Monographs on the Evaluation of Carcinogenic Risks to Humans*, Vol. 49, *Chromium, Nickel and Welding*, Lyon (in press)

International Labour Office (1921) *Cancer of the Bladder Among Workers in Aniline Factories* (Studies and Reports, Series F, No. 1), Geneva, pp. 2-26

Kazantzis, G., Lam, T.H. & Sullivan, K.R. (1988) Mortality of cadmium-exposed workers. A five-year update. *Scand. J. Work Environ. Health*, *14*, 220-223

Olsen, J.H., Dragsted, L. & Autrup, H. (1988) Cancer risk and occupational exposure to aflatoxins in Denmark. *Br. J. Cancer*, *58*, 392-396

Chapter 6. Complex exposures

Agents can be identified which are well-defined entities but are composed of a mixture of chemicals. Thus, although it is sometimes possible to attribute a carcinogenic risk to exposure to a substance, such as soot or, as is described later, tobacco smoke, the individual chemical or chemicals cannot be singled out.

In industrial settings, people are seldom exposed to a single chemical compound or entity, but rather to a large number of different chemical and physical agents. Technical chemical products are usually not chemically pure but may be crude mixtures of varying composition. When it is possible to show that people exposed during a certain process or industrial operation are at elevated risk for cancer, the causative agent may not be identifiable. In such cases, the risk for cancer may not be the same for workers in factories where apparently the same product is manufactured using similar, but not identical, processes. The risk for cancer is also likely to vary with modifications of technology and changes in exposure conditions over time, and evaluations of carcinogenic risk using epidemiological methods do not necessarily pertain to the situation in all industrial settings today. However, such evaluations are essential for a number of reasons, not least of which is that conditions in work places vary widely in different parts of the world, and processes long ago abandoned in industrialized countries may still be used in the less developed parts of the world.

Mixtures containing polycyclic aromatic hydrocarbons

One of the earliest observations of an association between an occupational hazard and human cancer was made more than two centuries ago by Percival Pott, who reported a high frequency of scrotal cancer in chimney sweeps. The coal soot responsible for these cancers was rich in polycyclic aromatic hydrocarbons, although this was not known until the carcinogenicity of dibenz[*a,h*]anthracene, the first such compound to be purified, was established in 1930. Benzo[*a*]pyrene was isolated from coal-tar in 1933.

Carcinogenicity to humans has now been established for **coal-tar pitches**, encountered in a number of industrial situations and by roofers (IARC, 1987); **coal-tars** (IARC, 1985a, 1987), used medicinally and also present in fossil fuel power plants and other industries; **untreated and mildly-treated mineral oils** (IARC, 1984a, 1987), used in the past in textile production and metal machining and by printing pressmen; **shale-oils** (IARC, 1985b, 1987), mined for years in Scotland, Estonia and the USA; and **soots** (IARC, 1985c, 1987), on which the early observations in chimney sweeps were made. All of these mixtures produce cancers of the skin, but many also increase the incidences of cancers at other sites, including the urinary and respiratory systems.

The evidence with regard to the carcinogenicity of other mixtures containing polycyclic aromatic hydrocarbons is less clear-cut, mainly because of a paucity of epidemiological data. Thus, **creosotes** are probably carcinogenic to humans (IARC, 1987), but no analytical epidemiological study on these compounds has been carried out. No epidemiological study of people exposed exclusively to **bitumens** (IARC, 1985d, 1987) has been carried out either, and the available studies on **carbon blacks** (IARC, 1984b, 1987) could not distinguish a clear association. However, experiments in animals with extracts of both bitumens and carbon blacks clearly showed a carcinogenic effect, indicating their possible carcinogenicity to humans.

Aluminium production

Working in the aluminum production industry has been associated notably with increased risks for lung cancer and bladder cancer. For both cancer sites, the risks increase with increasing exposures to pitch volatiles (tar), and these are considered to be the possible causative agent (IARC, 1984c, 1987).

Destructive distillation of coal

Case reports from the first half of the twentieth century suggested that tumours of the skin (including the scrotum), bladder and respiratory tract were associated with exposures in industries involving the destructive distillation of coal, such as **coal gasification** and **coke production** (IARC, 1984d, 1987). These early suggestions were corroborated by epidemiological studies based on death certificates. A series of analytical studies of the UK gas industry further confirmed the risk for tumours of the lung, bladder and scrotum in that industry. There appears to have been a relationship between elevated risk for tumours and work in retort houses used in early coal gasification processes. Substantial exposures to airborne polynuclear aromatic compounds, together with concomitant exposures to a variety of other contaminants, have been reported to have occurred in the retort houses. More recent epidemiological studies have confirmed the risks for cancers of the lung and kidney in coke production workers. Increasing risk for dying from lung cancer is strongly associated with duration and intensity of exposure to coke-oven fumes and to increasing exposure to coal-tar pitch volatiles. A possible causative agent of the lung cancer seen in coal gasification and coke production workers is thus coal-tar fume.

Iron and steel founding

Several studies from around the world have consistently shown an elevated risk for lung cancer associated with certain exposures in iron and steel founding, although the carcinogenic agents in the work environment that are responsible have not been identified. Polycyclic aromatic hydrocarbons, silica, metal fumes and formaldehyde, for example, are all found in such work places. Elevated risks for leukaemia and cancers of the digestive system and genitourinary system have also been reported from this industry (IARC, 1984e, 1987).

Engine exhausts

Exhausts from internal combustion engines are complex mixtures containing literally thousands of chemical compounds. Epidemiological studies of people exposed occupationally to exhausts, such as railroad workers, truck and bus drivers and dockers, have indicated increased risks for cancers of the lung and urinary bladder. Although in some of the studies, it was difficult to distinguish exposures to diesel and to gasoline engine exhausts, more evidence was available with regard to workers exposed to diesel exhaust. It has been concluded that **diesel engine exhausts** are probably carcinogenic to humans and **gasoline engine exhausts** possibly so (IARC, 1989a).

Petroleum refining

Working in petroleum refineries is probably carcinogenic to humans. The evidence indicates that such workers have increased risks for skin cancer and leukaemia; for cancers at all other sites, the evidence is inadequate or not available. The specific exposures within the industry that entail the elevated risk for cancer cannot, at this time, be determined, since information on specific jobs or exposures is available in only a few of the published epidemiological studies. Skin cancers have been reported in particular among wax pressmen, and leukaemia among boiler makers and pipe fitters and workers exposed to benzene. A number of specific refinery streams were found to be carcinogenic to experimental animals (IARC, 1989b).

Boot and shoe manufacture and repair

Employment in this trade entails exposures that are carcinogenic to humans. Risks for nasal adenocarcinoma ten times greater than expected have been reported from studies in England and in Italy, and there is also evidence for an increased risk for other types of nasal cancer. The highest risks have been found among people working in the dustiest operations and with heavy exposure to leather dust, suggesting that exposure to leather plays a role in the association. Early surveys of death certificates showed an increased risk for bladder cancer among shoemakers and repairers; subsequent studies provided evidence of an increased risk associated with employment in the leather industry, although it was not possible to determine whether this risk was related to boot and shoemakers in particular or also to other occupational subgroups. More recent studies have also indicated increased risks for bladder cancer among boot and shoemakers and repairers. The occurrence of leukaemia among shoemakers after exposure to benzene is well documented (IARC, 1981a, 1987).

Furniture and cabinet making

Nasal adenocarcinomas are caused by exposures in the furniture- and cabinet-making industry. This finding stems from early observations of men working in the furniture industry in Buckinghamshire, UK; a number of epidemiological studies have confirmed the excess risk, which occurs mainly among people exposed to wood dust. Since woodworking machinists (who saw timber) and cabinet- and chairmakers (who shape, finish, sand and assemble furniture) experience similar risks, it is unlikely that the cancers are due to a chemical agent applied to the wood at a particular stage of the process; and, more probably, they are due to a substance in wood itself. Although nasal adenocarcinoma predominates, increased risks for other nasal cancers have also been suggested (IARC, 1981b, 1987).

Manufacture of isopropyl alcohol

Isopropyl alcohol is used as a chemical intermediate in the production of acetone and is used itself as a solvent. It is manufactured by a reaction of sulfuric acid with propylene gas from refinery exhausts. An older process in which this reaction was a lengthy procedure (the 'strong-acid' process) has been replaced in most western countries by a shorter reaction. The manufacture of isopropyl alcohol by the strong-acid process is causally associated with cancer in humans: an increased incidence of cancer of the paranasal sinuses has been observed among workers in factories where this process is undertaken, and there may have been an elevated risk for laryngeal cancer. The carcinogenic agent in this process that is responsible has not been identified, but diisopropyl sulfate, a process intermediate, and isopropyl oils, formed as by-products, have been suggested as candidates (IARC, 1987).

Mining

In the sixteenth century, Agricola described unusually high mortality from respiratory diseases in the region of the Erz mountains in eastern Europe where metal ores were mined. In 1879, Harting and Hesse reported on the lung cancer hazard of miners in Schneeberg; their report provided clinical and autopsy descriptions of intrathoracic neoplasms in miners, which they classified as lymphosarcoma, but which may have been small-cell carcinomas of the lung. In the present century, many reports have been published about increased frequencies of lung cancer among miners. The best documented is the increased risk among uranium miners. Increased risks have also been reported for miners of iron, fluorspar, asbestos, niobium, tin and unspecified metals. It is evident in some cases that the exposure that is causing cancer is radon and its decay products (IARC, 1988), but miners are also exposed to several other agents that cause cancer, such as silica, asbestos and other mineral fibres, nickel compounds, chromium compounds, arsenic compounds and diesel engine exhausts.

Painting

Painters are potentially exposed to a large variety of chemicals and complex mixtures which occur in their working environment, the type depending on the specific trade, time and place. Approximately 200 000 workers worldwide are employed in paint manufacture; the total number of professional painters is probably several million. Painters may be exposed to hydrocarbon and chlorinated solvents, polyesters, phenol–formaldehyde and polyurethane resins, various metals, and asbestos; thousands of chemical compounds are used in paint products. Benzene, a known leukaemogenic agent (see above), was widely used before it was banned in most industrialized countries in the 1960s. Chromium compounds are used commonly as paint pigments. Asbestos has been used as a filter and may occur in spackling and taping compounds. Exposure to silica may occur during the preparation of surfaces. A large number of studies based on national statistics, cohort studies and case–control studies have consistently shown an excess risk for lung cancer of approximately 40% among painters. The data on smoking habits in this occupational group indicate that an excess risk for lung cancer of this magnitude cannot be explained by smoking alone. Risks for cancers of the oesophagus, stomach and bladder were increased in many of the studies, but the excesses were generally smaller and more variable than those for lung cancer. An IARC working group concluded that occupational exposure as a painter is carcinogenic. The group could not specify the agents responsible for the carcinogenic effect; neither could the type of painting exposure in which the risk is greatest be distinguished (IARC, 1990a).

Rubber industry

Employment in the rubber industry entails exposures that are carcinogenic to humans. Although not necessarily all of the etiological factors can be specified, because of the variability and multiplicity of possible exposures within the industry, some have been identified. Workers employed in the industry before 1950 have a high risk for bladder cancer that is probably associated with exposure to aromatic amines. Leukaemias have been associated with exposure to solvents and with employment in back processing, tyre curing, synthetic rubber production and vulcanization. A high risk for lymphoma has been noted among workers exposed to solvents, for example in footwear departments and tyre plants. Other cancers have been reported as occurring in excess in workers in various production areas and departments, but the findings in different studies have not been consistent (IARC, 1982, 1987).

Textile manufacture

The textile manufacturing industry employs over ten million workers worldwide. Working in this industry entails potential exposure to a large number of chemicals, including dyes, solvents, oils, formaldehyde, resins, fumigants and flame retardants, and organic dusts. Some of these compounds are known or suspected carcinogens and, consequently, employment in the textile industry might carry a carcinogenic risk. Several epidemiological investigations of cancer risk among textile workers have shown an increased risk for cancers of the nasal cavity. In some studies, workers exposed during dusty operations appeared to be particularly at risk. Several studies have also shown moderately elevated risks for cancer of the bladder, especially in connection with the use of dyes; weavers also seemed to be at elevated risk. An IARC working group concluded that employment in the textile manufacturing industry entails exposures that are possibly carcinogenic (IARC, 1990b).

Welding

Although the number of welders varies from country to country, it has been estimated that 0.2–2% of the working population is involved in welding activities. Welding entails potential exposure to dusts, such as silica and asbestos; gases, such as nitrogen and other oxides, carbon monoxide and carbon dioxide; and metals, such as iron, chromium, nickel, manganese and aluminium. Welders may also be exposed to other chemical compounds present on the metal being welded, such as solvents from paints. The known and suspected carcinogens to which welders may be exposed include asbestos, arsenic, chromium, nickel, benzo[a]pyrene, beryllium, lead, silica, cadmium and trichloroethylene. The most consisting finding in epidemiological investigations is a 30–50% increased risk for lung cancer, although in some studies risks for other cancers, such as of the nose, larynx and kidney, have been observed. The increased risk could not be attributed with certainty to exposure to carcinogenic metals, like chromium and nickel, nor to exposure to asbestos, which occurs frequently during welding in shipyards, nor to exposure to other compounds (IARC, 1990c).

References

IARC (1981a) *IARC Monographs on the Evaluation of the Carcinogenic Risk of Chemicals to Humans*, Vol. 25, *Wood, Leather and Some Associated Industries*, Lyon, pp. 249-277

IARC (1981b) *IARC Monographs on the Evaluation of the Carcinogenic Risk of Chemicals to Humans*, Vol. 25, *Wood, Leather and Some Associated Industries*, Lyon, pp. 99-138

IARC (1982) *IARC Monographs on the Evaluation of the Carcinogenic Risk of Chemicals to Humans*, Vol. 28, *The Rubber Industry*, Lyon

IARC (1984a) *IARC Monographs on the Evaluation of the Carcinogenic Risk of Chemicals to Humans*, Vol. 33, *Polynuclear Aromatic Compounds, Part 2, Carbon Blacks, Mineral Oils and Some Nitroarenes*, Lyon, pp. 87-168

IARC (1984b) *IARC Monographs on the Evaluation of the Carcinogenic Risk of Chemicals to Humans*, Vol. 33, *Polynuclear Aromatic Compounds, Part 2, Carbon Blacks, Mineral Oils and Some Nitroarenes*, Lyon, pp. 35-85

IARC (1984c) *IARC Monographs on the Evaluation of the Carcinogenic Risk of Chemicals to Humans*, Vol. 34, *Polynuclear Aromatic Compounds, Part 3, Industrial Exposures in Aluminium Production, Coal Gasification, Coke Production, and Iron and Steel Founding*, Lyon, pp. 37-64

IARC (1984d) *IARC Monographs on the Evaluation of the Carcinogenic Risk of Chemicals to Humans*, Vol. 34, *Polynuclear Aromatic Compounds, Part 3, Industrial Exposures in Aluminium Production, Coal Gasification, Coke Production, and Iron and Steel Founding*, Lyon, pp. 65-99, 101-131

IARC (1984e) *IARC Monographs on the Evaluation of the Carcinogenic Risk of Chemicals to Humans*, Vol. 34, *Polynuclear Aromatic Compounds, Part 3, Industrial Exposures in Aluminium Production, Coal Gasification, Coke Production, and Iron and Steel Founding*, Lyon, pp. 133-190

IARC (1985a) *IARC Monographs on the Evaluation of the Carcinogenic Risk of Chemicals to Humans*, Vol. 35, *Polynuclear Aromatic Compounds, Part 4, Bitumens, Coal-tars and Derived Products, Shale-oils and Soots*, Lyon, pp. 83-159

IARC (1985b) *IARC Monographs on the Evaluation of the Carcinogenic Risk of Chemicals to Humans*, Vol. 35, *Polynuclear Aromatic Compounds, Part 4, Bitumens, Coal-tars and Derived Products, Shale-oils and Soots*, Lyon, pp. 161-217

IARC (1985c) *IARC Monographs on the Evaluation of the Carcinogenic Risk of Chemicals to Humans*, Vol. 35, *Polynuclear Aromatic Compounds, Part 4, Bitumens, Coal-tars and Derived Products, Shale-oils and Soots*, Lyon, pp. 219-241

IARC (1985d) *IARC Monographs on the Evaluation of the Carcinogenic Risk of Chemicals to Humans*, Vol. 35, *Polynuclear Aromatic Compounds, Part 4, Bitumens, Coal-tars and Derived Products, Shale-oils and Soots*, Lyon, pp. 39-81

IARC (1987) *IARC Monographs on the Evaluation of Carcinogenic Risks to Humans*, Suppl. 7, *Overall Evaluations of Carcinogenicity: An Updating of IARC Monographs Volumes 1-42*, Lyon

IARC (1988) *IARC Monographs on the Evaluation of Carcinogenic Risks to Humans*, Vol. 43, *Man-made Mineral Fibres and Radon*, Lyon, pp. 173-259

IARC (1989a) *IARC Monographs on the Evaluation of Carcinogenic Risks to Humans*, Vol. 46, *Diesel and Gasoline Engine Exhausts and Some Nitroarenes*, Lyon, pp. 41-185

IARC (1989b) *IARC Monographs on the Evaluation of Carcinogenic Risks to Humans*, Vol. 45, *Occupational Exposures in Petroleum Refining; Crude Oil and Major Petroleum Fuels*, Lyon, pp. 39-117

IARC (1990a) *IARC Monographs on the Evaluation of Carcinogenic Risks to Humans*, Vol. 47, Some Organic Solvents, Resin Monomers and Related Compounds, Pigments and Occupational Exposures in Paint Manufacture and Painting, Lyon (in press)

IARC (1990b) *IARC Monographs on the Evaluation of Carcinogenic Risks to Humans*, Vol. 48, Some Flame Retardants and Textile Chemicals, and Exposures in the Textile Manufacturing Industry, Lyon (in press)

IARC (1990c) *IARC Monographs on the Evaluation of Carcinogenic Risks to Humans*, Vol. 49, Chromium, Nickel and Welding, Lyon (in press)

Chapter 7. Drugs and exogenous sex hormones

Antineoplastic agents

One of the principal strategies in the chemotherapy of cancer has been the development of agents and of combinations of agents that kill tumour cells by interacting with their DNA. However, these agents are not specific to tumour cells, and their interaction with the DNA of normal cells may subsequently result in the development of second cancers, after the first cancer has been successfully treated. The very effectiveness of these drugs, whether used individually or as combinations such as MOPP (nitrogen mustard, procarbazine, prednisone and vincristine), has made the risk of developing a second cancer a problem of growing importance.

The use of a medication that is associated with an adverse effect must be considered in relation to its therapeutic efficacy. When they were introduced, cytotoxic agents were used mainly in patients with advanced neoplastic disease, who rarely survived without such therapy; thus, concern about later complications associated with use of these compounds was a minor consideration. However, successful treatment of advanced malignancy in some patients, the increasing proportion of patients given adjuvant chemotherapy and the use of some of these agents in the treatment of nonmalignant disease indicates a different approach to the assessment of risks and benefits.

The first experimental evidence that cytotoxic drugs used in the chemotherapy of cancer could themselves be carcinogenic was reported by Boyland and Horning (1949) and by Heston (1949, 1953). Since then, a number of commonly used cancer chemotherapeutic agents have been shown to be carcinogenic to both man and experimental animals (Table 12), causing mainly cancers of the haematopoietic and lymphatic systems.

Causal associations have been established between the subsequent appearance of leukaemia and treatment of breast cancer (with **chlorambucil** (IARC, 1981a, 1987), **cyclophosphamide** (IARC, 1981b, 1987) or **melphalan** (IARC, 1975a, 1987)), of cancer of the gastrointestinal tract (with 1-(2-chloroethyl)-3-(4-methylcyclohexyl)-1-nitrosourea (methyl-CCNU; IARC, 1987)), of Hodgkin's disease (with **MOPP and other combined chemotherapy including alkylating agents**; IARC, 1987), of lung cancer (with **1,4-butanediol dimethanesulfonate** (Myleran; IARC, 1974a, 1987) or cyclophosphamide, of multiple myeloma (with cyclophosphamide or melphalan), of non-Hodgkin's lymphoma (with cyclophosphamide) and of ovarian cancer (with chlorambucil, cyclophosphamide, melphalan or **treosulphan**; IARC, 1981c, 1987).

Not only leukaemias but also solid tumours are induced by some of the agents. Cyclophosphamide is toxic to the bladder mucosa, and many cases of bladder cancer have been reported following its administration for the treatment of various malignancies. Patients treated with Myleran for leukaemia have been found to develop carcinomas. Solid tumours, especially non-Hodgkin's lymphomas and lung cancer, but also sarcomas, melanoma, malignancies of the central nervous system and carcinomas of the thyroid and gastrointestinal system, have been reported after combined chemotherapy for Hodgkin's disease, although the results have not been consistent.

Table 12. Antineoplastic agents that have been evaluated by IARC working groups as carcinogenic (Group 1), probably carcinogenic (Group 2A) or possibly carcinogenic (Group 2B) to humans

Agent	First used clinically	Degree of evidence[a] Humans	Animals	Group	IARC Monograph Vol.	Page	Year
Adriamycin	1970s	I	S	2A	10	43	1976
Azacitidine	1970s	ND	S	2A	50		1990
Azaserine	1955	ND	S	2B	10	73	1976
N,N-Bis(2-chloroethyl)-2-naphthylamine (chlornaphazine)	1950s	S	L	1	4	119	1974
Bischloroethyl nitrosourea (BCNU)	1971	L	S	2A	26	79	1981
1,4-Butanediol dimethylsulphonate (Myleran)	1950s	S	L	1	4	247	1974
Chlorambucil	late 1950S	S	S	1	26	115	1981
1-(2-Chloroethyl-3-cyclohexyl-1-nitrosourea (CCNU)	late 1960s	I	S	2A	26	137	1981
1(2-Chloroethyl)-3-(4-methylcyclohexyl)-1-nitrosourea (Methyl-CCNU)	?	S	L	1	Suppl. 7	150	1987
Chlorozotocin	?	ND	S	2A	50		1990
Cisplatin	1970s	I	S	2A	26	151	1981
Cyclophosphamide	1960s	S	S	1	26	165	1981
Dacarbazine	1960s	I	S	2B	26	203	1981
Daunomycin	1965	ND	S	2B	10	145	1976
Melphalan	1950s	S	S	1	9	167	1975
Merphalan	1950s	ND	S	2B	9	167	1975
Mitomycin C	1959	ND	S	2B	10	171	1976
MOPP and other combined chemotherapy including alkylating agents	late 1960s	S	ND	1	26	311	1981
Nitrogen mustard	1950	L	S	2A	9	193	1975
Nitrogen mustard N-oxide	1950s	ND	S	2B	9	209	1975
Procarbazine hydrochloride	1960s	I	S	2A	26	311	1981
Streptozotocin	late 1960s	ND	S	2B	17	337	1978
Tris(1-aziridinyl) phosphine sulphate (Thiotepa)	1953	S	S	1	50		1990
Treosulphan	late 1960s	S	ND	1	26	341	1981
Trichlormethine	?	ND	S	2B	50		1990
Uracil mustard	1960s	I	S	2B	9	235	1975

[a] S, sufficient; L, limited; I, inadequate; ND, no data

Both leukaemia and solid tumours may also be induced in patients treated with these agents for nonmalignant disorders. N,N-**Bis(2-chloroethyl)-2-naphthyl-amine (chlornaphazine;** IARC, 1974b, 1987), used in some countries for the treatment of leukaemia and of Hodgkin's disease, is also used against polycythaemia vera. Its use has been limited, however, since the finding that in patients treated for the latter condition it gave rise to bladder cancer. Chlorambucil is used not only in the treatment of cancers of the breast and ovary, but also in juvenile arthritis, glomerulonephritis and polycythaemia vera. In several studies, it was shown that such patients had increased risks for developing a subsequent malignancy, and especially acute nonlymphocytic leukaemia. Another study (Kinlen, 1985) showed that they had an increased risk for developing non-Hodgkin's lymphoma. Cyclophosphamide can induce bladder cancer in patients treated for a variety of nonmalignant disorders. Squamous-cell carcinomas of the skin have been observed on skin surfaces not exposed to the sun after long-term application of **nitrogen mustard** (IARC, 1975b, 1987; the principal alkylating agent in leukaemogenic combination chemotherapy given for Hodgkin's disease) as a treatment for mycosis fungoides and psoriasis.

Radiotherapy is often used in conjunction with chemotherapy in the treatment of cancer. The two do not appear to have a synergistic effect in increasing the risk for leukaemia (Coleman *et al.*, 1988).

Other drugs

Epidemiological studies to determine the carcinogenicity to humans of several other chemically and therapeutically diverse pharmaceutical drugs have been hindered by a number of problems, including the fact that these preparations are often taken in conjunction with other drugs, apart from the usual problems of defining other exposures associated with diet and habits such as smoking and with occupation. One specific therapeutic treatment that has been shown to be causally associated with human cancer, apart from the antineoplastic agents, is **8-methoxypsoralen with ultra-violet A radiation** (IARC, 1987). The relationship was examined in several studies of patients treated with this combination for psoriasis or vitiligo, but the strongest evidence comes from a study of 1380 psoriatic patients: these persons had a risk for squamous-cell carcinoma of the skin which clearly increased with the dose of treatment they were given. The effect was found to be independent of other forms of therapy for their condition, such as ionizing radiation and topical application of coal-tar ointments.

It has also been possible to associate the use of **analgesic mixtures containing phenacetin** (IARC, 1987) with cancers of the urinary tract. Thus, there have been many case reports of renal pelvic and other urothelial tumours in patients who used large amounts of phenacetin-containing analgesics, and a number of case-control studies have corroborated these observations. In studies in which it was possible to distinguish groups of patients who had taken different doses, a dose-response relationship was seen. Since, in one study (but not in the others), use of analgesics that do not contain phenacetin appeared to increase the risk for cancer of the renal pelvis to the same extent as did use of those containing phenacetin, it is not possible to conclude that the carcinogenic effect was due only to phenacetin.

The immunosuppressive drug, **azathioprine**, which has been used widely to prevent rejection of transplanted organs, has been shown to induce non-Hodgkin's lymphoma, squamous-cell carcinoma of the skin and other tumours in treated patients. It is also used in the treatment of a variety of other diseases presumed to be related to the immune system, including rheumatoid arthritis and multiple sclerosis (IARC, 1981d, 1987). Another immunosuppressive agent, ciclosporin, also induces lymphoma in organ-transplant recipients (IARC, 1990).

There is sufficient evidence that several drugs cause cancer in experimental animals, although information on humans is lacking. These include pharmaceutical **coal-tar preparations** (IARC, 1985, 1987), used locally in a variety of skin disorders; **dantron**, a laxative (IARC, 1990); **griseofulvin**, an antifungal antibiotic (IARC, 1976, 1987); **5-methoxypsoralen** (IARC, 1986, 1987) and **8-methoxypsoralen** (IARC, 1980a, 1987), used in combination with long-wave ultra-violet radiation in the treatment of psoriasis; **methyl-** and **propylthiouracil** (IARC, 1974c), which, by their action on the synthesis of thyroid hormones, can be used to treat hyperthyroidism; **metronidazole** (IARC, 1977a, 1987), prescribed for amoebiasis, trichomoniasis and giardasis; **niridazole** (IARC, 1977b, 1987), an antischistosomal and anti-amoebic agent; **panfuran S** (IARC, 1980b, 1987), an antibacterial agent; **phenacetin** (IARC, 1980c, 1987), a widely used analgesic; **phenazopyridine** (IARC, 1980d, 1987), another analgesic, used primarily for pain associated with urinary disorders; **phenobarbital** (IARC, 1977c, 1987), a long acting sedative, hypnotic and anticonvulsant; **phenoxybenzamine** (IARC, 1980e, 1987), an adrenergic blocking agent used in the treatment of hypertension; and **phenytoin** (IARC, 1977d, 1987), an anticonvulsant and antiepileptic treatment.

Exogenous hormones

Steroid hormones are essential for the growth, differentiation and function of many tissues. It has been established by animal experimentation that modification of the hormonal environment, by surgical removal of endocrine glands, by pregnancy or by administration of steroids, can alter the 'spontaneous' occurrence of tumours or the occurrence of tumours induced by carcinogenic agents. Oestrogens and progestins are used in medical practice for a number of indications. These include contraception, the treatment of disorders of the menstrual cycle and endometrial tissue and of uterine bleeding, and as replacement therapy in patients with abnormal gonadal development and in women with menopausal symptoms. In obstetric practice, progestins have been used in the management of threatened abortion and to prevent premature labour.

Metastatic carcinoma of the prostate is treated with diethylstilboestrol and other oestrogenic compounds, and oestrogens are used to develop secondary female sex characteristics in transsexual males; androgens are used to suppress these characteristics in transsexual females. Androgens have also been used in the treatment of underdeveloped male gonads, various forms of anaemia, hypopituitary activity, chronic renal failure and menopausal symptoms, and in advanced mammary tumours in women. Sex hormones are also used in veterinary medicine and as supplements to foodstuffs to promote growth of animals destined for human consumption.

Tumours associated with therapeutic use of hormones occur most often in organs that are sensitive to the hormonal stimulus. It has been postulated, therefore, that the carcinogenic effect is related directly to the hormonal effect and is thus relatively independent of the chemical structure of the hormone. However, some of the synthetic oestrogenic hormones (diethylstilboestrol, dienoestrol, hexoestrol and chlorotrianisene) are not steroids, and their carcinogenic effect may be due to another action.

Several of the sex hormones that occur naturally in the body (**oestradiol 17β, oestrone, progesterone** and **testosterone**) and a number of synthetic steroid hormones (**ethinyloestradiol, mestranol, medroxyprogesterone acetate** and **norethisterone**) are carcinogenic to experimental animals (IARC, 1979a, 1987). In epidemiological studies, it has not usually been possible to study the effects of single hormones, since many are used in combination or several different treatments are used. Therefore, except for diethylstilboestrol, evaluations of carcinogenicity have been made in relation to the therapeutic goal of the treatment, i.e., for oestrogen replacement therapy, oral contraception (combined and sequential preparations) and androgenic (anabolic) steroid therapy.

Diethylstilboestrol is the only chemical carcinogen found to act in humans transplacentally. Despite the results of experimental studies and its doubtful therapeutic properties, it was used for about 20 years in pregnant women, usually as treatment for threatened abortion. Diethylstilboestrol induced vaginal and cervical carcinomas in the daughters of treated women ten to thirty years later, and possibly an increased risk for testicular cancer in their sons. In addition, the women themselves had an increased risk for developing breast cancer after treatment with diethylstilboestrol (IARC, 1979b, 1987).

Epidemiological studies have revealed a consistent, positive association between **oestrogen replacement therapy**, given to relieve symptoms of the climacteric, and the incidence of cancer of the endometrium. In several studies, the risk was found to be related to the total dose that the women had received, measured either as the duration of therapy or as the daily dose of oestrogen. Studies on the risk for developing breast cancer in women treated with oestrogen replacement therapy have given inconsistent results (IARC, 1987).

Use of **combined oral contraceptives** can cause both benign and malignant liver tumours, the risk increasing strongly the longer the preparations are used. Conversely, there is conclusive evidence that use of these agents protects against cancers of the ovary and endometrium. Several studies have indicated that women who used combined oral contraceptives early in their reproductive years have an increased risk for breast cancer, but this finding remains controversial. The situation with regard to cervical cancer is also unclear: although the risk appears to be increased in women who use combined oral contraceptives, it may well be that the association between use of oral contraceptives and sexual behaviour, and possibly a sexually transmitted infective agent, explains this increase in risk (IARC, 1987).

The finding that users of **sequential oral contraceptives** have a higher risk for developing endometrial cancer than non-users is in contrast to the finding for combined oral contraceptives, which appear to protect against this cancer. The risk increases with length of use, and was much higher in users of a preparation that contained a relatively large amount of a potent oestrogen, ethinyloestradiol, and only a weak progestin, dimethisterone (IARC, 1987).

The evidence that treatment with **anabolic steroids** can cause both benign and malignant liver tumours is quite strong, although no analytical epidemiological study has been carried out to test this situation, and the evidence comes entirely from case reports. A possible relationship with the development of prostatic cancer has been investigated, but at present no firm conclusion can be drawn in this respect (IARC, 1987).

References

Boyland, E. & Horning, E.S. (1949) The induction of tumours with nitrogen mustards. *Br. J. Cancer*, *3*, 118-123

Coleman, M., Easton, D.F., Horwich, A. & Peckham, M.J. (1988) Second malignancies and Hodgkin's disease - the Royal Marsden Hospital experience. *Radiother. Oncol.*, *11*, 229-238

Heston, W.E. (1949) Induction of pulmonary tumors in strain A mice with methylbis(β-chloromethyl)amine hydrochloride. *J. Natl Cancer Inst.*, *10*, 125-130

Heston, W.E. (1953) Occurrence of tumors in mice injected subcutaneously with sulphur mustard and nitrogen mustard. *J. Natl Cancer Inst.*, *14*, 131-140

IARC (1974a) *IARC Monographs on the Evaluation of Carcinogenic Risk of Chemicals to Man*, Vol. 4, *Some Aromatic Amines, Hydrazine and Related Substances, N-Nitroso Compounds and Miscellaneous Alkylating Agents*, Lyon, pp. 247-252

IARC (1974b) *IARC Monographs on the Evaluation of Carcinogenic Risk of Chemicals to Man*, Vol. 4, *Some Aromatic Amines, Hydrazine and Related Substances, N-Nitroso Compounds and Miscellaneous Alkylating Agents*, Lyon, pp. 119-124

IARC (1974c) *IARC Monographs on the Evaluation of Carcinogenic Risk of Chemicals to Man*, Vol. 7, *Some Anti-thyroid and related Substances, Nitrofurans and Industrial Chemicals*, Lyon, pp. 53-65, 67-76

IARC (1975a) *IARC Monographs on the Evaluation of Carcinogenic Risk of Chemicals to Man*, Vol. 9, *Some Aziridines, N-, S- and O-Mustards and Selenium*, Lyon, pp. 167-180

IARC (1975b) *IARC Monographs on the Evaluation of Carcinogenic Risk of Chemicals to Man*, Vol. 9, *Some Aziridines, N-, S- and O-Mustards and Selenium*, Lyon, pp. 193-207

IARC (1976) *IARC Monographs on the Evaluation of Carcinogenic Risk of Chemicals to Man*, Vol. 10, *Some Naturally Occurring Substances*, Lyon, pp. 153-161

IARC (1977a) *IARC Monographs on the Evaluation of Carcinogenic Risk of Chemicals to Man*, Vol. 13, *Some Miscellaneous Pharmaceutical Substances*, Lyon, pp. 113-122

IARC (1977b) *IARC Monographs on the Evaluation of Carcinogenic Risk of Chemicals to Man*, Vol. 13, *Some Miscellaneous Pharmaceutical Substances*, Lyon, pp. 123-130

IARC (1977c) *IARC Monographs on the Evaluation of Carcinogenic Risk of Chemicals to Man*, Vol. 13, *Some Miscellaneous Pharmaceutical Substances*, Lyon, pp. 157-181

IARC (1977d) *IARC Monographs on the Evaluation of Carcinogenic Risk of Chemicals to Man*, Vol. 13, *Some Miscellaneous Pharmaceutical Substances*, Lyon, pp. 201-225

IARC (1979a) *IARC Monographs on the Evaluation of the Carcinogenic Risk of Chemicals to Humans*, Vol. 21, *Sex Hormones (II)*, Lyon, pp. 49, 233-255, 257-278, 279-326, 343-362, 417-429, 441-460, 519-547

IARC (1979b) *IARC Monographs on the Evaluation of the Carcinogenic Risk of Chemicals to Humans*, Vol. 21, *Sex Hormones (II)*, Lyon, pp. 173-231

IARC (1980a) *IARC Monographs on the Evaluation of the Carcinogenic Risk of Chemicals to Humans*, Vol. 24, *Some Pharmaceutical Drugs*, Lyon, pp. 101-124

IARC (1980b) *IARC Monographs on the Evaluation of the Carcinogenic Risk of Chemicals to Humans*, Vol. 24, *Some Pharmaceutical Drugs*, Lyon, pp. 77-83

IARC (1980c) *IARC Monographs on the Evaluation of the Carcinogenic Risk of Chemicals to Humans*, Vol. 24, *Some Pharmaceutical Drugs*, Lyon, pp. 135-161

IARC (1980d) *IARC Monographs on the Evaluation of the Carcinogenic Risk of Chemicals to Humans*, Vol. 24, *Some Pharmaceutical Drugs*, Lyon, pp. 163-173

IARC (1980e) *IARC Monographs on the Evaluation of Carcinogenic Risk of Chemicals to Man*, Vol. 24, *Some Pharmaceutical Drugs*, Lyon, pp. 185-194

IARC (1981a) *IARC Monographs on the Evaluation of the Carcinogenic Risk of Chemicals to Humans*, Vol. 26, *Some Antineoplastic and Immunosuppressive Agents*, Lyon, pp. 115-136

IARC (1981b) *IARC Monographs on the Evaluation of the Carcinogenic Risk of Chemicals to Humans*, Vol. 26, *Some Antineoplastic and Immunosuppressive Agents*, Lyon, pp. 165-202

IARC (1981c) *IARC Monographs on the Evaluation of the Carcinogenic Risk of Chemicals to Humans*, Vol. 26, *Some Antineoplastic and Immunosuppressive Agents*, Lyon, pp. 341-347

IARC (1981d) *IARC Monographs on the Evaluation of the Carcinogenic Risk of Chemicals to Humans*, Vol. 26, *Some Antineoplastic and Immunosuppressive Agents*, Lyon, pp. 47-78

IARC (1985) *IARC Monographs on the Evaluation of the Carcinogenic Risk of Chemicals to Humans*, Vol. 35, *Polynuclear Aromatic Compounds, Part 4, Bitumens, Coal-tars and Derived Products, Shale-oils and Soots*, Lyon, pp. 83-159

IARC (1986) *IARC Monographs on the Evaluation of the Carcinogenic Risk of Chemicals to Humans*, Vol. 40, *Some Naturally Occurring and Synthetic Food Components, Furocoumarins and Ultraviolet Radiation*, Lyon, pp. 327-347

IARC (1987) *IARC Monographs on the Evaluation of Carcinogenic Risks to Humans*, Suppl. 7, *Overall Evaluations of Carcinogenicity: An Updating of IARC Monographs Volumes 1-42*, Lyon

IARC (1990) *IARC Monographs on the Evaluation of Carcinogenic Risks to Humans*, Vol. 50, *Some Pharmaceutical Drugs (II)*, Lyon (in press)

Kinlen, L.J. (1985) Incidence of cancer in rheumatoid arthritis and other disorders after immunosuppressive treatment. *Am. J. Med.*, 78, 44-49

Chapter 8. Radiation

Ionizing radiation

Radiation is said to be ionizing when it has the capacity to accelerate electrons in matter, either directly or indirectly. The part of the electromagnetic spectrum known as X- or γ-radiation (the name depends on the way in which it is produced) transfers photon energy directly to pre-existing electrons. Particles such as electrons, α–particles and neutrons transfer their kinetic energy to electrons, protons and atomic nuclei by a series of collisions along a linear track.

Human exposure to ionizing radiation is ubiquitous. The most important natural sources are radioactive nuclides in air, water, the food chain and minerals present near or at the surface of the Earth's crust, and the cosmic rays that bombard the Earth's atmosphere continually, creating new radioactive nuclides and γ-rays from interactions with the atoms of the atmosphere.

Before the twentieth century, natural sources were the only means by which human beings were exposed to ionizing radiation. However, the discovery of how to produce X-rays led immediately to their use in diagnostic and therapeutic medicine. Nuclear fission was achieved by scientists in the late 1930s, resulting first in the production of weapons of mass destruction, such as those which were exploded over Hiroshima and Nagasaki at the end of the Second World War, and subsequently in the development of electricity generation by nuclear reactors. Nevertheless, natural sources (so-called 'background') provide the greatest contribution to the radiation exposure of most of the Earth's population (see Figure 19).

The first cancers observed in association with exposure to radiation were skin carcinomas on the hands of radiologists (Upton, 1975), reported as early as seven years after Roentgen discovered X-rays in 1895. Several cases of what was probably leukaemia were noted 20–30 years later among workers exposed to radiation. By the 1930s, a few cases of bone cancer had been seen among young women who had ingested radium-containing paint by licking the brushes they used for painting clock and watch dials (Martland, 1931), and their numbers increased over the next few decades. The induction of sarcomas in laboratory animals exposed to radiation was reported in 1910 (Marie *et al.*, 1910, 1912), and many subsequent experiments clearly demonstrated the carcinogenicity of ionizing radiation (United Nations Scientific Committee on the Effect of Atomic Radiation, 1977).

Important epidemiological studies of radiation carcinogenesis have been carried out on the survivors of the atomic bombs in Hiroshima and Nagasaki, on a number of populations irradiated for medical reasons, and on underground miners who had been exposed to radon gas and its decay products. It is now accepted that ionizing radiation can induce cancer in any organ in which cancer occurs naturally. Organs differ substantially in their intrinsic susceptibility, in the latent period between exposure and appearance of a cancer and in the correlation with sex and with age at the time of exposure. Thus, no generalization can be

Figure 19. Sources of exposure to radiation[a]

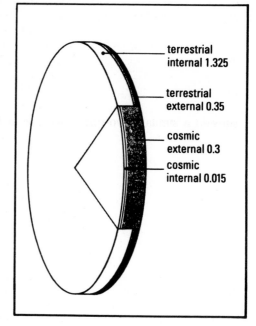

[a] From Lean (1985). A, average annual effective dose equivalents from natural and man-made sources of radiation; figures in millisievert. B, average annual effective dose equivalents from natural sources of radiation; figures in millisievert

made with regard to radiation-induced malignancies, and the sites are discussed separately below.

Leukaemia

The Atomic Bomb Casualty Commission was established in 1947 to study the long-term effects of the atomic bombing in 1945. At about the same time, it had become clear that bomb survivors were at increased risk for developing leukaemia (Ichimaru *et al.*, 1981; Kato & Schull, 1982); the increase was apparent for acute and chronic myeloid leukaemia and acute lymphocytic leukaemia, but not for chronic lymphocytic leukaemia. Among survivors who had received doses of ionizing radiation exceeding 10 cGy, there were about 62 deaths from radiation-induced leukaemia (39% of all cases) and 183 deaths from other cancers (10% of all cases) by the end of 1982. The peak in leukaemia incidence occurred seven to eight years after the bombing. The excess of leukaemia has been decreasing since that time, although it still remains significantly elevated (Finch, 1984).

Patients treated with X-rays for ankylosing spondylitis (a chronic progressive arthritis occurring mainly in young men) are also at increased risk for leukaemia (Smith & Doll, 1982; Darby *et al.*, 1987), beginning within two years of treatment. Above a certain level of exposure, however, the risk for leukaemia may not increase and may seem to decrease. This phenomenon was first seen in spondylitis patients but more recently also in women treated with radiotherapy for cancer of the cervix (Boice *et al.*, 1985). A proposed explanation, based on the results of experiments in animals, is that as dose increases more target cells are sterilized and are thus unable to give rise to a neoplasm.

A large study of children who died before age 10 in the 1950s (Stewart *et al.*, 1956) reported that the risk of leukaemia and other cancers in childhood was increased by diagnostic X-irradiation *in utero*. This assessment remains controversial (MacMahon, 1985). Two studies in twins (Mole, 1974; Harvey *et al.*, 1985), for whom the twin pregnancy itself was usually the reason for the X-ray showed a similar (two-fold) increase in leukaemia and cancer risk among the twins irradiated *in utero* compared to those not irradiated.

Cancer of the breast

Risk for breast cancer is elevated among atomic bomb survivors (Preston *et al.*, 1986), among patients who have been treated with X-rays for post-partum mastitis (Shore *et al.*, 1986), and among patients who had multiple fluoroscopies in the course of treatment for pulmonary tuberculosis (Baral *et al.*, 1977; Boice & Monson, 1977; Land *et al.*, 1980; Howe, 1984).

In women examined by fluoroscopy, the increased risk for breast cancer was observed only 15 years after first exposure for women who were under 25 at the time of treatment and after ten years for women exposed at 25 years or older (Howe, 1984); similar findings were reported in the study of mastitis patients.

Boice *et al.* (1979) reviewed the results of all these studies and showed that the risk for breast cancer increased linearly with dose and at the same rate per unit dose in all of the groups studied. The length of exposure had no effect on this rate (Shore *et al.*, 1986).

Among the atomic bomb survivors, the increase in risk was first observed among older women five to nine years after irradiation (Boice *et al.*, 1979); however, the carcinogenic effect of radiation on the breast appears to be greatest when exposure occurred around menarche and then decreases with increasing age at exposure up to age 40–49, after which there may have been no increase in risk. Information on people exposed to ionizing radiation before menarche is available only for survivors of the atomic bombs, but the numbers are currently too small to test whether the significantly increased risk in this group is of the same magnitude or larger than that observed in women who were aged 10–19 at the time of exposure (Tokunaga *et al.*, 1984).

Cancer of the lung

The risk for lung cancer is elevated in populations exposed to external γ- and X-radiation, such as the atomic bomb survivors (Preston *et al.*, 1986; Shimizu *et al.*, 1987) and patients treated for ankylosing spondylitis (Smith & Doll, 1982), and in underground miners whose bronchial mucosa was exposed to radon gas and its decay products. The studies of miners were reviewed in detail at the IARC (1988), and it was concluded that there was sufficient evidence that this occupational exposure caused lung cancer. Investigations on the effects of exposure to radon from natural sources in houses are being carried out in many countries.

Following exposure to radiation, the risk for lung cancer appears to increase with age in proportion to the risk among unexposed individuals; this observation was made for both atomic bomb survivors (Preston *et al.*, 1986) and for miners (Waxweiler *et al.*, 1981; International Commission for Radiation Protection, 1987). For both these populations, a greater risk for lung cancer was seen among people exposed later in life. Male and female survivors of the bomb show the same increase in absolute risk (Yamamoto *et al.*, 1987); the relative increase for women is three to four times larger than that for men since their rate of lung cancer is so much lower in the absence of exposure to radiation (Preston *et al.*, 1986).

Several attempts have been made to study the interaction between exposure to radiation and cigarette smoking in causing lung cancer. The studies of atomic bomb survivors suggest that the relationship is additive (Prentice *et al.*, 1983; Kopecky *et al.*, 1986), but data on underground miners in Colorado are more consistent with a multiplicative effect (Whittemore & McMillan, 1983; Hornung & Meinhardt, 1987).

Cancer of the thyroid

The risk for cancer of the thyroid is particularly difficult to quantify, owing to the low rate of fatality from this cancer and to the long latency before its appearance. The risk is elevated among atomic bomb survivors (Prentice *et al.*, 1982) and among people treated with radiotherapy as children, at the thymus and for tinea capitis (ringworm) (Ron & Modan, 1984; Shore *et al.*, 1984; Ron *et al.*, 1987). Iodine absorbed into the body concentrates in the thyroid gland, and its radioactive isotopes, such as iodine-131, have been used medically to treat hyperthyroidism and to diagnose thyroid disease, without increasing the risk for cancer of the thyroid (Hoffman, 1984; Holm, 1984), as irradiation of the thyroid cells is spread out in time. Single, brief external exposures to X- or γ-rays at the same level would be predicted to cause cancer, on the basis of results from experimental studies.

In the atomic bomb survivors, the risk for cancer of the thyroid had decreased by 30 years after exposure (Beebe *et al.*, 1977), but in other studies the increase in risk seems to persist for at least 30 years (Shore *et al.*, 1985). The data on children irradiated for ringworm indicate that exposure at six to fifteen years of age carries a somewhat higher risk than exposure at older ages. Among the atomic bomb survivors, the risk is greater for those exposed before the age of 20 than after.

Gastrointestinal cancers

An increased risk for stomach cancer has been observed among atomic bomb survivors (Shimizu *et al.*, 1987), especially for people exposed under the age of 20 (Preston *et al.*, 1986), and among patients treated with X-rays for ankylosing spondylitis (Smith & Doll, 1982). Atomic bomb survivors also had an increased risk for cancer of the colon, again especially after exposure when young. The incidence of rectal cancer was higher in women who had received radiation treatment for cancer of the cervix than in those who had not (Day & Boice, 1983; Boice *et al.*, 1988). These women had received doses to their tissues that were up to 100 times greater than those received by atomic bomb survivors, whose risk for this cancer does not appear to have increased.

Cancer of the liver

Patients who were injected for diagnostic purposes with very large doses of a colloidal preparation of thorium-232, Thorotrast, now an obsolete procedure, had a very high frequency of cancer of the liver (cholangiocellular carcinoma and haemangiosarcoma) and smaller increases in risk for leukaemia and for sarcoma of the bone (Van Kaick *et al.*, 1984). Thorotrast is deposited in phagocytic cells in very high concentrations, especially in the liver and bone marrow, and the nearby cells are intensely irradiated by α-particles. The tumours in the bone began to appear some 20 years after injection, but the risk probably continues throughout life.

Multiple myeloma

Multiple myeloma can be caused by irradiation of the bone marrow, like many kinds of leukaemia. A small increase in the risk for this neoplasia was observed in atomic bomb survivors (Shimizu *et al.*, 1987) and in patients treated with radiotherapy for cervical cancer (Boice *et al.*, 1985). The increase became evident much later than that of leukaemia, so that multiple myeloma is the most recent cancer to have been linked with exposure to radiation. Several studies have been carried out of cancer risk among workers involved in nuclear reactor research, the processing of nuclear fuels and nuclear weapons production, who are exposed chronically to relatively low doses of radiation; increases in risk for myeloma were seen, but no consistent increase in risks for cancers at other sites (Gilbert & Marks, 1979; Smith & Douglas, 1986; Gilbert *et al.*, 1989).

Cancer of the bone

Information about radiation-induced cancers of the bone comes from studies of women who were exposed to a mixture of radium isotopes while painting luminous dials (Rowland *et al.*, 1978) and of patients treated for various diseases by injections of radium-224 (Mays & Spiess, 1984). Radium deposited in body tissues causes cancer, by emitting α-particles. Whatever the route of exposure, radium is mostly transferred to bone. The first sarcomas of bone appear in less than ten years. In the dial painters, some cases occurred in the jaw bone nearly 60 years after exposure began; however, in the patients injected with radium, the pattern is closer to that of leukaemia induced by radiation. The explanation of this difference is that long-lived isotopes of radium-226 and radium-228 deposited in bone continue to irradiate it for decades, whereas irradiation of bone by radium-224, which has a half-life of only a few days, is much shorter. For the same total dose of radium-224, the risk for sarcoma of the bone was somewhat higher when many repeated weekly injections were given than when only a few were given (Spiess & Mays, 1973).

Other cancers

The risk for pancreatic cancer is increased in ankylosing spondylitis patients (Smith & Doll, 1982) and in women treated with radiation for cancer of the cervix (Day & Boice, 1983). Possible increases in risk for this cancer reported earlier in atomic bomb survivors (Kato & Schull, 1982) and in workers in the nuclear industry (Gilbert & Marks, 1979) were not confirmed by continued observation (Tolley *et al.*, 1983; Shimizu *et al.*, 1987).

The frequency of skin cancer (other than melanoma) was increased among radiologists and other people exposed occupationally to high levels of radiation at the beginning of this century (Matanoski *et al.*, 1984), among children given X-ray therapy for ringworm (Shore *et al.*, 1976), among children treated at the thymus with X-rays (Hempelmann *et al.*, 1975) and in uranium miners (International Commission for Radiation Protection, 1987).

Risks for cancers of the kidney and of the bladder were increased in both spondylitis patients (Smith & Doll, 1982) and atomic bomb survivors. For the latter, a clear dose–response relationship was observed (Preston *et al.*, 1986). A few cases of oesophageal cancer were also found in these two populations.

Quantitative and qualitative aspects

More quantitative information is available about radiation carcinogenesis than for any other human carcinogen. Both epidemiological and experimental studies have provided data on the shape of the dose-response curve for cancer induction following exposure to radiation, on the relative effects of different types of radiation and on the effect of prolonging exposure. Nevertheless, our understanding of the mechanisms underlying the process is still very incomplete. Furthermore, it is often necessary to be able to predict the number of cases of cancer that will result from exposure to radiation of a certain kind; when no data are available from observations of humans, extrapolation must be done on the basis of mathematical models. For example, suppose that one wished to predict the number of cancers in Europe that will result from exposure to radiation following the accident in Chernobyl in 1986. Data on atomic bomb survivors, underground miners and people who received medical irradiation are relevant, but substantial differences remain: the exposure after the Chernobyl accident was to low levels of radiation, involved the whole organism (due to intake of contaminated air, food and water) and has been spread over months or years. In contrast, exposure after the atomic bomb explosions was external and was predominantly completed within a few seconds; miners have protracted exposure, mainly to α-emitters absorbed through the lung, and radiation therapy is typically delivered in fractionated, high doses over several days or weeks.

Whether there is a threshold below which radiation is not carcinogenic has long been a subject of scientific debate (Upton, 1983). It has not been possible to demonstrate such a threshold in any organ, although, by definition, statistical error virtually precludes the demonstration of *absence* of effect. There is in any case little biological plausibility that there is a threshold. Thousands of animals are required to study experimentally the carcinogenic effect of doses of radiation that cause very small increases in the risk for cancer (see, for example: Ullrich & Storer, 1979a,b,c). In studies of human populations exposed to such low doses of ionizing radiation, the difficulties lie in accurate quantification of exposure and adequate control for the effect of confounding factors and of various other biases. Consequently, attempts to study the association between cancer risk and geographic variations in natural background radiation have provided somewhat equivocal results (Knox *et al.*, 1988).

The dose-response curve for radiation carcinogenesis appears to be well described by a linear curve at low levels of response to so-called high LET (linear energy transfer) types of radiation, such as α-particles and neutrons, and to be concave upwards for low LET radiation, such as γ- and X-rays (BEIR III: Committee on the Biological Effects of Ionizing Radiation, 1980; Mole, 1984). At very high levels of exposure, the probability of malignant transformation taking place reaches a plateau then eventually decreases, because of increased cell killing; tumour yield actually drops, as described above for leukaemia in general and as has been seen for myeloid leukaemia in mice (Mole & Major, 1983).

It is clear that some tissues are much more susceptible to radiation carcinogenesis than others, although we do not know why (Table 13). The bone marrow is a site of particular and rapidly manifested sensitivity, although the breast and thyroid are also highly sensitive to radiation.The recent detection of clusters of cases of leukaemia among children living near nuclear plants has been the subject of great scientific and public interest. A number of explanations have been advanced for the observed excess risks, such as a rare response to common viral infections occurring in rural populations with low herd immunity (Kinlen, 1988) or increased sensitivity to internally absorbed high-LET emitters in the environment. It now appears that the excess risk may be explained by occupational exposure of the father to very low doses of ionizing radiation in the period before conception of the child, supposedly through a mutagenic effect on germ cells (Gardner *et al.*, 1990).

An increased risk for cancers at various sites has been reported recently among persons who were exposed *in utero* to ionizing radiation from the atomic bombs dropped on Hiroshima and Nagasaki (Kato *et al.*, 1989; Yoshimoto *et al.*, 1988).

It appears, from studies in experimental animals of the relative carcinogenicity of different types and doses of radiation, that, in general, high LET radiation is substantially more carcinogenic than low LET radiation at low doses, and that protracted exposure to low LET radiation produces a smaller carcinogenic effect than an acute exposure to the same cumulated dose (Hall, 1978).

The atomic bomb survivors provided an important source of comparative information on the relative effectiveness for cancer induction of high LET (neutron) and low LET (γ) radiation. However, estimates of the doses of radiation recently underwent major revision, and the neutron component of the total dose received in Hiroshima is now seen to have been much less than was previously estimated, to the extent that the exposure in both Hiroshima and Nagasaki is now known to have been essentially due to γ-radiation (Preston & Pierce, 1987).

The only data on human exposure to high LET radiation now come from studies of miners exposed to α-particles. The results are consistent in showing that α-particles are much more efficient than γ- or X-rays in inducing lung cancer, although the relative effect has not been well quantified. Protraction of exposure over a long period – an issue of major importance in preventive measures to reduce occupational and environmental exposures – has been the focus of recent

Table 13. Excess cancer incidence (excluding leukaemia and bone cancer) per 10⁴ person-years and per Gy, 11–30 years after exposure[a]

Site	Age at exposure (years)					Age weighted average[b]
	0–9	10–19	20–34	35–40	>50	
Males						
Thyroid	2.20	2.40	2.20	2.20	2.20	2.20
Lung	0.00	0.54	2.45	5.10	6.79	3.64
Oesophagus	0.07	0.07	0.13	0.21	0.56	0.26
Stomach	0.40	0.40	0.77	1.27	3.35	1.53
Intestine	0.26	0.26	0.52	0.84	2.23	1.02
Liver	0.70	0.70	0.70	0.70	0.70	0.70
Pancreas	0.24	0.24	0.45	0.75	1.97	0.90
Urinary	0.04	0.23	0.50	0.92	1.62	0.81
Lymphoma	0.27	0.27	0.27	0.27	0.27	0.27
Other	0.62	0.38	1.12	1.40	2.90	1.52
All sites	4.80	5.29	9.11	13.66	22.59	12.85
Females						
Thyroid	5.80	5.80	5.80	5.80	5.80	5.80
Breast	0.00	7.30	6.60	6.60	6.60	5.82
Lung	0.00	0.54	2.45	5.10	6.79	3.94
Oesophagus	0.07	0.07	0.13	0.21	0.56	0.28
Stomach	0.40	0.40	0.77	1.27	3.35	1.68
Intestine	0.26	0.26	0.52	0.84	2.23	1.12
Liver	0.70	0.70	0.70	0.70	0.70	0.70
Pancreas	0.24	0.24	0.45	0.75	1.97	0.99
Urinary	0.04	0.23	0.50	0.92	1.62	0.88
Lymphoma	0.27	0.27	0.27	0.27	0.27	0.27
Other	0.62	0.38	1.12	1.40	2.90	1.64
All sites	8.40	16.19	19.31	23.86	32.79	23.10

[a] Estimated in BEIR III (1980)
[b] Average of age-specific coefficients, weighted according to the age distribution of the population of the USA

studies of employees in nuclear industries (see for example: Inskip *et al.*, 1987; Smith & Douglas, 1986), but the results are difficult to compare with those of the studies of acute exposure.

Note added in proof:

A report of the US National Academy of Sciences (BEIR V, 1990) slightly alters the above conclusions. It now appears that, even for low LET radiation, the dose-dependent excess of mortality from all cancers other than leukaemia shows no departure from linearity up to doses of 4 Sv. The dose-dependent excess of cancer is, furthermore, consistent with a relative risk model. Cancer risk estimates are now about three times larger than for solid cancers and about four times larger for leukaemia than those published in BEIR III.

For leukaemia, the effect of age of exposure is an important risk modifier: the risk is initially higher in those exposed below 20 years of age. The effect of age at exposure is also important for radiation-induced thyroid cancer risk, this risk being at least twice as large in children than in adults. Hormone balance is another important modifier of thyroid cancer risk.

Finally, radiation-related increases in cancer risk have also been noted for the following sites: brain and nervous system, parathyroid glands, salivary glands and prostate.

BEIR V: Committee on the Biological Effects of Ionizing Radiation (1990). *Health Effects of Exposure to Low Levels of Ionizing Radiation*, Washington DC, National Academy of Science.

Ultra-violet radiation

Most human exposure to ultra-violet (UV) radiation is from the sun, and the most highly exposed individuals are therefore those living nearest to the equator and, at any given latitude, those whose work or recreation takes them outdoors. Much lower levels of exposure result from certain types of fluorescent lighting. The carcinogenicity of UV radiation was discussed in a detailed appendix to a volume of *IARC Monographs* (IARC, 1986), which, unless otherwise stated, is the source used for writing this section.

Data from epidemiological studies are consistent in demonstrating a causal relationship between exposure to sunlight and cancers of the lip and skin. However, in these studies, exposure to sunlight, rather than specifically to UV radiation, was being measured, although the UV frequency range is presumed to be the active component of sunlight in view of its known tissue-damaging and mutagenic effects (Cole *et al.*, 1986). UV radiation produces skin and other external tumours in exposed experimental animals.

Case reports of non-melanocytic skin cancers in sailors and other outdoor workers first appeared a century ago; in the 1940s, descriptive studies from the USA clearly showed that, unlike any other cancer, the incidence of non-melanocytic skin cancer was higher in southern than in northern states. This has also been found in Canada and (inversely) in Australia (see Part I, p. 68). Other pieces of evidence that strongly support the role of sunlight in causing non-melanocytic skin cancer are its anatomical distribution (80% on the head and neck) and the finding that outdoor workers have a higher risk than indoor workers. Nevertheless, the few case-control studies of non-melanocytic skin cancer have been of uneven quality and have perhaps for this reason not demonstrated a risk as clearly as one might have expected. The evidence concerning lip cancer is far clearer: several well-executed case-control studies have shown that the risk is substantially increased among individuals who are exposed extensively to the sun because of their occupation.

For cutaneous melanoma, the epidemiological data are more complex (see Part I, p. 67). Unlike non-melanocytic skin cancer, the anatomical distribution is not predominantly on exposed areas of the skin (Elwood & Gallagher, 1983), and in several studies indoor workers had risks equal to or greater than that of outdoor workers (Lee & Strickland, 1980; Beral & Robinson, 1981; Cooke *et al.*, 1984). The gradient by latitude does, however, appear to hold, except in Europe, where the trend may be inversed by skin pigmentation: the highest rates occur in northern Europe, which is further from the equator but home to fair-skinned people.

Theories have been advanced that individuals who maintain suntans, through extensive recreational or occupational exposure, are at lower risk for melanoma than those who are exposed intermittently (Elwood & Hislop, 1982; Holman *et al.*, 1983). A recent review of relevant epidemiological studies indicates that there is now strong empirical support for the intermittent exposure hypothesis (Armstrong, 1988). This phenomenon could be due either to increased filtering of UV by tanned skin or to repeated stimulation of melanocytes during intermittent tanning. It appears that exposure in childhood or early adolescence may confer a greater risk than exposure in adult life (Holman & Armstrong, 1984). In some of the studies of indoor exposure to UV radiation (fluorescent lighting), an increase in risk for melanoma was observed, but at this stage it is not possible to exclude the effects of the intermittent exposure to the sun that indoor workers receive.

Electromagnetic fields

Exposure to extremely low frequency (ELF, 0–300 Hz) electromagnetic fields has been suspected only recently of increasing the risk for cancer, and particularly for acute myeloid leukaemia. A number of studies of men likely to have been exposed occupationally to ELF fields has shown greater than expected incidence of and mortality from leukaemia, particularly the acute myeloid form (Milham, 1982; Wright *et al.*, 1982; Coleman *et al.*, 1983; McDowall, 1983; Stern *et al.*, 1986), in the order of a 20% increase for all leukaemia and 45% for acute myeloid leukaemia (Coleman & Beral, 1988). In none of these studies was exposure to ELF electromagnetic fields assessed directly, however, and the occupational groups were defined in different ways: increased risks were not always found in the same group. Further, probable exposure in some jobs to other known or potential leukaemogens, such as benzene, was not fully taken into account. Despite these drawbacks, the consistency of the results obtained in several countries and for different occupational groups and using different study designs is notable, and the results probably indicate a true increase in risk for electrical workers. Studies in which detailed, direct assessment of exposure is undertaken are under way, and these should help to clarify whether the small increase in risk for leukaemia is related to exposure to ELF fields or to some other agent (Coleman & Cardis, 1990).

In several studies, leukaemia and cancer risk have been examined in both adults and children in relation to residential exposure to ELF fields. The results are less consistent than those of the occupational studies. In most, indirect measures of exposure were used, such as the nature of overhead wiring configurations near the home or the distance of such structures from the home, although such measures appear to correlate well with direct measurements of ELF fields (Wertheimer & Leeper, 1979, 1982; Tomenius, 1986; Savitz, 1987). In addition, all studies had major methodological deficiencies, particularly in the selection of control subjects representative of the population that gave rise to the cases. Small increases in risk for leukaemia were seen among children. The major problems in estimating risk are the ubiquity of the exposure and the difficulties in measuring it.

References

Armstrong, B.K. (1988) Epidemiology of malignant melanoma: intermittent or total accumulated exposure to the sun? *J. Dermatol. Surg. Oncol.*, *14*, 835-849

Baral, E., Larsson, L.E. & Mattson, B. (1977) Breast cancer following irradiation of the breast. *Cancer*, *40*, 2905-2910

Beebe, G.W., Kato, H. & Land, C.B. (1977) *Mortality Experience of Atomic Bomb Survivors, 1950-74. Life Span Study Report 8* (Radiation Effects Research Foundation Technical Report 1-77), Hiroshima, Radiation Effects Research Foundation

BEIR III: Committee on the Biological Effects of Ionizing Radiation (1980) *The Effects on Populations of Exposure to Low Levels of Ionizing Radiation*, Washington DC, National Academy of Sciences

Boice, J.D. & Monson, R.R. (1977) Breast cancer in women after repeated fluoroscopic examinations of the chest. *J. Natl Cancer Inst.*, *59*, 823-832

Boice, J.D., Land, C.E., Shore, R.E., Norman, J.E. & Tokunaga, M. (1979) Risk of breast cancer following low-dose radiation exposure. *Radiology*, *131*, 589-597

Boice, J.D., Jr and 35 others (1985) Cancer risk following radiation treatment for cervical cancer. An international collaboration among cancer registries. *J. Natl Cancer Inst.*, *74*, 955-975

Boice, J.D. Jr and 41 others (1988) Radiation dose and second cancer risk in patients treated for cancer of the cervix. *Radiat. Res.*, *116*, 3-55

Cole, C.A., Forbes, D. & Davies, R.E. (1986) An action spectrum for UV photocarcinogenesis. *Photochem. Photobiol.*, *43*, 275-284

Coleman, M. & Beral, V. (1988) A review of epidemiological studies of the health effects of living near or working with electricity generation and transmission equipment. *Int. J. Epidemiol.*, *17*, 1-13

Coleman, M. and 23 others (1990) Extremely low frequency electric and magnetic fields and human cancer risk. *Bioelectromagnetics* (in press)

Coleman, M., Bell, J. & Skeet, R. (1983) Leukemia incidence in electrical workers. *Lancet, i*, 982-983

Darby, S.C., Doll, R., Gill, S.K. & Smith, P.G. (1987) Long-term mortality after a single treatment course with X-rays in patients treated for ankylosing spondylitis. *Br. J. Cancer*, *55*, 179-190

Day, N.E. & Boice, J.D., eds (1983) *Second Cancer in Relation to Radiation Treatment for Cervical Cancer* (IARC Scientific Publications No. 52), Lyon, IARC

Elwood, J.M. & Gallagher, R.P. (1983) Site distribution of malignant melanoma. *Can. Med. Assoc. J.*, *128*, 1400-1404

Elwood, J.M. & Hislop, T.G. (1982) Solar radiation in the etiology of cutaneous malignant melanoma in Caucasians. *Natl Cancer Inst Monogr.*, *62*, 167-171

Finch, S.C. (1984) Leukemia and lymphoma in atomic bomb survivors. In: Boice, J.D. & Fraumeni, J.F., eds, *Radiation Carcinogenesis: Epidemiology and Biological Significance*, New York, Raven Press, pp. 37-44

Gardner, M.J., Snee, M.P., Hall, A.J., Powell, C.A., Downes, S. & Terrell, J.D. (1990) Results of case-control study of leukaemia and lymphoma among young people near Sellafield nuclear plant in West Cumbria. *Br. Med. J.*, *300*, 423-429

Gilbert, E.S. & Marks, S. (1979) An analysis of the mortality of workers in a nuclear facility. *Radiat. Res.*, *79*, 122-148

Gilbert, E.S., Peterson, G.R. & Buchanan, J.A. (1989) Mortality of workers at the Hanford site: 1945-1981. *Health Phys.*, *56*, 11-25

Hall, E.J. (1978) *Radiobiology for Radiologists*, Second Edition, Philadelphia, Harper & Row

Harvey, E.B., Boice, J.D., Jr, Honeyman, M. & Flannery, J.T. (1985) Prenatal X-ray exposure and childhood cancer in twins. *N. Engl. J. Med.*, *312*, 541-545

Hempelmann, L.H., Hall, W.J., Phillips, M., Cooper, R.A. & Ames, W.R. (1975) Neoplasms in persons treated with X-rays in infancy: fourth survey in 20 years. *J. Natl Cancer Inst.*, *55*, 519-530

Hoffman, D.A. (1984) Late effects of iodine-131 therapy in the United States. In: Boice, J.D. & Fraumeni, J.F., eds, *Radiation Carcinogenesis: Epidemiology and Biological Significance*, New York, Raven Press, pp. 173-280

Holm, L.E. (1984) Malignant disease following iodine-131 therapy in Sweden. In: Boice, J.D. & Fraumeni, J.F., eds, *Radiation Carcinogenesis: Epidemiology and Biological Significance*, New York, Raven Press, pp. 263-271

Holman, C.D.J., Armstrong, B.K. & Heenan, P.J. (1983) A theory of the etiology and pathogenesis of human cutaneous malignant melanoma. *J. Natl Cancer Inst.*, *71*, 651-656

Hornung, R.W. & Meinhardt, T.J. (1987) Quantitative risk assessment of lung cancer in US uranium miners. *Health Phys.*, *52*, 417-430

Howe, G.R. (1984) Epidemiology of radiogenic breast cancer. In: Boice, J.D. & Fraumeni, J.F., eds, *Radiation Carcinogenesis: Epidemiology and Biological Significance*, New York, Raven Press, pp. 119-129

IARC (1986) *IARC Monographs on the Evaluation of the Carcinogenic Risk of Chemicals to Humans*, Vol. 40, *Some Naturally Occurring and Synthetic Food Components, Furocoumarins and Ultraviolet Radiation*, Lyon, pp. 379-415

IARC (1988) *IARC Monographs on the Evaluation of Carcinogenic Risks to Humans*, Vol. 43, *Man-made Mineral Fibres and Radon*, Lyon, pp. 173-259

Ichimaru, M., Ishimaru, T., Mikami, M., Yamada, Y. & Ohkita, T. (1981) *Incidence of Leukemia in Atomic Bomb Survivors and Controls in a Fixed Cohort, Hiroshima and Nagasaki, October 1950-December 1978* (Radiation Effects Research Foundation Technical Report 13-81), Hiroshima, Radiation Effects Research Foundation

Inskip, H., Beral, V., Fraser, P., Booth, M., Coleman, D. & Brown, A. (1987) Further assessment of the effects of occupational radiation exposure in the United Kingdom Atomic Energy Authority mortality study. *Br. J. Ind. Med.*, *44*, 149-160

International Commission for Radiological Protection (1987) *Lung Cancer Risk from Indoor Exposures to Radon Daughters* (ICRP Publication 50), Oxford, Pergamon

Kato, H. & Schull, W.J. (1982) Studies of the A-bomb survivors. 7. Mortality, 1950-1978. Part I. Cancer mortality. *Radiat. Res.*, *90*, 395-432

Kato, H., Yoshimoto, Y. & Schull, W.J. (1989) Risk of cancer among children exposed to atomic bomb radiation *in utero*: a review. In: Napalkov, N.P., Rice, J.M., Tomatis, L. & Yamasaki, H., eds, *Perinatal and Multigeneration Carcinogenesis* (IARC Scientific Publications No. 96), Lyon, IARC, pp. 365-374

Kinlen, L. (1988) Evidence for an infective cause of childhood leukaemia: comparison of a Scottish new town with nuclear reprocessing sites in Britain. *Lancet, ii*, 1323-1327

Knox, E.G., Stewart, A.M., Gilman, E.A. & Kneale, G.W. (1988) Background radiation and childhood cancers. *J. Radiat. Prot.*, *8*, 9-18

Kopecky, K.J., Yamamoto, T., Fujikura, T., Tokuoka, S., Monzen, T., Nishimori, I., Nakashima, E. & Koto, H. (1986) *Lung Cancer, Radiation Exposure and Smoking among A-Bomb Survivors, Hiroshima and Nagasaki, 1950-1980* (Radiation Effects Research Foundation Technical Report 13-86), Hiroshima, Radiation Effects Research Foundation

Land, C.E., Boice, J.D., Shore, R.E., Norman, J.E. & Tokunaga, M. (1980) Breast cancer risk from low-dose exposures to ionizing radiation: results of parallel analysis of three exposed populations of women. *J. Natl Cancer Inst.*, *65*, 353-376

Lean, G., ed. (1985) *Radiation Doses, Effects, Risks*, Nairobi, United Nations Environment Programme, p. 14

Lee, J.A.H. & Strickland, D. (1980) Malignant melanoma: social status and outdoor work. *Br. J. Cancer*, *41*, 757-763

MacMahon, B. (1985) Prenatal X-ray exposure and twins. *N. Engl. J. Med.*, *312*, 576-577

Marie, P., Clunet, T. & Raulot-Lapointe, G. (1910) Contribution à l'étude du developpement des tumeurs malignes sur les ulcères de Roentgen. *Bull. Assoc. Fr. Etude Cancer, 3*, 404-426

Marie, P., Clunet, T. & Raulot-Lapointe, G. (1912) Nouveau cas de tumeur maligne provoquée par une radiodermite expérimentale chez le rat blanc. *Bull. Assoc. Fr. Etude Cancer, 5*, 125-135

Martland, H.S. (1931) The occurrence of malignancy in radioactive persons. *Am. J. Cancer, 15*, 2435-2516

Matanoski, G., Sartwell, P., Elliott, E., Tonascia, J. & Sternberg, A. (1984) Cancer risks in radiologists and radiation workers. In: Boice, J.D. & Fraumeni, J.F., eds, *Radiation Carcinogenesis: Epidemiology and Biological Significance*, New York, Raven Press, pp. 83-96

Mays, C.W. & Spies, H. (1984) Bone sarcomas in patients given radium-224. In: Boice, J.D. & Fraumeni, J.F., eds, *Radiation Carcinogenesis: Epidemiology and Biological Significance*, New York, Raven Press, pp. 241-252

McDowall, M.E. (1983) Leukemia mortality in electrical workers in England and Wales. *Lancet, i*, 246

Milham, S. (1982) Mortality from leukemia in workers exposed to electrical and magnetic fields. *New Engl. J. Med.*, *307*, 249

Mole, R.H. (1974) Antenatal irradiation and childhood cancer: causation or coincidence. *Br. J. Cancer, 30,* 199-208

Mole, R.H. (1984) Dose-response relationships. In: Boice, J.D. & Fraumeni, J.F., eds, *Radiation Carcinogenesis: Epidemiology and Biological Significance*, New York, Raven Press, pp. 403-420

Mole, R.H. & Major, I.R. (1983) Myeloid leukemia frequency after protracted exposure to ionizing radiation: experimental confirmation of the flat dose-response found in ankylosing spondylitis after a single treatment course with X-rays. *Leuk. Res., 7,* 295-300

Prentice, R.L., Kato, H., Yoshimoto, K. & Mason, M.W. (1982) Radiation exposure and thyroid cancer incidence among Hiroshima and Nagasaki residents. *Natl Cancer Inst. Monogr., 62,* 207-212

Prentice, R.L., Yoshimoto, Y. & Mason, M.W. (1983) Relationship of cigarette smoking and radiation exposure to cancer mortality in Hiroshima and Nagasaki. *J. Natl Cancer Inst., 70,* 611-622

Preston, D.L. & Pierce, D.A. (1987) *The Effects of Changes in Dosimetry on Cancer Mortality Risk Estimates in the Atomic Bomb Survivors* (Radiation Effects Research Foundation Technical Report 9-87), Hiroshima, Radiation Effects Research Foundation

Preston, D.L., Kato, H., Kopecky, K.J. & Fujita, S. (1986) *Life Span Study Report 10, Part 1: Cancer Mortality among A-Bomb Survivors in Hiroshima and Nagasaki, 1950-1982* (Radiation Effects Research Foundation Technical Report 1-86), Hiroshima, Radiation Effects Research Foundation

Ron, E. & Modan, B. (1984) Thyroid and other neoplasms following childhood scalp irradiation. In: Boice, J.D. & Fraumeni, J.F., eds, *Radiation Carcinogenesis: Epidemiology and Biological Significance*, New York, Raven Press, pp. 139-151

Ron, E., Kleinerman, R.A., Boice, J.D., Jr, LiVolsi, V.A., Flannery, J.T. & Fraumeni, J.F., Jr (1987) A population-based case-control study of thyroid cancer. *J. Natl Cancer Inst., 79,* 1-12

Rowland, R.E., Stehney, A.F. & Lucas, H.F., Jr (1978) Dose-response relationships for female radium dial painters. *Radiat. Res., 76,* 368-383

Savitz, D. (1987) *Case-control Study of Childhood Cancer and Residential Exposure to Electric and Magnetic Fields.* Report to the New York State Department of Health Power Lines Project

Shimizu, Y., Kato, H., Schull, W.J., Preston, D.L., Fujita, S. & Pierce, D.A. (1987) *Life Span Study Report 11, Part 1: Comparison of Risk Coefficients for Site-specific Cancer Mortality Based on the DS86 and T65DR Shielded Kerma and Organ Doses* (Radiation Effects Research Foundation Technical Report 12-87), Hiroshima, Radiation Effects Research Foundation

Shore, R.E., Albert, R.E. & Pasternak, B.S. (1976) Follow-up study of patients treated by X-ray epilation for tinea capitis: resurvey of post-treatment illness and mortality experience. *Arch. Environ. Health, 31,* 21-28

Shore, R.E., Woodard, E.D. & Hempelmann, L.H. (1984) Radiation-induced thyroid cancer. In: Boice, J.D. & Fraumeni, J.F., eds, *Radiation Carcinogenesis: Epidemiology and Biological Significance*, New York, Raven Press, pp. 131-138

Shore, R.E., Woodard, E., Hildreth, N., Dvoretsky, P., Hempelmann, L. & Pasternak, B. (1985) Thyroid tumours following thymus irradiation. *J. Natl Cancer Inst., 74,* 1177-1184

Shore, R.E., Hildreth, N., Woodard, E.D., Dvoretsky, P., Hempelmann, L. & Pasternak, B. (1986) Breast cancer among women given X-ray therapy for acute postpartum mastitis. *J. Natl Cancer Inst., 77,* 689-696

Smith, P.G. & Doll, R. (1982) Mortality among patients with ankylosing spondylitis after a single treatment course with X-rays. *Br. Med. J., 248,* 449-460

Smith, P.G. & Douglas, A.J. (1986) Mortality of workers at the Sellafield plant of British Nuclear Fuels. *Br. Med. J., 293,* 845-854

Spiess, H. & Mays, C.W. (1973) Protraction effect on bone sarcoma-induction of 224Ra in children and adults. In: Sanders, C.L., Busch, R.H., Ballon, J.E. & Mahlum, D.D., eds, *Radionuclides Carcinogenesis* (AEC Symposium Series 29, CONF-720505), Springfield, Virginia, National Technical Information Service, pp. 437-450

Stern, F.B., Waxweiler, R.A., Beaumont, J.J., Lee, S.T., Rinsky, R.A., Zumwalde, R.D., Halperin, W.E., Bierbaum, P.J., Landrigan, P.J. & Murray, W.E., Jr (1986) A case-control study of leukemia at a naval nuclear shipyard. *Am. J. Epidemiol.*, *123*, 980-992

Stewart, A., Webb, J., Giles, D. & Hewitt, D. (1956) Malignant disease in childhood and diagnostic irradiation *in utero*. *Lancet*, *2*, 447

Teppo, L., Pukkala, E., Hakama, M., Hakulinen, T., Herva, A. & Saxén, E. (1980) Way of life and cancer incidence in Finland. A municipality-based ecological analysis. *Scand. J. Soc. Med., Suppl. 19*, 50-54

Tokunaga, M., Land, C.E., Yamamoto, T., Asano, M., Tokuoka, S., Ezaki, H., Nishimori, I. & Fujikura, T. (1984) Breast cancer among atomic bomb survivors. In: Boice, J.D. & Fraumeni, J.F., eds, *Radiation Carcinogenesis: Epidemiology and Biological Significance*, New York, Raven Press, pp. 45-56

Tolley, H.D., Marks, S., Buchanan, J.A. & Gilbert, E.S. (1983) A further update of the analysis of mortality of workers in a nuclear facility. *Radiat. Res.*, *95*, 211-213

Tomenius, L. (1986) 50 Hz electromagnetic environment and the incidence of childhood tumours in Stockholm county. *Bioelectromagnetics*, *7*, 191-207

Ullrich, R.L. & Storer, J.B. (1979a) Influence of γ irradiation on the development of neoplastic disease in mice. I. Reticular tissue tumors. *Radiat. Res.*, *80*, 303-316

Ullrich, R.L. & Storer, J.B. (1979b) Influence of γ irradiation on the development of neoplastic disease in mice. II. Solid tumors. *Radiat. Res.*, *80*, 317-324

Ullrich, R.L. & Storer, J.B. (1979c) Influence of γ irradiation on the development of neoplastic disease in mice. III. Dose rate effects. *Radiat. Res.*, *80*, 325-342

United Nations Scientific Committee on the Effects of Atomic Radiation (1977) *Sources and Effects of Ionizing Radiation*, New York, United Nations

Upton, A.C. (1975) Physical carcinogenesis: radiation history and sources. In: Becker, F.F., ed., *Cancer: A Comprehensive Treatise*, New York, Plenum, pp. 387-403

Upton, A.C. (1983) Environmental standards for ionizing radiation: theoretical basis for dose-response curves. *Environ. Health Perspect.*, *52*, 31-39

Van Kaick, G., Muth, H., Kal, A., Immich, H., Liebermann, D., Lorenz, D., Lorenz, W.J., Lührs, H., Scheer, K.E., Wagner, G., Wegener, K. & Wesch, H. (1984) Results of the German thorotrast study. In: Boice, J.D. & Fraumeni, J.F., eds, *Radiation Carcinogenesis: Epidemiology and Biological Significance*, New York, Raven Press, pp. 253-262

Waxweiler, R.J., Roscoe, R.J., Archer, V.E., Thun, M.J., Wagoner, J.K. & Lundin, F.E., Jr (1981) Mortality follow-up through 1977 of the white underground uranium miners cohort examined by the United States Public Health Service. In: Gomez, M., ed., *Radiation Hazards in Mining: Control, Measurement and Medical Aspects*, New York, Society of Mining Engineers of the American Institute of Mining, Metallurgical and Petroleum Engineers, pp. 823-880

Wertheimer, N. & Leeper, E. (1979) Electrical wiring configuration and childhood cancer. *Am. J. Epidemiol.*, *109*, 273-284

Wertheimer, N. & Leeper, E. (1982) Adult cancer related to electrical wires near the home. *Int. J. Epidemiol.*, *11*, 345-355

Whittemore, A.S. & McMillan, A. (1983) Lung cancer mortality among US uranium miners: a reappraisal. *J. Natl Cancer Inst.*, *71*, 489-499

Wright, W.E., Peters, J.M. & Mack, T.M. (1982) Leukemia in workers exposed to electrical and magnetic fields. *Lancet*, *i*, 1160-1161

Yamamoto, T., Kopecky, K.J., Fujikura, T., Tukuoka, S., Monzen, T., Nishimori, I., Nakashima, E. & Kato, H. (1987) Lung cancer incidence among A-bomb survivors in Hiroshima and Nagasaki, 1950-1980. *J. Radiat. Res.*, *28*, 156-171

Yoshimoto, Y., Kato, H. & Schull, W.J. (1988) Risk of cancer among children exposed *in utero* to A-bomb radiations: 1950-84. *Lancet*, *ii*, 665-669

Chapter 9. Tobacco

Tobacco has been consumed in a variety of ways for centuries in many parts of the world. Wider access to tobacco was made possible towards the end of the nineteenth century when cigarettes began to be produced industrially, and production expanded enormously during the twentieth century. Cigarettes have become by far the most common form in which tobacco is used throughout the world, and consumption has been increasing steadily in most regions, although in a few western countries the sales of cigarettes have become stable or even declined in recent years.

The fact that tobacco smoking causes lung cancer has been recognized ever since the studies in the UK and the USA at the beginning of the 1950s (Doll & Hill, 1950; Wynder & Graham, 1950). In the following, we review briefly the evidence accrued since those early studies on the causal relationship between smoking and the occurrence of lung cancer, but the major part is devoted to a description of the epidemiological evidence that factors such as age, age at starting to smoke, cessation of smoking, the composition of the cigarettes smoked and interactions with other exposures modify the incidence of lung cancer. We describe the evidence that tobacco also causes cancer in other body organs, and that different forms of tobacco smoking – cigars, pipes, *bidis* – are all carcinogenic. We also review current evidence for the carcinogenicity of 'passive' exposure to cigarette smoke. More detailed summaries of studies on these aspects of tobacco smoking are given in an IARC monograph (IARC, 1985a), and only studies not referenced in that monograph are cited here.

In many parts of the world, tobacco is chewed or snuffed. These practices have been common for centuries in Asia, Africa and other areas and have seen a recrudescence in western countries recently. The carcinogenic effects of these forms of tobacco consumption are also described, based mainly on the IARC monograph on this subject (IARC, 1985b).

Lung cancer and cigarette smoking

The increases in the incidence of and mortality from lung cancer observed in most populations of the world can be related reasonably clearly to patterns of tobacco consumption, as described in Part I (p. 62). A considerable number of investigations conducted in different countries, on different subsets of the general population and with different designs have consistently reported an increase in the occurrence of lung cancer among smokers in comparison with nonsmokers. The results of some of the major cohort studies are summarized in Table 14. All of these investigations show a clear-cut dose–response relationship between the amount smoked daily and the subsequent risk for lung cancer, with a risk about 20 times higher for smokers of one pack a day for 30 years or more, as compared to nonsmokers. The association has been shown particularly for squamous-cell carcinoma of the bronchi, the histological type that has increased dramatically in incidence among males during this century; small-cell and oat-cell carcinomas

-169-

and adenocarcinomas also occur more frequently among smokers than among nonsmokers. Cigarette smoke induces malignant tumours of the respiratory tract in experimental animals, and it contains chemicals known to produce cancer in animals and humans.

Table 14. Risks of male cigarette smokers for dying from lung cancer relative to nonsmokers, in some major cohort studies

Country	No. of subjects in study	Daily no. of cigarettes	Relative risk[a]	Reference
USA	440 558	0	1.0	Hammond (1966)
		1-9	4.6	
		10-19	7.5	
		20-39	13.1	
		$\geq$40	16.6	
Japan	122 261	0	1.0	Hirayama (1974)
		1-9	1.9	
		10-14	3.5	
		15-24	4.1	
		25-49	4.6	
		$\geq$50	5.7	
Sweden	27 342	0	1.0	Cederlöf *et al.*
		1-7	2.1	(1975)
		8-15	8.0	
		$\geq$16	12.6	
UK	34 440	0	1.0	Doll & Peto (1976)
		1-14	7.8	
		15-24	12.7	
		$\geq$25	25.1	

[a] Ratio between the occurrence rate of cancer among smokers and that among nonsmokers

Cancers in other organs

Tobacco smoking is causally associated not only with cancer of the lung but also with cancers of the upper respiratory tract (lip, oral cavity, pharynx, larynx), upper digestive tract (oesophagus), pancreas, bladder and renal pelvis. In the cohort and case–control studies, dose–response relationships between the number of cigarettes smoked and risks for developing cancers at these sites have been found consistently.

Tobacco smoking (particularly of cigarettes) is an important cause of cancers of the bladder and renal pelvis, and the relationships of risk with duration and intensity of smoking are similar to those for lung cancer, although the risks are lower (Rebelakos *et al.*, 1985; Claude *et al.*, 1986; Hartge *et al.*, 1987; Iscovich *et al.*, 1987; Schifflers *et al.*, 1987). Table 15 gives the results of only a few of the investigations, all of which showed consistent findings.

Table 15. Risks for cancer of the bladder of male cigarette smokers relative to those for nonsmokers

Country	Daily no. of cigarettes	Relative risk[a]	Reference
USA	Nonsmokers	1.0	Wynder & Goldsmith
	1-10	1.4	(1977)
	11-20	2.4	
	21-30	2.7	
	31-40	2.3	
	≥ 41	3.3	
Canada	Nonsmokers	1.0	Howe *et al.* (1980)
	< 10	2.6	
	10-20	3.8	
	> 20	5.1	
Italy	Nonsmokers	1.0	Vineis *et al.* (1984)
	1-14	4.0	
	15-29	5.7	
	≥ 30	10.1	
USA	Nonsmokers	1.0	Morrison *et al.* (1984)
	< 1 pack/day	1.4	
	1-< 2 packs/day	3.2	
	2+ packs/day	4.7	
UK	Nonsmokers	1.0	Morrison *et al.* (1984)
	< 1 pack/day	1.9	
	1-< 2 packs/day	3.2	
	≥ 2 packs/day	4.0	
Japan	Nonsmokers	1.0	Morrison *et al.* (1984)
	< 1 pack/day	1.6	
	1-< 2 packs/day	2.1	
	≥ 2 packs/day	2.8	
USA	< 20 cigarettes/day	1.8	Hartge *et al.* (1987)
	20-39 cigarettes/day	2.6	
	> 40 cigarettes/day	2.6	

[a] Ratio between the occurrence rate of cancer among smokers and that among nonsmokers

In nondrinking male cigarette smokers, the risk for developing cancer of the oral cavity is about double that of nondrinking nonsmokers. Elevations of ten fold or more have been seen for cancer of the larynx (De Stefani *et al.*, 1987; Tuyns *et al.*, 1988) and a five- to six-fold increase for cancer of the oesophagus (Tuyns *et al.*, 1977; Victora *et al.*, 1987; Table 16).

Cancer of the pancreas has been associated with cigarette smoking in several different studies, the risk among smokers being two to three times that of nonsmokers. Table 17 gives the results of two case–control investigations that show the dose–response relationship. In a more recent study (Mack *et al.*, 1986), an increased risk was found both in current smokers and in ex-smokers who had stopped smoking fewer than ten years previously, with a dose–response relationship: relative risks were 4.3 and 5.7 in smokers of <1 pack and >1 pack daily, respectively.

Table 16. Risks for cancers of the upper digestive and respiratory tracts in male smokers relative to that of nonsmokers who drink little or no alcohol

Site	Amount smoked	Relative risk	Reference
Larynx	1-15 g tobacco/day	3.0	Wynder *et al.* (1976)
	16-34 g tobacco/day	6.0	
	35+ g tobacco/day	7.0	
	1-15 cigarettes[a]	2.0	Burch *et al.* (1981)
	15-29 cigarettes	3.9	
	≥30 cigarettes	7.6	
Intrinsic larynx	1-9 cigarettes/day	1.7	Elwood *et al.* (1984)
	10-19 cigarettes/day	2.1	
	20-29 cigarettes/day	4.0	
	≥30 cigarettes/day	3.9	
Oesophagus	10-19 g tobacco/day	3.4	Tuyns *et al.* (1977)
	≥20 g tobacco/day	5.1	
Endolarynx	0 cigarette/day	1.0	Tuyns *et al.* (1988)
	1-7 cigarettes/day	2.4	
	8-15 cigrettes/day	6.7	
	16-25 cigarettes/day	13.7	
	≥26 cigarettes/day	16.4	
Hypolarynx/ Epilarynx	0 cigarette/day	1.0	Tuyns *et al.* (1988)
	1-7 cigarettes/day	4.2	
	8-15 cigarettes/day	10.8	
	16-25 cigarettes/day	15.8	
	≥26 cigarettes/day	16.1	

[a] x 10 000 lifetime consumption

Table 17. Risks for cancer of the pancreas in cigarette smokers relative to that for nonsmokers

Daily no. of cigarettes	Relative risk		Reference
	Males	Females	
0	1.0	1.0	Wynder *et al.* (1983)
1-10	0.9	1.8	
11-20	2.1	1.5	
21-30	2.3	2.0	
≥31	3.0		
0	1.0		Whittemore *et al.* (1983)
1-9	1.0		
10-19	2.1		
20-29	2.4		
≥30	2.5		

Cancer of the cervix has been associated with cigarette smoking in a number of studies (La Vecchia *et al.*, 1986). The general level of risk in smokers compared to nonsmokers is of the order of 2.0, after taking account of other risk factors for the disease, although these factors are difficult to control for adequately.

The risk for cancer of the kidney has been found to be elevated among cigarette smokers, and a causal nature of this association may be plausible. Cancers of the nasal cavity and paranasal sinuses have been associated with smoking in three studies (Brinton *et al.*, 1984; Fukuda *et al.*, 1987; Hayes *et al.*, 1987). Cancers of the stomach and liver are seen, but whether they are related causally to tobacco smoking is still uncertain (Austin & Cole, 1986; Austin *et al.*, 1986; Severson, 1987).

Forms of tobacco smoking

Most of the evidence summarized above relates to cigarette smoking, yet in many parts of the world other forms of tobacco are used, ranging from pipes, cigars and cigarillos in the western world, to *bidis* and other traditional forms of smoking tobacco, especially in parts of Asia.

In most studies of lifelong pipe and cigar smokers, the risk for dying from lung cancer is intermediate between that of nonsmokers and that of smokers both of pipes or cigars and cigarettes (mixed smokers) (Benhamou *et al.*, 1986). In other studies in western Europe where smoking only of pipes or cigars is common, the risk has been shown to be at the same level as that for cigarette smokers. Pipe smoking has for long been associated with cancer of the lip, and pipe and cigar smoking appear to induce approximately the same risks for oral, pharyngeal, laryngeal and oesophageal cancer as does cigarette smoking, but a lower risk for bladder cancer than cigarettes.

The relationship between *bidi* smoking and lung cancer risk has been evaluated in two case–control studies in Bombay, India, which show significant increases in the risk for lung cancer, with dose–response relationships. Another study in Bombay indicated that people who smoked *bidis* had a higher risk for oral cavity cancer than those who smoked cigarettes.

Cancer of the cervix has been associated with cigarette smoking in a number of studies (La Vecchia *et al.*, 1986). The general level of risk in smokers compared to nonsmokers is of the order of 2.0, after taking account of other risk factors for the disease, although these factors are difficult to control for adequately.

Role of age at start, duration and cessation of smoking

The annual death rate from lung cancer in people aged 55–64 is about three times higher for those who started smoking at age 15 than for those who started at age 25, for smokers of 21–39 cigarettes/day. Other studies have shown that people who started smoking at around 15–20 years of age have a higher relative risk for getting lung cancer than those who start at 25 or later, taking account of the total duration of smoking and the amount smoked daily.

Duration of smoking appears to be an extremely critical factor. A maximal impact on the incidence of lung cancer in a population occurs when that population has attained a maximal prevalence of smoking which has continued throughout most of the lifespan of the smokers. This effect has been identified by studying specific birth cohorts (see Part I, p. 62). The consequence is that, for many populations (especially those of the developing countries), the full impact of current smoking rates on future lung cancer risk will not be seen for many years.

When a person stops smoking, his excess risk for lung cancer remains, but some studies suggest that his risk may approximate that of nonsmokers with time (see Part IV, p. 307). Similar effects of cessation of smoking have been shown for cancers of the bladder (Vineis *et al.*, 1988; Hartge *et al.*, 1987) and larynx (Tuyns *et al.*, 1988).

Role of gender

Although rates for tobacco-associated cancers are almost invariably lower in females than in males, the difference is due predominantly to a different distribution of the intensity and duration of cigarette smoking. Thus, in countries where cigarette smoking was taken up extensively by women around the time of the Second World War, there have been major and accelerating increases in mortality from lung cancer among women, with a progressive reduction in male:female sex ratios. In the USA, for example, lung cancer is now overtaking breast cancer as the leading cause of death from cancer among women, whereas in countries where cigarette smoking was taken up more recently by women at later ages, hardly any increase has been detected.

Males and females do not appear to have differential susceptibility to the induction of lung cancer by cigarettes. Thus, Garfinkel and Stellman (1988) demonstrated equivalent effects in females to males for equivalent amounts smoked.

Similar effects are seen for cancers at other sites: although the risk for bladder cancer due to cigarette smoking is lower in females than in males, this effect appears to be related to differences in amount smoked or age at start.

Role of cigarette composition

Over the last two decades, cigarette design has changed considerably, affecting smoke composition and the yields of what is commonly known as 'tar'. 'Tar' consists in fact of all solid particles in cigarette smoke with diameters greater than 0.1 μm and some of the vapours and gases trapped within the particles. The changes in the composition of cigarettes include the introduction of filters to remove a certain amount of 'tar', porous paper to increase air flow and changes in type of tobacco. Because of the importance of duration of smoking, it is unlikely that the full effects of these changes on disease rates have yet been seen, as few of the people who are now developing smoking-associated disease will have been able to smoke only cigarettes with 'low tar' levels. However, some studies do suggest greater risks for lung cancer among people who smoked only the types of cigarettes that were available until the late 1950s than among people who smoked mainly filter or low-tar cigarettes. Similar reductions in risk for smokers of filter compared to non-filter cigarettes have been demonstrated for bladder cancer (Hartge *et al.*, 1987; IARC, 1987) and laryngeal cancer (Tuyns *et al.*, 1988). Wynder and Stellman (1979) also evaluated the effect of long-term use of filter cigarettes on the risk for laryngeal cancer. After adjusting for duration and quantity of tobacco use and alcohol consumption, the relative risk for users of nonfilter cigarettes *versus* that of long-term (ten years or more) users of filter cigarettes was 1.5 in men and 4.0 in women.

If this effect is strong, there should be a corresponding reduction in the rates of lung cancer in countries where tar levels have been reduced (largely in western Europe, the Nordic countries, North America and Australasia). Of particular interest are the major reductions in lung cancer rates occurring in England and Wales and in Finland, where tobacco usage had reached its peak by 1960 and remained constant thereafter, and where lung cancer rates in people of all ages would have also been expected to remain constant or to continue to rise. In Finland, mortality from lung cancer from about 1968 was reduced in men of all ages under 50, and some reduction in men aged 55–64 was also seen. In England and Wales, mortality from lung cancer in men began to decline in about 1955 in those aged 35–39, in men aged 40–54 five years later, in men aged 55–59 ten years later and in men aged 60–64 fifteen years later (Wald *et al.*, 1988), showing a mixture of effects on birth cohort and on people of all ages. During the same period, complex changes in cigarette usage were occurring. In males under the age of 40, cigarette consumption was approximately constant over the period 1950–75, but there was a reduction among older men and in men under the age of 40 in 1976–85. In addition, changes in the type of tobacco smoked and a switch to the use of filter cigarettes brought about a 30% reduction in the average amount of tar delivered per cigarette between 1955 and 1975 and a further 25% reduction between 1975 and 1985 (Wald *et al.*, 1988). This change, coupled with the stability of cigarette consumption by younger men, results in an effect of lowering tar levels on the reduction in mortality from lung cancer.

Following the Clean Air Act in the UK in 1956, there was a substantial reduction in air pollution, which may have had some effect on lung cancer rates, although the amount is difficult to quantify. The effect of this reduction is discussed further below (p. 229).

Interaction with other exposures

Alcohol consumption, exposure to asbestos and exposure to ionizing radiation have been studied in several investigations in relation to their interaction with the carcinogenic effects of smoking. Table 18 shows that the risks for laryngeal cancer among smokers increase considerably with increasing levels of alcohol consumption, suggesting a multiplication of the separate risks for the two exposures. These are discussed in detail on p. 305. Similar patterns have been found for cancers of the oral cavity and of the pharynx. The results of other studies, however, are at variance with these patterns, some indicating a lower and others a higher joint effect of the two exposures, in comparison with the effect represented by a multiplication of the respective risks (Saracci, 1987).

In evaluating the proportion of oesophageal cancer due to consumption of alcohol and of tobacco, respectively, the results of several large studies were analysed; their combined effects are discussed on p. 299. The joint effects of exposure to ionizing radiation and tobacco smoking are discussed on p. 158.

An example of the multiplicative effect of joint exposure to asbestos and cigarette smoking is given in Table 19, based on a cohort study of 17 800 insulation workers. Other studies of this interaction give less clear-cut results. It is noteworthy, however, from the point of view of public health, that quitting smoking can considerably lower the risk for lung cancer among people who were exposed to asbestos in the past.

Table 18. Risks for cancer of the hypopharynx/epilarynx and of the endolarynx according to daily consumption of tobacco and alcohol[a]

Alcohol consumption (g ethanol/day)	Tobacco consumption (no. of cigarettes/day)			
	0-7	8-15	16-25	26+
Hypopharynx/epilarynx				
0-40	1.0	4.6	13.9	4.9
41-80	3.0	15.6	19.5	18.4
81-120	5.5	27.5	48.2	37.6
≥121	14.7	71.6	67.8	135.5
Endolarynx				
0-40	1.0	6.7	12.7	11.5
41-80	1.6	5.9	12.2	18.5
81-120	2.3	10.7	21.0	23.5
≥121	3.8	12.2	31.5	43.2

[a] From Tuyns *et al.* (1988); risks are expressed relative to those of people who consume 0-40 g ethanol/day and 0-7 g tobacco/day

Table 19. Joint effects on mortality from lung cancer of cigarette smoking and exposure to asbestos in male insulation workers[a]

Category of exposure	Mortality rates from lung cancer (per 100 000 per year)	Risk[b]
Smoking plus asbestos	601.6	53.2
Asbestos only (nonsmokers)	58.4	5.2
Smoking only (not exposed to asbestos)	122.6	10.8
Nonsmokers not exposed to asbestos	11.3	1.0

[a] From Hammond *et al.* (1979)
[b] Relative to that of nonsmokers not exposed to asbestos

Passive exposure to environmental tobacco smoke

Attention was first directed to the potential carcinogenicity of tobacco smoke released into the ambient air (environmental tobacco smoke; ETS) by two studies showing an increased risk for lung cancer in-nonsmoking women married to smoking men (Hirayama, 1981; Trichopoulos *et al.*, 1981). The topic has subsequently been the object of a number of epidemiological investigations and has been under continuous discussion and review. In 1986, a US National Research Council Report made a summary estimate on the basis of the results of ten case-control studies and three cohort studies of the relative increase in risk for lung cancer in nonsmoking spouses of smokers of 20–50%. This estimate remains essentially unchanged by the results of eight subsequent case–control investigations. It should be noted, however, that it is difficult to measure exposure to ETS and to be sure that self-declared nonsmokers actually do not smoke. An evaluation of the carcinogenic risk deriving from exposure to ETS must include other sources of evidence as well. For instance, it is known that sidestream smoke, the smoke formed in between puffs and emitted into the air, contains higher concentrations of *N*-nitroso compounds and aromatic amines than mainstream smoke, the smoke taken in by smokers. Given that persons exposed passively to ETS are exposed to many of the same components that cause cancer in smokers and that a quantitative, nonthreshold relationship between dose and effect is observed for exposure to tobacco smoke, it can be reasonably inferred that passive exposure to ETS gives rise to some risk for cancer (Saracci & Riboli, 1989).

Tobacco chewing and snuffing

Use of 'smokeless' tobacco is an important cause of cancer of the oral cavity. The evidence, derived largely from case–control studies but increasingly also from cohort studies, indicates that long-term users of quids (plugs) containing tobacco are at substantially increased risk for developing oral cancer. Use of small packets of snuff, which are retained between the cheek and the gum, has increased recently, especially among young males; it is estimated that in the USA, up to 17% of boys aged 11–15 regularly use this type of product. Risks two to three times higher than among those who do not have this habit have also been reported for cancers of the pharynx, larynx and oesophagus. Tobacco-specific *N*-nitrosamines are possibly implicated, as they are found in relatively high concentrations in the saliva of tobacco and betel-quid chewers. Some studies from South Africa support the hypothesis that nasal inhalation of snuff increases the risks for cancers of the nasal cavity and of the paranasal sinuses, while studies in both South Africa and North America suggest that oral use of snuff may also increase the risk for nasal cancer.

Betel-quid and areca-nut chewing

The habit of chewing betel quid (betel leaf, areca nut and lime) is at least two thousand years old. Reports of an association between oral cancer and the habit of chewing betel quid started to appear in the medical literature during the late nineteenth century. In many parts of the world, particularly in the Indian subcontinent, tobacco is added to the quid; whether chewing betel quids that do not contain tobacco is carcinogenic has been the subject of some controversy. The evidence summarized here is considered in more detail in the monograph on this topic (IARC, 1985b), in which relevant references are given.

Epidemiological evidence comes from several, mainly indirect, sources. In Papua New Guinea, where most people chew betel quids that do not contain tobacco, the oral cavity is the most common site of cancer. It has been found further that the occurrence of oral cancer correlated well with the known distribution of the betel chewing habit and that the site in the mouth at which most of the cancer cases occurred was consistent with the reported site distribution among betel chewers in other parts of the world. In Malaysia, oral cancer is common in the Indian community but rare among Malays: both chew betel quids, but Indians add tobacco to their quid whereas Malays do not. Similarly, in two studies in other parts of Asia, the habit of chewing betel quid without tobacco did not seem to increase the risk for oral cancer.

A large study was conducted of patients with cancers of the oral cavity, pharynx and oesophagus in Bombay, India. Although the number of cases who claimed to chew betel quid without tobacco was much smaller than that of cases who chewed with tobacco or of non-chewers, the risks for cancers of the oral cavity and pharynx were similar in the two groups of chewers. For oesophageal cancer, however, the risk was higher for people who chewed betel quid without tobacco than for those who added tobacco. The explanation given was that chewers of betel quid without tobacco habitually swallow most of the liquid, in contrast to those who add tobacco. In Pakistan, there seemed to be a significantly increased risk for oral cancer associated with the habit of chewing betel quid without tobacco.

References

Austin, H. & Cole, P. (1986) Cigarette smoking and leukaemia. *J. Chronic Dis.*, *39*, 417-421

Austin, H., Delzell, E., Grufferman, S., Levine, R., Morrison, A.S., Stolley, P.D. & Cole, P. (1986) A case-control study of hepatocellular carcinoma and the hepatitis B virus, cigarette smoking, and alcohol consumption. *Cancer Res.*, *46*, 962-966

Benhamou, S., Benhamou, E. & Flamant, R. (1986) Lung cancer risk associated with cigar and pipe smoking. *Int. J. Cancer*, *37*, 825-829

Brinton, L.A., Blot, W.J., Becker, J.A., Winn, D.M., Browder, J.P., Farmer, J.C., Jr & Fraumeni, J.F., Jr (1984) A case-control study of cancers of the nasal cavity and paranasal sinuses. *Am. J. Epidemiol.*, *119*, 896-906

Burch, J.D., Howe, G.R., Miller, A.B. & Semenciw, R. (1981) Tobacco, alcohol, asbestos, and nickel in the etiology of cancer of the larynx: a case-control study. *J. Natl Cancer Inst.*, *67*, 1219-1224

Cederlöf, R., Friberg, L., Hrubec, Z. & Lorich, U. (1975) *The Relationship of Smoking and Some Social Covariables to Mortality and Cancer Morbidity. A Ten Year Follow-up in a Probability Sample of 55,000 Swedish Subjects, Age 18-69*, Part 1 and Part 2, Stockholm, Department of Environmental Hygiene, Karolinska Institute

Claude, J., Kunze, E., Frentzel-Beyme, R., Paczkowski, K., Schneider, J. & Schubert, H. (1986) Life-style and occupational risk factors in cancer of the lower urinary tract. *Am. J. Epidemiol.*, *124*, 578-589

De Stefani, E., Correa, P., Oreggia, F., Leiva, J., Rivero, S., Fernandez, G., Deneo-Pellegrini, H., Zavala, D. & Fontham, E. (1987) Risk factors for laryngeal cancer. *Cancer*, *60*, 3087-3091

Doll, R. & Hill, A.B. (1950) Smoking and carcinoma of the lung. Preliminary report. *Br. Med. J.*, *ii*, 739-748

Doll, R. & Peto, R. (1976) Mortality in relation to smoking: 20 years' observations on male British doctors. *Br. Med. J.*, *ii*, 1525-1536

Elwood, J.M., Pearson, J.C.G., Skippen, D.H. & Jackson, S.M. (1984) Alcohol, smoking, social and occupational factors in the aetiology of cancer of the oral cavity, pharynx and larynx. *Int. J. Cancer*, *34*, 603-612

Fukuda, K., Shibata, A. & Harada, K. (1987) Squamous cell cancer of the maxillary sinus in Hokkaido, Japan: a case-control study. *Br. J. Ind. Med.*, *44*, 263-266

Garfinkel, L. & Stellman, S.D. (1988) Smoking and lung cancer in women: findings in a prospective study. *Cancer Res.*, *48*, 6951-6955

Hammond, E.C. (1966) Smoking in relation to the death rates of one million men and women. *Natl Cancer Inst. Monogr.*, *19*, 127-204

Hammond, E.C., Selikoff, I.J. & Seidman, H. (1979) Asbestos exposure, cigarette smoking and death rates. *Ann. N.Y. Acad. Sci.*, *330*, 473-490

Hartge, P., Silverman, D., Hoover, R., Schairer, C., Altman, R., Austin, D., Cantor, K., Child, M., Key, C., Marrett, L.D., Mason, T.J., Meigs, J.W., Myers, M.H., Narayana, A., Sullivan, J.W., Swanson, G.M., Thomas, D. & West, D. (1987) Changing cigarette habits and bladder cancer risk: a case-control study. *J. Natl Cancer Inst.*, *78*, 1119-1125

Hayes, R.B., Kardaun, J.W.P.F. & de Bruyn, A. (1987) Tobacco and sinonasal cancer: a case-control study. *Br. J. Cancer*, *56*, 843-846

Hirayama, T. (1974) Epidemiology of lung cancer based on population studies. In: Finkel, A.J. & Duel, W.C., eds, *Clinical Implications of Air Pollution Research*, Acton, MA, Publishing Sciences Group, pp. 69-78

Hirayama, T. (1981) Non-smoking wives of heavy smokers have a higher risk of lung cancer. A study from Japan. *Br. Med. J.*, *282*, 183-185

Howe, G.R., Burch, J.D., Miller, A.B., Cook, G.M., Estève, J., Morrison, B., Gordon, P., Chambers, L.W., Fodor, G. & Winsor, G.M. (1980) Tobacco use, occupation, coffee, various nutrients, and bladder cancer. *J. Natl Cancer Inst.*, *64*, 701-713

IARC (1985a) *IARC Monographs on the Evaluation of the Carcinogenic Risk of Chemicals to Humans*, Vol. 38, *Tobacco Smoking*, Lyon

IARC (1985b) *IARC Monographs on the Evaluation of the Carcinogenic Risk of Chemicals to Humans*, Vol. 37, *Tobacco Habits Other than Smoking; Betel-quid and Areca-nut Chewing; and Some Related Nitrosamines*, Lyon

IARC (1987) *IARC Monographs on the Evaluation of Carcinogenic Risks to Humans*, Suppl. 7, *Overall Evaluations of Carcinogenicity: An Updating of IARC Monographs Volumes 1-42*, Lyon, pp. 359-362

Iscovich, J., Castelletto, R., Estève, J., Muñoz, N., Colanzi, R., Coronel, A., Deamezola, I., Tassi, V. & Arslan, A. (1987) Tobacco smoking, occupational exposure and bladder cancer in Argentina. *Int. J. Cancer*, *40*, 734-740

LaVecchia, C., Franceschi, S., De Carli, A., Fasoli, M., Gentile, A. & Tognoni, G. (1986) Cigarette smoking and the risk of cervical neoplasia. *Am. J. Epidemiol.*, *123*, 22-29

Mack, T.M., Yu, M.C., Hanisch, R. & Henderson, B.E. (1986) Pancreas cancer and smoking, beverage consumption, and past medical history. *J. Natl Cancer Inst.*, *76*, 49-60

Morrison, A.S., Buring, J.E., Verhoek, W.G., Aoki, K., Leck, I., Ohno, Y. & Obata, K. (1984) An international study of smoking and bladder cancer. *J. Urol.*, *131*, 650-654

Rebelakos, A., Trichopoulos, D., Tzonou, A., Zavitsanos, X., Velonakis, E. & Trichopoulou, A. (1985) Tobacco smoking, coffee drinking, and occupation as risk factors for bladder cancer in Greece. *J. Natl Cancer Inst.*, *75*, 455-461

Saracci, R. (1987) The interactions of tobacco smoking and other agents in cancer etiology. *Epidemiol. Rev.*, *9*, 175-193

Saracci, R. & Riboli, E. (1989) Passive smoking and lung cancer: current evidence and ongoing studies at the International Agency for Research on Cancer. *Mutat. Res.*, *222*, 117-127

Schifflers, E., Jamart, J. & Renard, V. (1987) Tobacco and occupation as risk factors in bladder cancer: a case-control study in southern Belgium. *Int. J. Cancer*, *39*, 287-292

Severson, R.K. (1987) Cigarette smoking and leukemia. *Cancer*, *60*, 141-144

Trichopoulos, D., Kalandidi, A., Sparros, L. & MacMahon, B. (1981) Lung cancer and passive smoking. *Int. J. Cancer*, *27*, 1-4

Tuyns, A.J., Péquignot, G. & Jensen, O.M. (1977) Oesophageal cancer in Ille et Villaine in relation to alcohol and tobacco consumption. Multiplicative risks (in French). *Bull. Cancer*, *64*, 45-60

Tuyns, A.J., Estève, J., Raymond, L., Berrino, F., Benhamou, E., Blanchet, F., Boffetta, P., Crosignani, P., del Moral, A., Lehmann, W., Merletti, F., Péquignot, G., Riboli, E., Sancho-Garnier, H., Terracini, B., Zubiri, A. & Zubiri, L. (1988) Cancer of the larynx/hypopharynx, tobacco and alcohol. *Int. J. Cancer*, *41*, 483-491

Victora, C.G., Muñoz, N., Day, N.E., Barcelos, L.B., Peccin, D.A. & Braga, N.M. (1987) Hot beverages and oesophageal cancer in southern Brazil: a case-control study. *Int. J. Cancer*, *39*, 710-716

Vineis, P., Estève, J. & Terracini, B. (1984) Bladder cancer and smoking in males: types of cigarettes, age at start, effect of stopping and interaction with occupation. *Int. J. Cancer*, *34*, 165-170

Vineis, P., Estève, J., Hartge, P., Hoover, R., Silverman, D.T. & Terracini, B. (1988) Effects of timing and type of tobacco in cigarette-induced bladder cancer. *Cancer Res.*, *48*, 3849-3852

Wald, N., Kiryluk, S., Darby, S., Pike, M. & Peto, R. (1988) *UK Smoking Statistics*, Oxford, Oxford University Press

Whittemore, A.S., Paffenbarger, R.S., Jr, Anderson, K. & Halpern, J. (1983) Early precursors of pancreatic cancer in college men. *J. Chronic Dis.*, *36*, 251-256

Wynder, E.L. & Goldsmith, R. (1977) The epidemiology of bladder cancer. A second look. *Cancer*, *40*, 1246-1268

Wynder, E.L. & Graham, E.A. (1950) Tobacco smoking as a possible etiologic factor in bronchogenic carcinoma. A study of six hundred and eighty-four proved cases. *J. Am. Med. Assoc.*, *143*, 329-336

Wynder, E.L. & Stellman, S.D. (1979) The impact of long-term filter cigarette usage on lung and larynx cancer risk: a case-control study. *J. Natl Cancer Inst.*, *62*, 471-477

Wynder, E.L., Covey, L.S., Mabuchi, K. & Mushinski, M. (1976) Environmental factors in cancer of the larynx. A second look. *Cancer*, *38*, 1591-1601

Wynder, E.L., Hall, N.E.I. & Polansky, M. (1983) Epidemiology of coffee and pancreatic cancer. *Cancer Res.*, *43*, 3900-3906

Chapter 10. Alcohol drinking

During the first few decades of this century, it was suggested on the basis of anecdotal evidence that excessive consumption of alcoholic beverages might be associated with an increased risk for cancer. Thus, in Paris, France, some 80% of cases of oesophageal and cardial stomach cancer were observed to be in alcoholics, most of whom were absinthe drinkers; and national statistics from various countries showing the numbers of deaths in different occupational groups showed high risks for cancers at several sites among persons employed in the production and distribution of alcoholic beverages, who presumably have easier access to them than other people. These initial observations have since been corroborated by numerous studies of alcohol consumption and cancer occurrence in individuals, and there is now overwhelming evidence that intake of alcohol increases the risk for cancer in humans.

There is consistent, strong evidence that drinking alcoholic beverages increases the risk for developing cancers of the oral cavity, pharynx, larynx, oesophagus and liver. There is no indication that the effect is dependent on type of beverage. It is clear that the risks for these cancers are multiplied in people who also smoke. Evidence for the carcinogenic risks associated with drinking alcohol was reviewed in a recent IARC monograph (IARC, 1988), on which the following is based and which gives the relevant references.

Cancers of the oral cavity and pharynx

Increased risks for dying from oro-pharyngeal cancer have been observed among persons in occupations in which there are possibilities for drinking large amounts of alcohol, such as brewery workers, and among alcoholics, whereas populations in which the majority of people abstain from drinking alcohol, such as Seventh-day Adventists and Mormons in the USA, have lower risks for cancers at these sites than the general population. Thus, among a large number of Danish brewery workers, who were not alcoholics but who had an above-average consumption of beer, the incidence of pharyngeal cancer was twice as high as that in the general population. Many of the studies show that the risks for cancers of the mouth and pharynx increase with increasing consumption of alcohol. The multiplicative interaction between alcohol and tobacco in inducing cancer of the mouth was noted in some of the early studies in the USA and was confirmed in the large study on cancers of the hypopharynx/epilarynx conducted in Europe (see Table 18).

Cancer of the larynx

In most studies of alcoholics, the risk for laryngeal cancer has been found to be increased in comparison to nonalcoholics. Among the Danish brewery workers, the risk was twice as high as that of the general population.

The role of alcohol in causing laryngeal cancer has been investigated in detail in a number of case-control studies in which the part of the risk that is due to tobacco smoking could be estimated. In the USA, the risk was found to increase with the amount of whisky taken daily, from 1.2–1.7 for people who drank one to six shots a day to 2.3–5.6 for those who drank seven shots or more per day. Later studies from the USA, Canada, Denmark and Uruguay corroborated the finding that the risk for laryngeal cancer increases with increasing daily consumption of alcohol. The interaction between alcohol and tobacco was again found to be multiplicative.

Cancer of the oesophagus

A high prevalence of alcoholism among patients with oesophageal cancer was noted early on in a number of different countries. Further, the risk for this disease was also seen to be increased among persons employed in the production and distribution of alcoholic beverages. Alcoholics almost invariably have a higher risk than the general population. The study of nonalcoholic brewery workers in Denmark again showed a two-fold increase in risk over that expected. Unfortunately, in none of these studies was information on tobacco smoking available.

Clear dose–response relationships have been observed for oesophageal cancer with the amount of alcohol consumed daily. In an early study, the risk among drinkers of seven or more units of whisky per day was approximately 25 times higher than that of light drinkers, and a dose–response relationship was also seen for beer consumers. The relationship between increasing risk for oesophageal cancer and increasing consumption of alcohol was confirmed in two large studies carried out in northern France (Table 20). A multiplication of risk was seen in heavy drinkers who also smoked heavily. Associations between alcohol consumption and cancer of the oesophagus were also found in studies in Singapore, Uruguay, Brazil and Switzerland.

Table 20. Relative risks for oesophageal cancer in relation to average daily alcohol consumption by males in Brittany and Normandy, France[a]

Alcohol consumption (g ethanol/day)	All males	Nonsmokers	
		Males	Females
0-40	1.0	1.0	1.0
41-80	4.0	3.8	5.6
81-120	6.3	10.1	11.0
≥121	30.9	101.0	-

[a] Risks are relative to those of persons who drank 0-40 g alcohol/day and smoked 0-9 g of tobacco/day

Primary liver cancer

An increased frequency of primary liver cancer has been observed in people with a high alcohol intake in a number of studies, although not consistently. Thus, of four cohort studies of the general population, two showed a significantly increased risk for this cancer among drinkers of alcoholic beverages, whereas in a third study, an increase was seen only in a subgroup of persons. Associations between high intake of alcoholic beverages and liver cancer were seen in eight of ten cohort studies and six of ten case–control studies. An analysis of the results of the ten cohort studies showed that alcoholics have a 50% greater risk for primary liver cancer than nonalcoholics. A particularly strong association between consumption of alcoholic beverages and primary liver cancer was demonstrated in a cohort study of blood donors who had antibodies against hepatitis B surface antigen. A major problem in establishing a relationship between alcohol drinking and liver cancer is that primary liver cancer is often misdiagnosed, and might therefore be overlooked as a cause of death, which is attributed to some other disease. Furthermore, in only a few studies have other risk factors for primary liver cancer been taken into consideration. However, in studies in which potential confounding due to hepatitis B virus, tobacco smoking and aflatoxin was explored, it did not alter the findings qualitatively.

Cancers at other sites

The evidence that the risk for *cancer of the stomach* is increased in people with a high consumption of alcohol is conflicting: in only two case–control studies was a strong association found, and in one of these only for people who drank vodka before breakfast! It is not known to what extent dietary and socioeconomic factors play a role in increasing the risk for this cancer.

In studies in many countries, correlations have been observed between the frequency of *cancer of the rectum* and beer consumption; however, in other studies, no such association was seen. The results with regard to *cancer of the colon* are less clear, and most of the studies that showed a relationship with the occurrence of rectal cancer have shown no association with cancer of the colon.

The results of 29 studies on *cancer of the pancreas* suggest that consumption of alcoholic beverages is unlikely to be related to the induction of cancer at this site.

The situation with regard to *breast cancer* is unclear, although, overall, the risk for breast cancer appears to be increased in women who drink heavily, and dose–response relationships have been observed in some recent studies. The consistency of this positive association makes it unlikely that the relationship is due to chance or to biases in the methods used in the studies; when confounding due to currently recognized risk factors for breast cancer was taken into account, the risks were still increased. The modest elevation in risk is potentially important because of the high incidence of breast cancer in many countries.

Overall, studies on cancers of the urinary bladder, kidney, lung, ovary, prostate and lymphatic and haematopoietic system show no association with consumption of alcoholic beverages. Little or no information is available on whether alcohol drinking affects the frequency of cancers at other sites.

Reference

IARC (1988) *IARC Monographs on the Evaluation of Carcinogenic Risks to Humans*, Vol. 44, *Alcohol Drinking*, Lyon, IARC

Chapter 11. Viruses and other biological agents

Viruses

Viruses may be associated with human cancer through a number of different mechanisms. Some viruses can directly transform a normal cell into a malignant one; since their continued presence is necessary for maintenance of the malignant state, the viral genome is transcribed in the cancer cells. Other viruses may be necessary only in the early phase of cell transformation, and their presence may not be required in later stages. This mechanism has been proposed for the role of herpes simplex virus-type 2 (HSV-2) in carcinoma of the cervix. Thus, at an early stage, HSV-2 infection is known to induce mutations in the cellular genome, but this viral imprint may subsequently disappear. In such cases, therefore, even though the virus might cause cancer, malignant cells may not harbour viral genomic sequences. It is not unusual that a viral infection precedes development of disease by several decades.

An apparent contradiction is that, although some viruses cause cancer directly by their presence in malignant cells, the presence of a virus in malignant cells does not necessarily mean that it is causally associated with the cancer. Many viruses remain latent within cells, and they may well be only 'passengers' who have nothing to do with the malignant process. This possibility cannot be excluded for some of the apparent associations described below, including that between Epstein–Barr virus and nasopharyngeal carcinoma.

Hepatitis B virus

Several epidemiological studies and laboratory investigations have established that there is a strong and specific association between infection with hepatitis B virus (HBV) and hepatocellular carcinoma (HCC) (Beasley *et al.*, 1981). The association is restricted to the chronically active forms of HBV infection, which are characterized by the presence in serum of the hepatitis B surface antigen (HBsAg); this is referred to as 'carrier status'. There does not appear to be any association with the presence of hepatitis B antibodies alone, so that past exposure is not a risk factor.

The epidemiology of the association of HCC with HBV, reviewed by Muñoz and Linsell (1982) and Muñoz and Bosch (1987), comprises three types of study. Correlation studies have demonstrated that, in general, there is a positive correlation between the incidence of or mortality from HCC and the prevalence of HBsAg carriers in a population (Szmuness, 1978; see also Part I, p. 59). Case–control studies in high-risk populations of Africa and south-east Asia and in populations with an intermediate risk for HCC, such as in Greece, have produced estimates of the relative risk associated with the presence of HBsAg in the range of 10–20 (Prince *et al.*, 1975; Lingao *et al.*, 1981; Trichopoulos *et al.*, 1987). In Europe and the USA, where the incidence of HCC and the prevalence of HBsAg are very low, the relative risk is higher (Tabor *et al.*, 1977; Yu *et al.*, 1983; see also Table 21).

In several cohort studies, shown in Table 22, the incidence of HCC among HBsAg carriers was found to be seven to over 100 times higher than that among a non-carrier control population. It is reasonable to assume that the relative risks observed in the cohort studies conducted in Japan and the USA are underestimates, since the method of follow-up used may have resulted in some of the cases going undetected. In contrast to the case–control studies, the prospective cohort studies provide unequivocal evidence that HBV infection precedes the development of HCC and does not appear simply as a consequence of the tumour. The relative risks estimated in these studies are among the highest observed in studies of cancer etiology. Besides being very strong, the association between HBV and HCC is also specific, because HBV is not associated with other cancers (Prince *et al.*, 1975; Beasley *et al.*, 1981) or with metastatic liver cancer (Trichopoulos *et al.*, 1978)

Two types of laboratory investigations have provided valuable information about the possible mechanism by which HBV may lead to HCC. Hybridization experiments using cloned, purified DNA from HBV have shown that it can be integrated into the genome of liver-cell lines derived from HCC (Edman *et al.*, 1980), into the genome of malignant liver cells from patients with HCC (Shafritz *et al.*, 1981; Hino *et al.*, 1985) and into the genome of liver cells of long-term symptomatic and asymptomatic HBsAg carriers (Shafritz *et al.*, 1981). The integration of HBV into DNA of patients without HCC indicates that integration itself is not sufficient for the development of HCC.

Viruses that closely resemble human HBV have been identified in three animal species: the woodchuck hepatitis virus, the ground squirrel hepatitis virus and the Chinese domestic duck virus (Summers, 1981). The woodchuck virus produces a chronic, persistent infection in woodchucks which eventually progresses to chronic active hepatitis and HCC. Moreover, integration of this virus into DNA has been demonstrated in the genomes of liver cells of woodchucks with HCC, providing a remarkable parallel to HBV and HCC. The oncogenic potential of the other two animal viruses remains to be established.

The strength, specificity and consistency of the association between HBV and HCC in several human populations, together with the clear evidence that the HBV infection precedes the development of HCC and the evidence for biological plausibility provided by laboratory investigations, indicate that the association is causal. Ultimate proof of causality will be provided by the demonstration that elimination of HBV infection by vaccination prevents HCC. Vaccination is under way in the Gambia and in China, and mass vaccination campaigns among neonates have been initiated in countries at high risk of HBV infection (Chen *et al.*, 1987; Gambia Hepatitis Study Group, 1987). These persons will be followed up for the required time to investigate the occurrence of HCC.

Herpes simplex virus-type 2

Epidemiological studies of cervical cancer have demonstrated a clear association between a woman's risk for contracting the disease and the number of sexual partners she, or her current partner, have had. This association strongly

Table 21. Case-control studies of carriers of hepatitis B virus surface antigen (HBsAg) and frequency of hepatocellular carcinoma (HCC)

Study population	No. of subjects		HBsAg+ (%)		Relative risk (95% confidence interval)	Attributable risk (%)	Reference
	HCC cases	Controls	HCC cases	Controls			
High-risk areas							
Senegal	165	328	61.2	11.3	12.4 (7.7–19.3)	56.3	Prince et al. (1975)
South Africa	289	213	61.6	11.3	12.6 (7.7–20.1)	56.7	Kew et al. (1979)
Hong Kong	107	107	82.0	18.0	21.3 (10.1–45.9)	78.5	Lam et al. (1982)
China	50	50	86.0	22.0	17.0 (4.3–99.4)	77.9	Yeh et al. (1985)
Philippines	104	84	70.0	18.0	10.83 (5.3–20.9)	63.9	Lingao et al. (1981)
Intermediate-risk area							
Greece	194	451	45.9	7.3	10.7 (6.8–16.6)	41.6	Trichopoulos et al. (1987)
Low-risk area							
USA	34	38	14.7	0.0	(1.5–∞)	–	Yarrish et al. (1980)
USA	86	161	17.9	0.0	(10.0–∞)	–	Austin et al. (1986)

suggests that a sexually transmitted agent is involved, and viruses have been considered as the most likely candidates. The viruses that most commonly infect the uterine cervix are HSV-2, human papilloma virus (HPV) and cytomegalovirus.

Table 22. Cohort studies of carriers of hepatitis B surface antigen (HBsAg) and hepatocellular carcinoma (HCC)

Study population	No. of subjects		HCC risk[a]		Reference
	Total	HBsAg+	RR or SMR (95% CI)	Attributable risk (%)	
Taiwan (1981)	22 707	3454	104.0 (51-212)	93.9	Beasley *et al.*
Japan	32 177	496	10.4 (5.0-19.1)	12.7	Iijima *et al.* (1984)
Japan, Osaka (1984)	-	8646	6.6 (4.0-10.2)	10.1[b]	Oshima *et al.*
USA, New York City	-	6850	9.7 (2.0-28.4)	1.0[c]	Prince & Alcabes (1982)
England & Wales	-	3934	42.0 (14.0-100.0)	4.0[c]	Hall *et al.* (1985)

[a] RR, relative risk; SMR, standardized mortality ratio; CI, confidence interval
[b] On the basis of a prevalence rate of HBsAg in the general population of 2.0%
[c] On the basis of a prevalence rate of HBsAg in the general population of 0.1%

Numerous case–control studies have been conducted in several geographic areas comparing the frequency of HSV-2 antibodies in women with cervical cancer and in control women. Although in most studies antibodies to HSV-2 have been found more frequently among cases than among controls, the interpretation of these results is difficult, because the serological tests used could not distinguish antibodies specific to HSV-2 but mainly antibodies common to HSV-1 and HSV-2 (Muñoz, 1978). However, in a cohort study of 10 000 women in which a technique to detect HSV-2-specific antibodies was used, no difference in the prevalence of these antibodies was found between the women who subsequently developed cervical cancer and the control women; unfortunately, the numbers involved in this study are too small for the results to be conclusive (Vonka *et al.*, 1984). Similar results were obtained in a smaller group of women (1134) enrolled in a prospective study of the development of cervical cancer in women exposed to diethylstilboestrol *in utero* (Adam *et al.*, 1985). Armstrong *et al.* (1986) suggested an association between HSV-2 infection and the current increase in the frequency of cervical intraepithelial neoplasia (CIN) among young women in Australia.

The inconclusive results of these epidemiological studies are compounded by the fact that molecular, immunological and other experimental studies have not provided clear-cut evidence that HSV-2 has oncogenic potential (Vonka *et al.*, 1987). In an attempt to reconcile the suggestive evidence derived from some of the epidemiological studies with the generally negative experimental observations, a 'hit-and-run' effect was postulated, in which HSV-2 only triggers malignancy and is not necessary at later stages (zur Hausen, 1982; Galloway & McDougall, 1983). This suggestion was followed by the presentation of a hypothesis that HSV-2 and HPV act synergistically (zur Hausen, 1986), and some supporting evidence – that viral sequences of both HSV and HPV are found simultaneously in human genital tumours – was reported subsequently (di Luca *et al.*, 1987).

Human papilloma virus

Human papilloma virus (HPV) has long been suspected of being associated with cervical cancer, but assessment of the association was hampered by the fact that the virus cannot be grown *in vitro*. This made difficult the development of appropriate laboratory tests to detect markers of HPV in human tissues and in serum. Since the DNA of HPV can now be cloned in bacteria, however, more than 60 different types of HPV have been identified, and their DNA can now be sought in cancerous and normal tissues using techniques of DNA hybridization (Orth *et al.*, 1978; zur Hausen, 1987). Serological tests to detect antibodies to these different types of HPV are still under development.

The epidemiological evidence linking HPV to cervical cancer and other genital tumours was reviewed by Muñoz *et al.* (1988). It comprises four types of data. In more than 30 reports, HPV-DNA was found in cervical specimens from patients with cervical cancer, from patients with various stages of CIN and, in some series, from women with morphologically normal cervices. The results suggest that HPV-16 and, to a lesser extent, HPV-18 are associated with advanced CIN or invasive carcinoma, while HPV-6 and -11 are found more often in association with lower-grade CIN and condylomata. In the absence of an appropriate group of controls, these results are difficult to interpret, and bias, chance or confounding cannot be ruled out.

In one ecological study, the prevalence of HPV-6/11 and of HPV-16/18 was determined in cervical scrapes from case series of women in Greenland and Denmark, using hybridization *in situ*, by examiners who did not know the disease status of the women. Unexpectedly, the prevalence of HPV-16/18 was 1.5 times higher in Denmark, where there is a six-fold lower incidence of cervical cancer than in Greenland (Kjaer *et al.*, 1989). However, in a subsequent study in Brazil, the prevalence of HPV-16/18 was higher in Recife than in São Paulo, correlating well with the incidence of cervical cancer, which is two times higher in Recife than in São Paulo (Villa & Franco, 1989). In addition, in neither of the studies was the prevalence of HPV infection correlated with the number of sexual partners or average age at first sexual intercourse, the main risk factors for cervical cancer.

Two studies have been reported in which prevalence of infection with HPV, as assessed by hybridization, was compared in cases and controls. In both, an increased risk for cancer of the cervix was found in association with infection with HPV types 16 and 18 (Reeves *et al.*, 1989; Schmauz *et al.*, 1989). In a larger study (Reeves *et al.*, 1989), infection with types 6 and 11 was also associated with cervical cancer, in contrast with the results of most series of case reports. However, as filter in-situ hybridization was used in this study (a method of low sensitivity and specificity), it is possible that cross-reactivity occurred. As in the two population surveys, prevalence of infection with HPV types 16 and 18 in the control group did not vary with age, educational level, months since last Pap smear, number of sexual partners, age at first intercourse or number of live births – all of which were considered to be risk factors for cervical cancer in these studies. These findings could suggest transmission routes for infection with HPV types 16 and 18 other than through sexual intercourse.

Three small cohorts of women with cytological evidence of HPV infection or CIN and in whom the presence of HPV-DNA was assessed by hybridization tests have been followed up. The probability of progression to more advanced CIN was greater in those infected with HPV types 16 or 18 than in those with types 6 or 11 (Campion *et al.*, 1986; Schneider *et al.*, 1987; Syrjänen *et al.*, 1987). However, there remain some uncertainties in respect of these studies, including how the subjects were selected, the timing of the hybridization tests, and whether exposure to HPV and disease assessment were ascertained without knowledge of the case status of the subjects. Some of these cohorts are being followed up, and several large case–control studies are in progress.

Other types of HPV, such as 31, 33, 35 and 39, have also been observed in women with cervical neoplasia, but little information is available about their prevalence. At present, the epidemiological evidence linking HPV infection to cervical cancer is limited both by the design of studies carried out to date and by uncertainty concerning the most appropriate means of assessing HPV infection. There is, however, substantial laboratory evidence suggesting the oncogenic potential of HPV: the HPV genome is integrated into cellular DNA in most invasive cancers, in high-degree CIN lesions and in cell lines derived from cervical cancers, and HPV-16 and other strains can transform cell lines *in vitro* (Storey *et al.*, 1988; Shah & Gissmann, 1989).

Epstein–Barr virus

The Epstein–Barr virus (EBV) was isolated from malignant Burkitt's lymphoma (BL) cells in 1964 (Epstein *et al.*, 1964), and was thus the first virus to be associated with a human cancer. Sero-epidemiological surveys have shown that it is one of the most common, widespread human viruses, affecting populations in all parts of the world (Henle & Henle, 1985). Infection usually occurs early in life (before five years of age), and 98% of the adult population in most parts of the world is infected. Infection by this virus is usually asymptomatic and persists throughout life. When infection is delayed until the second decade of life or later, as in many countries with high socioeconomic levels, EBV may cause infectious mononucleosis (Henle & Henle, 1979). It is assumed that the main route by which EBV is transmitted is through close salivary contact.

The blood target for EBV is the B lymphocytes. *In vitro*, infection of B lymphocytes by EBV leads to continuous stimulation of the cells, proliferation and immortalization of these cells into permanent cell lines. *In vivo*, the virus is thought to replicate in epithelial cells of the oropharynx (Rickinson *et al.*, 1985).

Burkitt's lymphoma

In some areas of Africa, BL is the most frequent tumour found in children, with annual incidence rates as high as ten cases per 100 000 (Magrath, 1983; see also Part I, p. 83).

BL is a well-defined pathoclinical entity comprising an undifferentiated, monoclonal lymphoma composed of malignant B cells. BL cells consistently show translocations between chromosome 8 and chromosome 14 or, less frequently chromosome 22 or 2 (Lenoir & Bornkamm, 1987). These translocations appear to result in activation of a cellular oncogene, *c-myc* (Leder *et al.*, 1983), and may represent an important step in the malignant process.

Markers of EBV (DNA or antigens) are found in 96% of tumours from people living in endemic areas in Africa, but in only 15% of so-called sporadic cases (Henle & Henle, 1985; Lenoir & Bornkamm, 1987). Thus, EBV does not seem to be implicated in the 4% of cases of BL in Africa in which no marker of EBV is found or in the 85% of cases of sporadic BL elsewhere. The results of a large seroepidemiological study conducted in Uganda (de-Thé *et al.*, 1978) was interpreted as indicating an association between high antibody titres to EBV and the development of BL. The causal role of EBV in tumours containing the EBV genome is thus supported by the epidemiological survey, but the molecular basis of EBV-induced B-cell proliferation is not yet understood and there is no formal proof at the molecular level that EBV genes are critical in the development of BL.

Other EBV-associated B-cell lymphomas

B-Cell lymphomas occur more frequently in people with depressed immunological systems. Most such lymphoproliferations are (at least at the beginning of the disease) polyclonal B-cell malignancies (arising in several cells, in contrast to BL). They are classified as diffuse lymphomas not of the BL type (Ziegler *et al.*, 1984; Kalter *et al.*, 1985) and represent proliferation of EBV-infected B-cells a long time after primary infection of individuals in whom T-cell functions have been impaired. These malignancies are observed in organ transplant recipients, who are treated with immune suppressants, and in patients with virus-induced immunodeficiencies, such as acute immune deficiency syndrome (AIDS), or genetic immunodeficiencies. EBV is implicated in those lymphomas because viral markers are detected in the proliferating cells.

Nasopharyngeal carcinoma

Nasopharyngeal carcinoma (NPC) occurs in all populations of the world but its incidence shows wide variation: it is very frequent in southern Chinese populations, rare in Europe and of intermediate incidence in Eskimos and in North Africa (see Part I, p. 53).

The presence of EBV-DNA in biopsies from NPC was first described in 1970 (zur Hausen & Schulte-Holthausen, 1970), and the association between EBV and undifferentiated and poorly differentiated carcinomas of the nasopharynx is consistent and is independent of the incidence in the population considered (Henle & Henle, 1985). Differentiated carcinomas are not associated with the virus. The association is based on the detection of viral markers (DNA or nuclear antigens) in the malignant epithelial cells (Wolf *et al.*, 1973). The EBV serology of NPC patients shows a characteristic spectrum that differs from that seen in patients with BL or infectious mononucleosis, or in the normal population (Henle *et al.*, 1979). A study in China suggested that NPC patients have elevated levels of immunoglobulin A antibodies to viral capsid antigen (Zeng *et al.*, 1982), but the study suffers from severe limitations.

Studies of migrant populations (see p. 54) strongly suggest the concomitant influence of environmental factors, such as diet (see p. 213), in the etiology of NPC.

Human T-lymphotropic virus-type 1

Despite the many demonstrations of cancers associated with retroviruses, a class of RNA viruses, in chicken, mice, cats, ungulates and non-human primates, intensive investigations in the late 1950s through to the late 1970s failed to identify a human retrovirus. The first report of a human retrovirus was that of Poiesz *et al.* (1980), who isolated human T-lymphotropic virus-type 1 (HTLV-1) from the lymphocytes of a patient with a variant form of cutaneous T-cell lymphoma. Since then, three further human retroviruses have been identified (Clark *et al.*, 1986). One is the HTLV-2, associated with hairy-cell leukaemia; the other two are the human immunodeficiency viruses I and II (HIV-I and -II), associated with AIDS. Thus, four human retroviruses have now been associated with disease.

Adult T-cell leukaemia-lymphoma (ATL) is a malignancy of mature T lymphocytes linked to infection with HTLV-1. The disease was first recognized clinically in Japan in the 1970s (Takatsuki *et al.*, 1977) and later in the Caribbean basin. It is characterized by a rapid progression and high fatality; 10-20% of patients may have indolent disease, but they also eventually enter an acute phase with rapid progression to death. HTLV-1 is prevalent in only certain geographical areas. The highest prevalences (5–15%) are found in parts of Japan (Takatsuki *et al.*, 1977). The Caribbean basin is another endemic area, with a seropositivity rate of about 5% in Jamaica and Haiti, 2–3% in Trinidad (Bartholomew *et al.*, 1985) and 1–2% in Martinique and Guadeloupe (Schaffar-Deshayes *et al.*, 1984). Prevalences in other continents are very low (<0.1%), but HTLV-1 infection is probably present in Africa.

Antibodies to HTLV-1 are present in 80–90% of cases of ATL (Hinuma *et al.*, 1982), and viral DNA sequences are integrated in malignant cells of ATL patients. ATL affects women and men about equally, at a median age of onset of 40–45 years. In Kyushu, Japan, the estimated annual incidence of ATL is 3.5 per 100 000 (Tajima & Kuroishi, 1985), and that in Jamaica is 1.5 per 100 000 (Gibbs *et al.*, 1987). It is highly probable that the virus is transmitted from mother to child during breast feeding (Hino *et al.*, 1985). Sexual transmission has been documented (Kajiyama *et al.*, 1986). This does not explain the progressive rise in seropositivity throughout life.

There is a long latent period between exposure to HTLV-1 and the development of leukaemia, as suggested by studies of migrants (Blattner *et al.*, 1986; Bartholomew *et al.*, 1987). Laboratory investigations have suggested that the virus plays an initiating role in malignant development; oncogene activation through chromosomal translocations may play a critical role in the progression process. HTLV-1 infection is thus predominantly silent, without clinical manifestation, and leukaemias occur in only less than 0.1% of seropositive individuals. Other risk factors have not yet been identified.

Human immunodeficiency viruses

The sudden appearance of opportunistic infections and generalized Kaposi's sarcoma in homosexual males in the USA in the 1980s was the first manifestation of the AIDS epidemic (Barré-Sinoussi *et al.*, 1983; Gallo *et al.*, 1984). The occurrence of high-grade non-Hodgkin's lymphoma was noted a little later. The virus responsible for AIDS, now termed HIV, was discovered soon afterwards. Both Kaposi's sarcoma and non-Hodgkin's lymphoma (small noncleaved cell lymphoma, immunoblastic sarcoma and primary lymphoma of the brain) form part of the clinical definition of AIDS (Centers for Disease Control, 1987); in Africa, the presence of disseminated Kaposi's sarcoma (not the usual endemic form) has been considered sufficient to make a clinical diagnosis of AIDS (World Health Organization, 1986). Other malignancies that have been noted in association with AIDS include Hodgkin's disease, oral cancer, colonic cancer, pancreatic cancer and testicular cancer; however, the magnitude of the excess risk, if any, is unknown. The only estimates of relative risk available are for a population presumed to be at high risk – young single males in San Francisco (Biggar *et al.*, 1987): the risks were extremely high for Kaposi's sarcoma (over 2000) and non-Hodgkin's lymphoma (4.2), but those for hepatoma and Hodgkin's disease were not significantly elevated.

The increased risk for certain cancers in HIV-infected subjects may be the result of immunosuppression: iatrogenically immunosuppressed individuals are at high risk for a similar range of unusual cancers (Penn, 1986; and see pp. 148 *et seq.*). However, some AIDS-related cancers – notably Hodgkin's disease – are not seen in immunosuppressed individuals, and HIV seropositive individuals appear to be at increased risk for non-Hodgkin's lymphoma and Kaposi's sarcoma even in the absence of measurable immunodeficiency (Ziegler *et al.*, 1984; Safai *et al.*, 1985). The role of cofactors (possibly other infectious agents) is suggested by the fact that the risk for Kaposi's sarcoma is greater in persons infected with HIV sexually than in persons infected intravenously (Curran *et al.*, 1985). It has also been reported that the frequency of Kaposi's sarcoma in both homosexually and intravenously transmitted cases of AIDS is declining (Des Jarlais *et al.*, 1987).

Other viruses

Cytomegalovirus (CMV) has been associated with Kaposi's sarcoma – both the endemic and the epidemic type associated with AIDS (see above). The original studies found higher titres of antibodies in Kaposi's sarcoma cases than in controls. More recently, CMV-DNA has been found in a variable proportion of tumour samples (Giraldo *et al.*, 1985). However, because of the ubiquity of CMV infection and the considerable homology between human DNA and the CMV genome, a causal link between CMV and Kaposi's sarcoma remains speculative.

Parasitic diseases

Schistosomiasis

Schistosomiasis remains one of the most widespread parasitic infections of man (Doumenge *et al.*, 1987). The geographic distribution of the different types of the causative parasite, *Schistosoma haematobium*, *S. japonicum*, *S. mansoni* and *S. intercalatum* is shown in Figure 20.

Figure 20. Global distribution of schistosomiasis[a]

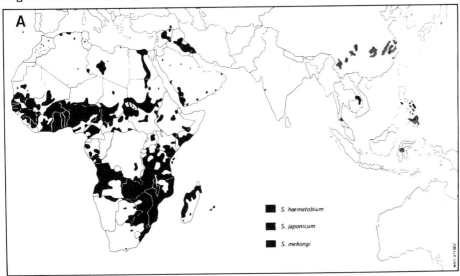

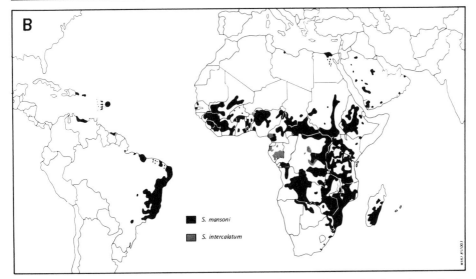

[a] From Doumenge *et al.* (1987) A, due to *Schistosoma haematobium* and *S. japonicum*; B, due to *S. mansoni* and *S. intercalatum*

A causal association between infection of the urinary bladder by the parasitic flatworm *S. haematobium* and cancer of that organ was first postulated near the beginning of this century (Ferguson, 1911), and the hypothesis has been supported by clinical and experimental observations. Bladder cancers associated with schistosomiasis are mainly of the squamous-cell type and rarely metastasize, in contrast to transitional-cell carcinomas which are the predominant type elsewhere.

The link is established firstly from the observation of elevated rates of bladder cancer in areas where infection is endemic, and secondly by the high proportion of bladder cancer cases in which there is evidence of present or past infection. Ferguson (1911) reported 'infestation' by *S. haematobium* in 29 of 39 men autopsied after bladder cancer, as compared to a rate of 40% in a general autopsy series of 600. Mustacchi and Shimkin (1958) assessed current infection with *S. haematobium* and bladder pathology among 1472 new in-patients at a general hospital in Egypt and estimated that the risk for bladder cancer in infected patients was about 2.5 times greater than that of uninfected patients, after taking into account age, sex and area of residence. Gelfand *et al.* (1967), in a small case–control study of bladder cancer in Rhodesia (Zimbabwe), used the degree of calcification in the bladder as a measure of long-term infection with *S. haematobium* and examined rectal biopsy specimens for *S. haematobium* ova. Relative risks of 15 and 6.5, respectively, can be estimated from their data for the association between bladder cancer and these two measures of infection, although these calculations are based on only 31 case–control pairs.

The areas principally affected are Iraq, Egypt and south-east Africa (Malawi, Mozambique, Zambia, Zimbabwe). In these areas, *Schistosoma* eggs are found more frequently in association with squamous-cell than with transitional-cell cancers (Al-Fouadi & Parkin, 1984; Kitinya *et al.*, 1986). The mechanisms involved in this association are not entirely clear. Chronic inflammation and urinary retention were originally suggested, but rather more specific hypotheses include alteration of liver function by hepatic schistosomiasis, leading to production and excretion of carcinogenic tryptophan metabolites, and the production of nitrosamines from precursors in urine by chronic bacterial infection, which may complicate schistosomiasis (el Aaser & el Merzabani, 1983). This last hypothesis has received some support from the finding of low levels of nitrosamines in the urine of young Egyptian men, and the finding that concomitant exposure of baboons to low doses of *N*-nitroso-*N*-butyl-*N*-butanolamine and infection with *S. haematobium* resulted in papillary growth and some carcinomas, at a much higher rate than in controls (Hicks, 1982).

The association of schistosomiasis with other cancers is much more questionable. *S. mansoni* and *S. japonicum* cause a form of cirrhosis, and a link with primary liver cancer has been sought, generally with negative results (Cheever, 1978; Inaba *et al.*, 1984). *S. japonicum*, which is endemic in parts of south-east Asia (Figure 20), gives rise to chronic schistosomal colitis, which has been suggested to enhance the probability of developing colonic cancer (Chen *et al.*, 1981; Zhao, 1981). In China, there is a strong geographical correlation between mortality from schistosomiasis (due to *S. japonicum*) and mortality from cancer of the colon and rectum (Doll, 1988); and a case–control study showed a positive association with rectal (but not colonic) cancer (Xu & Su, 1984). In an autopsy series in Ibadan, Nigeria (Edington *et al.*, 1970), lymphoreticular tumours were found three times more commonly in subjects with evidence of schistosomiasis than in those without.

Liver flukes

A causal relationship between infection with the liver flukes *Clonorchis sinensis* and *Opisthorchis viverrini* and primary cholangiocarcinoma is highly likely (Schwartz, 1980; Flavell, 1981). The evidence is based upon the close geographical relationship between cholangiocarcinoma (elsewhere a rare tumour) and infestation with these flukes, and the association of the two conditions at autopsy. Formal epidemiological proof is difficult to obtain because of the very high prevalence of infection in endemic areas, and because onset of the disease (cholangiocarcinoma) results in obstructive jaundice and hence loss of the marker of infection (excretion of eggs in the faeces; see, e.g., Kurathong, 1985).

The flukes are acquired by eating fresh-water and raw fish, an intermediate host which contains the metacercariae of the parasites. *O. viverrini* is confined to a well-defined area of north-east Thailand where infestation is highly prevalent; *C. sinensis* is found in southern China, the Democratic People's Republic of Korea, the Republic of Korea and Japan. The mechanisms by which these flukes induce cancer are unknown. They infest the intrahepatic bile ducts and give rise to hyperplasia and metaplasia of the epithelium. A strongly increased endogenous synthesis of *N*-nitrosamines has been observed in subjects infected with *O. viverrini* in Thailand (Srivanatakul *et al.*, 1990). Experimental studies in hamsters have shown that the ability of *N*-nitrosodimethylamine to induce cholangiocarcinoma is greatly enhanced in the presence of *Opisthorchis* infection (Thamavit *et al.*, 1978; Flavell & Lucas, 1982).

References

el Aaser, A.A. & el Merzabani, M.M. (1983) Etiology of bladder cancer. In: el Sebai, I. & Hoogstraten, B., eds, *Bladder Cancer*, Vol. 1, *General Review* (CRC Series on Experiences in Clinical Oncology), Boca Raton, Florida, CRC Press, pp. 39-58

Adam, E., Kaufman, R.H., Adler-Storthz, K., Melnick, J.L. & Dreesman, G.R. (1985) A prospective study of association of herpes simplex virus and human papillomavirus infection with cervical neoplasia in women exposed to diethylstilboestrol in utero. *Int. J. Cancer, 35*, 19-26

Al-Fouadi, A. & Parkin, D.M. (1984) Cancer in Iraq: seven years' data from the Baghdad Tumour Registry. *Int. J. Cancer, 34*, 207-213

Armstrong, B.K., Allen, O.V., Brennan, B.A., Fruzynski, I.A., de Klerk, N.H., Waters, E.D., Machin, J. & Gollow, M.M. (1986) Time trends in prevalence of cervical cytological abnormality in women attending a sexually transmitted diseases clinic and their relationship to trends in sexual activity and specific infections. *Br. J. Cancer, 54*, 669-675

Austin, H., Delzell, E., Grufferman, S., Levine, R., Morrison, A.S., Stolley, P.D. & Cole, P. (1986) A case–control study of hepatocellular carcinoma and the hepatitis B virus, cigarette smoking, and alcohol consumption. *Cancer Res., 46*, 962-966

Barré-Sinoussi, F., Chermann, J.C., Rey, F., Nugeyre, M.T., Chamaret, S., Gruest, J., Dauguet, C. & Axler-Blin, C. (1983) Isolation of a T-lymphotrophic retrovirus from a patient at risk for acquired immunodeficiency syndrome (AIDS). *Science, 220*, 868-871

Bartholomew, C., Charles, W., Saxinger, C., Blattner, W., Robert-Guroff, M., Raju, C., Ratan, P., Ince, W., Quamina, D., Basdeo-Maharaj, K. & Gallo, R.C. (1985) Racial and other characteristics of human T-cell leukemia/lymphoma (HTLV-1) and AIDS (HTLV-III) in Trinidad. *Br. Med. J.*, *290*, 1243-1246

Bartholomew, C., Saxinger, W.C., Clark, J.W., Gail, M., Dudgeon, A., Mahabir, B., Hull-Drysdale, B., Cleghorn, F., Gallo, R.C. & Blattner, W.A. (1987) Transmission of HTLV-I and HIV among homosexual men in Trinidad. *J. Am. Med. Assoc.*, *257*, 2604-2608

Beasley, R., Lin, C., Hwang, L.Y. & Chien, C.S. (1981) Hepatocellular carcinoma and hepatitis B virus. A prospective study of 22,707 men in Taiwan. *Lancet*, *ii*, 1129-1133

Biggar, R.J., Horm, J., Goedart, J.J. & Melbye, M. (1987) Cancer in a group at risk of acquired immunodeficiency syndrome (AIDS) through 1984. *Am. J. Epidemiol.*, *126*, 578-586

Blattner, W.A., Nomura, A., Clark, J.W., Ho, G.Y., Nakao, Y., Gallo, R. & Robert-Guroff, M. (1986) Models of transmission and evidence for viral latency from studies of human T-cell lymphotropic virus type I in Japanese migrant populations in Hawaii. *Proc. Natl Acad. Sci. USA*, *83*, 4895-4898

Campion, M.J., Cuzick, J., McCance, D.J. & Singer, A. (1986) Progressive potential of mild cervical atypia: prospective cytological, colposcopic, and virological study. *Lancet*, *i*, 237-240

Centers for Disease Control (1987) Revision of the CDC surveillance case definition for acquired immunodeficiency syndrome (AIDS). *Morb. Mortal. Weekly Rep.*, *36*, 1-13

Cheever, A.W. (1978) Schistosomiasis and neoplasia. *J. Natl Cancer Inst.*, *61*, 13-18

Chen, D.S., Hsu, N.H.M., Sung, J.L., Hsu, T.C., Hsu, S.T., Kuo, Y.T., Lo, K.L. & Shih, Y.T. (1987) A mass vaccination program in Taiwan against hepatitis B virus infection in infants of hepatitis B surface antigen-carrier mothers. *J. Am. Med. Assoc.*, *257*, 2597-2603

Chen, M.C., Chuang, C.Y., Wang, F.P., Chang, P.Y., Chen, Y.J., Tang, Y.C. & Chou, S.C. (1981) Colorectal cancer and schistosomiasis. *Lancet*, *i*, 971-973

Clark, J.W., Blattner, W.A. & Gallo, R.C. (1986) Human T-cell leukemia viruses and T-cell lymphoid malignancies. In: Petersdorf, R.Q., Adams, R.D., Braunwald, E. *et al.*, eds, *Update VII, Harrison's Principles of Internal Medicine*, New York, McGraw-Hill, pp. 29-48

Curran, J.W., Morgan, W.M., Hardy, A.M., Jaffe, H.W., Darrow, W.W. & Dowelle, W.R. (1985) The epidemiology of AIDS: current status and future prospects. *Science*, *229*, 1352-1357

Des Jarlais, D.C., Stoneburner, R., Thomas, P. & Friedman, S.R. (1987) Declines in proportion of Kaposi's sarcoma among cases of AIDS in multiple risk groups in New York City. *Lancet*, *ii*, 1024-1025

Doll, R. (1988) Epidemiology - the prevention of cancer: some recent developments. *J. Cancer Res. Clin. Oncol.*, *114*, 447-458

Doumenge, J.P., Mott, M.E., Cheung, C., Villanave, D., Chapuis, O., Perrin, M.F. & Reaud-Thomas, G., eds (1987) *Atlas of the Global Distribution of Schistosomiasis*, Geneva, World Health Organization

Edington, G.M., von Lichtenberg, F., Nwabuebo, I., Taylor, J.R. & Smith, J.H. (1970) Pathological effects of schistosomiasis in Ibadan, western state of Nigeria. I. Incidence and intensity of infection: distribution and severity of lesions. *Am. J. Trop. Med. Hyg.*, *19*, 982-995

Edman, J.C., Gray, P., Valenzuela, P., Rall, L.B. & Rutter, W.J. (1980) Integration of hepatitis B virus sequences and their expression in a human hepatoma cell line. *Nature*, *286*, 535-538

Epstein, M.A., Achong, B.G. & Barr, Y.M. (1964) Virus particles in cultured lymphoblasts from Burkitt's lymphoma. *Lancet*, *i*, 702-703

Ferguson, A.R. (1911) Associated bilharziasis and primary malignant disease of the urinary bladder, with observations in a series of forty cases. *J. Pathol. Bacteriol.*, *16*, 76-94

Flavell, D.J. (1981) Liver-fluke infection as an aetiological factor in bile duct carcinoma of man. *Trans. R. Soc. Trop. Med. Hyg.*, *75*, 814-824

Flavell, D.J. & Lucas, S.B. (1982) Potentiation by the human liver fluke, *Opisthorchis viverrini*, of the carcinogenic action of *N*-nitrosodimethylamine upon the biliary epithelium of the hamster. *Br. J. Cancer, 46*, 985-989

Gallo, R.C., Salahuddin, S.Z. & Popovic, M. (1984) Frequent detection and isolation of cytopathic retroviruses (HTLV-III) from patients with AIDS and at risk for AIDS. *Science, 224*, 500-503

Galloway, D.A. & McDougall, J.K. (1983) The oncogenic potential of herpes simplex viruses: evidence for a 'hit-and-run' mechanism. *Nature, 302*, 21-24

Gambia Hepatitis Study Group (1987) The Gambia hepatitis intervention study. *Cancer Res., 47*, 5782-5787

Gelfand, M., Weinberg, R.W. & Castle, W.M. (1967) Relation between carcinoma of the bladder and infestation with *Schistosoma haematobium*. *Lancet, i*, 1249-1251

Gibbs, W.N., Lofters, W.S., Campbell, N., Hanchard, B., LaGrenade, L., Cranston, B., Hendriks, J., Jaffe, E.S., Saxinger, C. & Robert-Guroff, M. (1987) Non-Hodgkin's lymphoma in Jamaica and its relation to adult T-cell leukemia lymphoma. *Ann. Intern. Med., 106*, 361-368

Giraldo, G., Beth, E. & Kyalwazi, S.K. (1985) Role of cytomegalovirus in Kaposi's sarcoma. In: Williams, A.O., O'Connor, G.T., de-Thé, G.B. & Johnson, C.A., eds, *Virus-associated cancers in Africa* (IARC Scientific Publications No. 63), Lyon, IARC, pp. 583-606

Hall, A.J., Winter, P.D. & Wright, R. (1985) Mortality of hepatitis B positive blood donors in England and Wales. *Lancet, i*, 91-93

zur Hausen, H. (1982) Human genital cancer: synergism between two virus infections and synergism between a virus infection and initiating events. *Lancet, ii*, 1370-1372

zur Hausen, H. (1986) Intracellular surveillance of persisting viral infections. Human genital cancer results from deficient cellular control of papillomavirus gene expression. *Lancet, ii*, 489-491

zur Hausen, H. (1987) Papillomaviruses in human cancer. *Cancer, 59*, 1692-1696

zur Hausen, H. & Schulte-Holthausen, H. (1970) Presence of EB virus nucleic acid homology in a virus-free line of Burkitt tumour cells. *Nature, 227*, 245-248

Henle, G. & Henle, W. (1979) The virus as the etiologic agent of infectious mononucleosis. In: Epstein, M.A. & Achong, B.G., eds, *The Epstein-Barr Virus*, Berlin (West), Springer, pp. 297-320

Henle, W. & Henle, G. (1985) Epstein-Barr virus and human malignancies. *Adv. Viral Oncol., 5*, 201-238

Henle, W., Henle, G. & Lennette, E.T. (1979) The Epstein-Barr virus. *Sci. Am., 241*, 48-59

Hicks, R.M. (1982) Nitrosamines as possible aetiological agents in bilharzial bladder cancer. In: Magee, P.N., ed., *Nitrosamines and Human Cancer* (Banbury Report 12), Cold Spring Harbor, NY, CSH Press, pp. 455-471

Hino, S., Yamaguchi, K., Katamine, S., Sugiyama, H., Amagasaki, T., Kinoshita, K., Yoshida, Y., Doi, H., Tsuji, Y. & Miyamoto, T. (1985) Mother-to-child transmission of human T-cell leukemia virus type-1. *Jpn. J. Cancer Res. (Gann), 76*, 474-480

Hinuma, Y., Komoda, H., Chosa, T., Kondo, T., Kohakura, M., Takenaka, T., Kikuchi, M., Ichimaru, M., Yunoki, S., Sato, I., Matsuo, R., Takiuchi, Y., Uchino, H. & Hanaoka, M. (1982) Antibodies to adult T-cell leukemia virus-associated antigen (ATLA) in sera from patients with ATL and controls in Japan: a nation-wide sero-epidemiologic study. *Int. J. Cancer, 29*, 631-635

Iijima, T., Saitoh, N., Nobutomo, K., Nambu, M. & Sakuma, K. (1984) A prospective cohort study of hepatitis B surface antigen carriers in a working population. *Gann, 75*, 571-573

Inaba, Y., Maruchi, N., Matsuda, M., Yoshihara, N. & Yamamoto, S. (1984) A case–control study on liver cancer with special emphasis on the possible aetiological role of schistosomiasis. *Int. J. Epidemiol., 13*, 408-412

Kajiyama, W., Kashiwagi, S., Ikematsu, H., Hayashi, J., Nomura, H. & Okochi, K. (1986) Intrafamilial transmission of adult T-cell leukemia virus. *J. Infect. Dis., 154*, 851-857

Kalter, S.P., Riggs, S.A., Cabanillas, F., Butler, J.J., Hagemeister, F.B., Mansell, P.W., Newell, G.R., Velasquez, W.S., Salvador, P., Barlogie, B., Rios, A. & Hersh, E.M. (1985) Aggressive non-Hodgkin's lymphoma in immunocompromised homosexual males. *Blood, 66*, 655-659

Kew, M.C., Gear, A.J., Baumgarten, I., Dusheiko, G.M. & Maier, G. (1979) Histocompatibility antigens in patients with hepatocellular carcinoma and their relationship to chronic hepatitis B virus infection in these patients. *Gastroenterology*, *77*, 537-539

Kitinya, J.N., Laurén, P.A., Eshleman, L.G., Paljärvi, L. & Tanaka, K. (1986) The incidence of squamous and transitional cell carcinomas of the urinary bladder in Northern Tanzania in areas of high and low levels of endemic Schistosoma haematobium infection. *Trans. R. Soc. Trop. Med. Hyg.*, *80*, 935-939

Kjaer, S.K., de Villiers, E.M., Haugaard, B.J., Christensen, R.B., Teisen, C., Moller, K.A., Poll, P., Jensen, H., Vestergaard, B.F., Lynge, E. & Jensen, O.M. (1988) Human papillomavirus, herpes simplex virus and cervical cancer incidence in Greenland and Denmark. A population-based cross-sectional study. *Int. J. Cancer*, *41*, 518-524

Kjaer, S.K., Teisen, C., Haugaard, B.J., Lynge, E., Christensen, R.B., Møller, K.A., Jensen, H., Poll, P., Vestergaard, B.F., de Villiers, E.M. & Jensen, O.M. (1989) Risk factors for cervical cancer in Greenland and Denmark: a population based cross sectional study. *Int. J. Cancer*, *44*, 40-47

Kurathong, S. (1985) *Opisthorchis viverrini* infection and cholangiocarcinoma. A prospective, case-controlled study. *Gastroenterology*, *89*, 151-156

Lam, K.C., Ho, J.C. & Yeung, R.T. (1982) Spontaneous regression of hepatocellular carcinoma: a case study. *Cancer*, *50*, 332-336

Leder, P., Battey, J., Lenoir, G.M., Moulding, C., Murphy, W., Potter, H., Stewart, T. & Taub, R. (1983) Translocations among antibody genes in human cancer. *Science*, *222*, 765-771

Lenoir, G.M. & Bornkamm, G.W. (1987) Burkitt's lymphoma, a human cancer model for the study of the multistep development of cancer: proposal for a new scenario. *Adv. Viral Oncol.*, *7*, 173-206

Lingao, A.L., Domingo, E.O. & Nishioka, K. (1981) Hepatitis B virus profile of hepatocellular carcinoma in the Philippines. *Cancer*, *48*, 1590-1595

diLuca, D., Rotola, A., Pilotti, S., Monini, P., Caselli, E., Rilke, F. & Cassai, E. (1987) Simultaneous presence of herpes simplex and human papilloma virus sequences in human genital tumors. *Int. J. Cancer*, *40*, 763-768

Magrath, I. (1983) Burkitt's lymphoma: clinical aspects and treatment. In: Molander, D.W., ed., *Diseases of the Lymphatic System, Diagnosis and Therapy*, New York, Springer, pp. 103-139

Muñoz, N. (1978) Viruses and carcinogenesis of the uterine cervix. In: Veronesi, U., Perussia, A., Di Re, F. & Emmanuelli, H., eds, *Le Neoplasie dell'apparato Genitale Feminile*, Milan, Casa Editrice Ambrosiana, pp. 83-87

Muñoz, N. & Bosch, F.X. (1987) Epidemiology of hepatocellular carcinoma. In: Okuda, K. & Ishak, K.G., eds, *Neoplasms of the Liver*, Tokyo, Springer, pp. 3-19

Muñoz, N., Bosch, F.X. & Kaldor, J.M. (1988) Does human papillomavirus cause cervical cancer? The state of the epidemiological evidence. *Br. J. Cancer*, *57*, 1-5

Muñoz, N. & Linsell, A. (1982) Epidemiology of primary liver cancer. In: Correa, P. & Haenszel, W., eds, *Epidemiology of Cancer of the Digestive Tract*, The Hague, Martinus Nijhoff, pp. 161-195

Mustacchi, P. & Shimkin, M.B. (1958) Cancer of the bladder and infestation with Schistosoma haematobium. *J. Natl Cancer Inst.*, *20*, 825-842

Orth, G., Jablonska, S., Favre, M., Croissant, O., Jarzabek-Chorzelska, M. & Rzesa, G. (1978) Characterization of two types of human papillomaviruses in lesions of epidermodysplasia verruciformis. *Proc. Natl Acad. Sci. USA*, *75*, 1537-1541

Oshima, A., Tsukuma, H., Hiyama, T., Fujimoto, I., Yamano, H. & Tanaka, M. (1984) Follow-up study of HBs Ag-positive blood donors with special reference to effect of drinking and smoking on development of liver cancer. *Int. J. Cancer*, *34*, 775-779

Penn, I. (1986) The occurrence of malignant tumours in immunosuppressed states. *Prog. Allergy*, *37*, 259-300

Poiesz, B.J., Ruscetti, F.W., Gazdar, A.F., Bunn, P.A., Minna, J.D. & Gallo, R.C. (1980) Detection and isolation of type C retrovirus particles from fresh and cultured lymphocytes of a patient with cutaneous T-cell lymphoma. *Proc. Natl Acad. Sci. USA*, *77*, 7415-7419

Prince, A.M. & Alcabes, P. (1982) The risk of development of hepatocellular carcinoma in hepatitis B virus carriers in New York. Preliminary estimate using death-records matching. *Hepatology*, *2*, 15S-20S

Prince, A.M., Szmuness, W., Michon, J., Demaille, J., Diebolt, G., Linhard, J., Quenum, C. & Sankale, M. (1975) A case/control study of the association between primary liver cancer and hepatitis B infection in Senegal. *Int. J. Cancer*, *16*, 376-383

Reeves, W.C., Caussy, D., Brinton, L.A., Brenes, M.M., Montalvan, P., Gomez, B., de Britton, R.C., Morice, E., Gaitan, E., de Lao, S.L. & Rawls, W.E. (1987) case–control study of human papillomaviruses and cervical cancer in Latin America. *Int. J. Cancer*, *40*, 450-454

Reeves, W.C., Brinton, L.A., Garcia, M., Brenes, M.M., Herrero, R., Gaitan, E., Tenorio, P., de Britton, R.C. & Rawls, W.E. (1989) Human papillomavirus infection and cervical cancer in Latin America. *New Engl. J. Med.*, *320*, 1437-1441

Rickinson, A.B., Yao, Q.Y. & Wallace, L.E. (1985) The Epstein-Barr virus as a model of virus-host interactions. *Br. Med. Bull.*, *41*, 75-79

Safai, B., Johnson, K.G., Myskowski, P.L., Koziner, B., Yang, S.Y., Cunningham-Rundles, S., Godbold, J.H. & Dupont, B. (1985) The natural listing of Kaposi's sarcoma in the acquired immunodeficiency syndrome. *Ann. Intern. Med.*, *103*, 744-750

Schaffar-Deshayes, L., Chavance, M., Monplaisir, N., Courouce, A.M., Gessain, A., Blesonski, S., Valette, I., Feingold, N. & Levy, J.P. (1984) Antibodies to HTLV-1 p24 in sera of blood donors, elderly people and patients with hemopoietic diseases in France and in French West Indies. *Int. J. Cancer*, *34*, 667-670

Schmauz, R., de Villiers, E.-M., Dennin, R., Lwanga, S.K. & Owor, R. (1989) Multiple infections in cases of cervical cancer from a high-incidence area in tropical Africa. *Int. J. Cancer*, *43*, 805-809

Schneider, A., Oltersdorf, T., Schneider, V. & Gissmann, L. (1987) Distribution pattern of human papilloma virus 16 genome in cervical neoplasia by molecular in situ hybridization of tissue sections. *Int. J. Cancer*, *39*, 717-721

Schwartz, D.A. (1980) Helminths in the induction of cancer: *Opisthorchis viverrini*, *Chlonorchis sinensis* and cholangiocarcinoma. *Trop. Geogr. Med.*, *32*, 95-100

Shafritz, D.A., Shouval, D., Sherman, H.I., Hadziyannis, S.J. & Kew, M.C. (1981) Integration of hepatitis B virus DNA into the genome of liver cells in chronic liver disease and hepatocellular carcinoma. *New Engl. J. Med.*, *305*, 1067-1073

Shah, K.V. & Gissmann, L. (1989) Experimental evidence on oncogenicity of papillomaviruses. In: Muñoz, N., Bosch, F.X. & Jensen, O.M., eds, *Human Papillomavirus and Cervical Cancer* (IARC Scientific Publications No. 94), Lyon, IARC, pp. 105-111

Srivanatakul, P., Ohshima, H., Khlat, M., Parkin, M., Sukaryodhin, S., Brouet, I. & Bartsch, H. (1990) Endogenous nitrosamines and liver flukes as risk factors for cholangiocarcinoma in Thailand. In: O'Neill, I.K., Chen, J.S. & Bartsch, H., eds, *Relevance to Human Cancer of N-Nitroso Compounds, Tobacco Smoke and Mycotoxins* (IARC Scientific Publications No. 105), Lyon, IARC (in press)

Storey, A., Pim, D., Murray, A., Osborn, K., Banks, L. & Crawford, L. (1988) Comparison of the *in vitro* transforming activity of human papillomavirus types. *EMBO J.*, *7*, 1815-1820

Summers, J. (1981) Three recently described animal virus models for human hepatitis B virus. *Hepatology*, *1*, 179-183

Syrjänen, K., Mäntyjärvi, R., Väyrynen, M., Syrjänen, S., Parkkinen, S., Yliskoski, M., Saarikoski, S. & Castrén, O. (1987) Evolution of human papillomavirus infections in the uterine cervix during a long-term prospective follow-up. *Appl. Pathol.*, *5*, 121-135

Szmuness, W. (1978) Hepatocellular carcinoma and the hepatitis B virus: evidence for a causal association. *Prog. Med. Virol.*, *24*, 40-69

Tabor, E., Gerety, R.J., Vogel, C.L., Bayley, A.C., Anthony, P.P., Chan, C.H. & Barker, L.F. (1977) Hepatitis B virus infection and primary hepatocellular carcinoma. *J. Natl Cancer Inst.*, *58*, 1197-1200

Tajima, K. & Kuroichi, T. (1985) Estimation of rate of incidence of ATL among ATLV (HTLV-1) carriers in Kyushu, Japan. *Jpn. J. Clin. Oncol.*, *15*, 423-430

Takatsuki, K., Uchiyama, T., Sagawa, K. & Yodoi, J. (1977) Adult T-cell leukemia in Japan. In: Seno, S., Takaku, K. & Irino, S., eds, *Topics in Hematology*, Amsterdam, Excerpta Medica, pp. 73-77

Thamavit, W., Bhamarapravit, N., Sahaphong, S., Vajrasthira, S. & Angsubhakorn, S. (1978) Effects of dimethylnitrosamine on induction of cholangiocarcinoma in *Opisthorchis viverrini*-infected Syrian golden hamsters. *Cancer Res.*, *38*, 4634-4639

de-Thé, G., Geser, A., Day, N.E., Tukei, P., Williams, E., Beri, D., Smith, P., Dean, A., Bornkamm, G., Feorino, P. & Henle, W. (1978) Epidemiological evidence for causal relationship between Epstein-Barr virus and Burkitt's lymphoma from Uganda prospective study. *Nature*, *274*, 756-761

Trichopoulos, D., Tabor, E., Gerety, R.J., Xirouchaki, E., Sparros, L., Muñoz, N. & Linsell, C.A. (1978) Hepatitis B and primary hepatocellular carcinoma in a European population. *Lancet*, *ii*, 1217-1219

Trichopoulos, D., Day, N.E., Kaklamani, E., Tzonou, A., Muñoz, N., Zavitsanos, X., Koumantaki, Y. & Trichopoulou, A. (1987) Hepatitis B virus, tobacco smoking and ethanol consumption in the etiology of hepatocellular carcinoma. *Int. J. Cancer*, *39*, 45-49

Villa, J.L. & Franco, M. (1989) Epidemiologic correlates of cervical neoplasia and risk of human papillomavirus infection in asymptomatic women in Brazil. *J. Natl Cancer Inst.*, *81*, 332-340

Vonka, V., Kanka, J., Jelinek, I., Subrt, I., Suchanek, A., Havrankova, A., Vachal, M., Hirsch, I., Domorazkova, E., Zavadova, J., Richterova, V., Naprstkova, J., Dvorakova, V. & Svoboda, B. (1984) Prospective study on the relationship between cervical neoplasia and herpes simplex type-2 virus. I. Epidemiological characteristics. *Int. J. Cancer*, *33*, 49-60

Vonka, V., Kanka, J. & Roth, Z. (1987) Herpes simplex type 2 virus and cervical neoplasia. *Adv. Cancer Res.*, *48*, 149-191

Wolf, H., zur Hausen, H. & Becker, V. (1973) EB viral genomes in epithelial nasopharyngeal carcinoma cells. *Nature (New Biol.)*, *224*, 245-247

World Health Organization (1986) Acquired immunodeficiency syndrome (AIDS). *Weekly Epidemiol. Rec.*, *61*, 69-73

Xu, Z. & Su, D.L. (1984) *Schistosoma japonicum* and colorectal cancer: an epidemiological study in the People's Republic of China. *Int. J. Cancer*, *34*, 315-318

Yarrish, R.L., Werner, B.G. & Blumberg, B.S. (1980) Association of hepatitis B virus infection with hepatocellular carcinoma in American patients. *Int. J. Cancer*, *26*, 711-715

Yeh, F.S., Mo, C.C., Luo, S., Henderson, B.E., Tong, M.J. & Yu, M.C. (1985) A serological case–control study of primary hepatocellular carcinoma in Guangxi, China. *Cancer Res.*, *45*, 872-873

Yu, M.C., Mack, T., Hanisch, R., Peters, R.L., Henderson, B.E. & Pike, M.C. (1983) Hepatitis, alcohol consumption, cigarette smoking, and hepatocellular carcinoma in Los Angeles. *Cancer Res.*, *43*, 6077-6079

Zeng, Y., Zhang, L.G., Li, H.Y., Jan, M.G., Zhang, Q., Wu, Y.C., Wang, Y.S. & Su, G.R. (1982) Serological mass survey for early detection of nasopharyngeal carcinoma in Wuzhou City, China. *Int. J. Cancer*, *29*, 139-141

Zhao, E.S. (1981) Cancer of the colon and schistosomiasis. *Proc. R. Soc. Med.*, *74*, 645

Ziegler, J.L., Beckstead, J.A., Volberding, P.A., Abrams, D.I., Levine, A.M., Lukes, R.J., Gill, P.S., Burkes, R.L., Meyer, P.R., Metroka, C.E., Mouradian, J., Moore, A., Riggs, S.A., Butler, J.J., Cabanillas, F.C., Hersh, E., Newell, G.R., Laubenstein, L.J., Knowles, D., Odajnyk, C., Raphael, B., Koziner, B., Urmacher, C. & Clarkson, B. (1984) Non-Hodgkin's lymphoma in 90 homosexual men. *New Engl. J. Med.*, *311*, 565-570

Chapter 12. Diet

Experiments on laboratory animals carried out in the early 1930s indicated that diet can influence the process of carcinogenesis. In his pioneering work, Tannenbaum (1942a,b) showed an increased number of breast tumours in animals fed a high-calorie or high-fat diet as compared to the yield in animals on normal diets.

The first epidemiological studies indicating that diet could play a role in human cancer started to appear in the 1960s, and their number has increased rapidly. Studies are available today concerning the effect of diet on female breast cancer and cancers of the digestive tract, endometrium, prostate and other less common sites such as the larynx and nasopharynx. Although some of these studies indicate that consumption of certain foods or nutrients either reduces or increases the risk for cancer, there is still substantial disagreement about the conclusions that can be drawn from these extensive but often contradictory data.

Methodological issues in studies of diet and cancer

Some of the uncertainties are due to the particular difficulties encountered in investigating the issue of diet and cancer in both epidemiological studies on humans and experimental studies on laboratory animals. Animal models to simulate the effect of diet on the frequency of cancers in humans have been criticized from several points of view. Hill (1989) argues that contrasting theories about, for instance, dietary fat and large-bowel cancer can be proved or disproved depending on the animal model that is selected. Epidemiological studies have provided strong evidence that certain life-style factors (e.g., tobacco and alcohol) and several environmental and industrial chemicals cause cancer, but it has been less easy to demonstrate the importance of diet. The main problems reside in the inherent difficulty of measuring human diets. Some of these difficulties are outlined briefly in order to illustrate the strengths and limitations of the epidemiological and experimental data.

Firstly, the information on dietary habits used in virtually all published studies on diet and cancer covers only a limited period. In case–control studies, data on diet are usually available for a few years prior to diagnosis of cases and for an equivalent period for controls. In the few prospective cohort studies that have been done, information on diet was collected only once – at the time the subjects were enrolled – and no information was gathered on changes that may have occurred during the follow-up period.

Secondly, diet comprises a very complex mixture of foods and beverages, which must be translated into terms of nutrient composition. Food composition tables published by national organizations are based (at best) on average national data and represent only an approximation of the diet of a real subject in a particular time and place. It has been shown that errors in measurement vary substantially for different nutrients and different dietary methods. In addition, the effects of certain nutrients are correlated simply because they are present in the same food items (e.g., animal protein and saturated fat, vitamin C and β-carotene, fibre and complex carbohydrates). This problem, which is usually referred to as 'multicolinearity between nutrients', adds to the difficulty of distinguishing between causal and spurious associations in the statistical analysis of epidemiological studies.

Lastly, as mentioned above, increase in risk associated with specific food items and nutrients is likely to be low. This does not deny the possibility that dietary habits as a whole could be responsible for substantial differences in cancer risk, but it further emphasizes the need for and the difficulty of evaluating whole diet, taking into account energy providing nutrients (fat, carbohydrates, protein and alcohol) as well as other components (e.g, vitamins, mineral salts, chemical contaminants).

Dietary assessment methods

A variety of methods has been used in nutritional studies, from the simplest self-administered questionnaire, consisting of a few questions, to use of complex dietary diaries in which all foods consumed must be weighed and described.

In cancer epidemiology, methods based on keeping diaries of individual diets have generally not been used owing to practical problems. The methods that have been used can, for simplicity, be grouped into three types: (i) brief questionnaires on the usual frequency of consumption of either a short list of foods (20–30 items) or a detailed list of foods, dishes and beverages, with additional questions on seasonal consumption or dietary changes during life, administered by an interviewer or self-administered; (ii) food frequency questionnaires with estimated portion size, which require subjects to estimate the usual amounts consumed of each food and beverage, using pictures or models; and (iii) dietary history during a given period of life obtained by a trained interviewer, using lists of foods with open questions and estimates of portion size.

The simplest food frequency methods cannot be used to estimate intake of nutrients like fat, protein and carbohydrate or energy intake. In some studies, simple questionnaires have been used to derive indices of these components of diet, and in others some foods have been assumed to be indicators of specific nutrients; for example, meat and dairy products have been used as indicators of fat consumption, and fresh vegetables and fruits as indicators of vitamin C and β-carotene intake. Dietary history and, to a lesser degree, food frequency methods provide quantitative estimates of food consumption which can be used to compute nutrient intake by means of food composition tables. The validity and precision of estimates of individual intake provided by the three types of method vary substantially in relation not only to the method itself but also to the dietary habits of the subjects, their ability to answer questions and the skill of the interviewer.

Short food frequency questionnaires usually provide the least reliable information, while dietary history and food frequency questionnaires with estimated portion size can provide estimates of individual diet which correlate moderately well with better methods, such as the long-term weighted diet diary.

The dietary factors potentially involved in the etiology of human cancer are discussed within two broad categories: first, factors that may increase the risk for cancer and, second, those that may confer protection.

Dietary factors that may increase the risk for cancer

Dietary fat

Correlation studies of incidence of and mortality from cancers of the large bowel, breast and prostate in different populations around the world show a strong association with average per-caput consumption of fat, and particularly of saturated fat; however, case–control and prospective cohort studies conducted on subjects within the same population have provided variable results: some showed increased risks for cancers of the large bowel, breast and prostate in association with a high intake of fat, while others found no association.

One explanation for these variable results is that only total fat has been considered in most epidemiological studies. Dietary fat and the fat incorporated in the human body comprise a large family of compounds.

Depot fat and structural lipids are the two forms in which lipids are found in the cells of adult humans and of edible animals. Adipose cells contain large amounts of neutral depot fat, mainly triglycerides, in their cytoplasm, and structural lipids are an essential component of cell membranes, including phospholipids and glycolipids. The basic constituents of both forms are fatty acids. In triglycerides, three fatty acids are attached to one molecule of glycerol ester; in phospholipids, there are usually two fatty acids in each molecule; and in glycolipids one fatty acid per molecule. Fatty acids are composed of long chains of carbon atoms with the basic formula $CH_3(CH_2)_n COOH$; in the human body, they have an even number of carbon atoms – between four and 24 – and varying degrees of saturation. In saturated fatty acids, all carbon-to-carbon bonds are single ($-CH_2-CH_2-$); in monounsaturates, there is one double bond ($-CH=CH-$); and in polyunsaturates, there are two or more double bonds. A perceptible feature of degree of saturation is that saturated fatty acids are solids at temperatures of about $20\,^\circ C$ (e.g., butter, lard), while mixtures rich in mono- and polyunsaturated fatty acids are liquid (e.g., olive oil, fish oil). An additional classification of mono- and polyunsaturated fatty acids indicates the position of the first carbon atom with a double bond, and there is a growing interest in the relative intake of δ unsaturated fats of the two families, n-3 (or ω-3) and n-6 (or ω-6), so called because the first carbon atom is in the third or sixth position, respectively. These two families of fatty acids are precursors of two types of δ prostaglandins that seem to have opposite effects on risk for cardiovascular disease, and the hypothesis has been put forward that they may modify individual susceptibility to some cancers.

Colorectal cancer

Table 23 summarizes the results of epidemiological studies on diet and colorectal cancer. Of the studies based on a dietary method which allowed the estimation of fat intake, five case–control studies, conducted in Puerto Rico (Martinez *et al.*, 1979), Canada (Miller *et al.*, 1983), the UK (Bristol *et al.*,

Table 23. Main results of case–control and cohort studies on risk for colorectal cancer and diet[a]

Protein	Fat	Fibre	Vitamin A	Vitamin C	Meat	Vegetables	Starches	Calories	Reference
					+	+	+[b]		Haenszel et al. (1973)
+	+				+	−			Phillips (1975)
		−			NA				Modan et al. (1975)
						−			Graham et al. (1978)
	(+)	(−)			(+)				Dales et al. (1979)
	+	+			+				Martinez et al. (1979)
					NA	NA[c]			Haenszel et al. (1980)
+	+	NA	NA	NA	+[d]			+	Jain et al. (1980)
+	+	NA	NA	NA	+[d]			+	Miller et al. (1983)
	+				+	−			Manousos et al. (1983)
NA	+	NA	NA	NA	NA	NA	+/−[e]	+	Bristol et al. (1985)
NA	NA	−	NA	−	NA		NA	NA	Macquart-Moulin et al. (1986)
		+	+/NA[f]	NA	−			+	Potter & McMichael (1986)
	(+)	−	−	−	+/−[g]	−	−[i]		Kune et al. (1987)
NA	NA/−[h]	−	+		NA	−		NA	Tuyns et al. (1988)
+	+	−						+	Slattery et al. (1988)
					+	−			Young & Wolf (1988)
	+	−						+	Graham et al. (1988)

Case–control studies

Table 23 (contd)

	Protein	Fat	Fibre	Vitamin A	Vitamin C	Meat	Vege-tables	Starches	Calories	Reference
Cohort studies										
						-	-	-[b]		Hirayama (1981)
	NA	-/+[j]				NA	NA	NA		Stemmermann et al. (1984)
					NA	NA	NA			Phillips & Snowdon (1985)
Studies on polyps										
	NA	+	-		NA	NA	NA	-	NA	Hoff et al. (1986)
	NA	NA	-/NA[k]		NA	NA	NA	-[i]	NA	Macquart-Moulin et al. (1987)

[a] +, increased risk; -, decreased risk; NA, no association; ( ), not statistically significant; blank, not studied
[b] Rice only
[c] Decreased risk for high consumption of peas, bracken, leeks
[d] Risk increased for rectal cancer but not for colon cancer
[e] +, sugar depleted in fibre; -, 'natural sugar'
[f] Risk increased for cereal fibre and for vegetable fibre
[g] Risk increased for high consumption of beef and decreased for high consumption of pork
[h] Risk decreased for high intake of polyunsaturated fat
[i] Polysaccharides only
[j] Risk decreased for colon cancer and slightly increased for rectal cancer
[k] Risk decreased for vegetable and fruit fibre; NA for other fibres

1985) and the USA (Graham *et al.*, 1988; Slattery *et al.*, 1988), showed a statistically significant increase in risk for colorectal cancer associated with high fat intake. In a study carried out in Australia, a weak association was found (Kune *et al.*, 1987); and in a study conducted in the USA (Dales *et al.*, 1979), there was a nonsignificant increase in risk which became statistically significant when subjects reporting high fat/low fibre intake were compared with those reporting a low fat/high fibre diet. In contrast, in two case–control studies conducted in France (Macquart-Moulin *et al.*, 1986) and Australia (Potter & McMichael, 1986), no association was found; and in one study conducted in Belgium (Tuyns *et al.*, 1988), a reduced risk was observed in association with high intake of polyunsaturated fat, and particularly linoleic acid, primarily from vegetable oils and margarine. This finding is similar to that of Macquart-Moulin *et al.* (1986) in France, who found a reduced risk associated with consumption of vegetable oil.

The results of three prospective cohort studies shed no further light on this issue. Hirayama (1981), in a large study in Japan, found a decreased risk for colorectal cancer among people who reported frequent consumption of meat. In the cohort study of Stemmerman *et al.* (1984), meat eating was associated with a decreased risk for colon and an increased risk for rectal cancer; however, there may have been misclassification of individual fat intake, since diet was measured by means of a single 24-h recall at the time of the study. In a cohort study of Seventh-day Adventists, Phillips and Snowdon (1985) found no association between consumption of meat and risk for colorectal cancer, while in a previous small case–control study of subjects belonging to the same religious group they had found an increased risk with fat intake (Phillips, 1975).

Several etiological mechanisms have been postulated to explain how fat, and particularly saturated fat, could increase the risk for colorectal cancer (Hill, 1981; Trichopoulos & Polychronopoulou, 1986) and for cancer in general. A considerable volume of work has been devoted to the effect of saturated fat on the metabolism of biliary acids and on the composition of the bacterial flora of the large bowel. Biliary secretion of acid and neutral steroids may be increased by a high-fat diet, and this may lead to modifications in bacterial flora and bacterial enzymatic activity (Hill *et al.*, 1971; Reddy *et al.*, 1975); or such diets may themselves modify bacterial flora. An increase in the number of anaerobic bacteria able to dehydroxylate primary bile acids would increase the absolute amounts of secondary bile acids and degraded neutral steroids. Secondary bile acids have been shown to increase cancer yields in some experiments on laboratory animals (Hill, 1985).

Female breast cancer

Until the mid-1970s, the hypothesis that a high-fat diet was a causal factor in breast cancer was supported mainly by the results of experimental animal studies and a few epidemiological observations. Since then, more than 20 epidemiological investigations have been reported in the literature, five of which were prospective cohort and the remainder case–control studies. In 1982, the Working Group on Diet and Cancer convened by the US National Research Council concluded that the evidence supporting a causal link between fat intake and cancer was particularly convincing for cancer of the breast. The Committee recommended that consumption of total and of saturated fat be reduced. Although this recommendation is widely considered to be sensible from the point of view of public health, there is still substantial disagreement on the interpretation of the scientific evidence. Studies published since 1982 have brought no solution to the issue. The evidence that fat intake is related to risk for breast cancer has been reviewed critically by several authors (Goodwin & Boyd, 1987; Skegg, 1987; Williams & Dickerson, 1987; Berrino & Panico, 1989).

Epidemiological studies on fat and breast cancer are summarized in Table 24. Of nine case–control studies in which fat intake was measured, three showed a statistically increased risk for breast cancer associated with intake of total fat or saturated fat (Miller *et al.*, 1978; Sarin *et al.*, 1985; Toniolo *et al.*, 1989). In three other case–control studies, there was some suggestion of an association, which either did not reach statistical significance (Hirohata *et al.*, 1985, 1987) or was limited to subgroups of the investigated subjects (Lubin *et al.*, 1986). In three further studies, there was no association (Nomura *et al.*, 1978; Graham *et al.*, 1982; Kolonel *et al.*, 1983).

In the other eight case–control studies, diet was measured by simple methods, most often of the food frequency type, and total fat intake could not be estimated. In these studies, the frequency of consumption of meat and dairy produce was used as the indicator of fat intake. Seven studies showed statistically significant or borderline significant increased risks for breast cancer related to more frequent consumption of milk and dairy products. Frequent meat consumption was found to be associated with increased risk in two studies, and in three other studies there was a suggestion of a weaker association.

The results of five prospective studies have been published; in the only two in which fat intake measured, no association was found. In particular, the results of the prospective study on US nurses (Willett *et al.*, 1987) lend no support to the hypothesis that breast cancer is related to dietary fat intake. This study involved more than 100 000 women, whose dietary habits were investigated by means of a self-administered food frequency questionnaire. It has been suggested that the absence of an association is due to the fact that this population has a reduced range of fat intake and to the use of a method relying on standard food portion size instead of asking the women to estimate their own usual food portion size. However, the methods used in most epidemiological studies on this issue are probably no better. The issue of range of consumption in relation to the detectability of risk cannot be discarded, particularly in view of the positive results seen in countries where a substantial proportion of women have diets quite low in fat (Toniolo *et al.*, 1989).

The possible mechanisms linking dietary fat intake to breast cancer are not clear, although several hypotheses have been formulated some of which have received empirical support from investigations in humans and animals. Fat may increase the risk for breast cancer by interfering with hormonal regulation, which is widely accepted to be involved in the occurrence of breast cancer (see p. 240). High fat and high calorie intake may lead to obesity, which has consistently been found to increase the risk for breast cancer in post-menopausal women, although obesity has been found to be inversely related to the risk for breast cancer in

Table 24. Main results from case–control and prospective studies on diet and risk for breast cancer[a]

Controls[b]	No. of cases	Total or saturated fat	Vegetable fat	Animal protein	Meat	Milk and dairy products	Fruit and/or vegetables	Reference
Case-control studies								
P, H	77				–	(+)		Phillips (1975)
P	86	NA			+	+		Nomura et al. (1978)
P	400	+	–*		+	+		Miller et al. (1978)
P	577			+	+	+		Lubin et al. (1981)
H	2024	NA					–*	Graham et al. (1982)
H, P	268	NA						Kolonel et al. (1983)
H	368				NA	+		Talamini et al. (1984)
F	328				(+)		+*	Zemla (1984)
H	68	+						Sarin et al. (1985)
H, P	212	(+)	(–)					Hirohata et al. (1985)
H	1010	+*			NA	+	NA	Lê et al. (1986)
H, P	818						–	Lubin et al. (1986)
P	861				+*	+*	–*	Hislop et al. (1986)
H	120		(–)		NA	NA	–	Katsouyanni et al. (1986)
H, P	344	(+)	NA					Hirohata et al. (1987)
P	250	+	NA	+	(+)	+	NA	Toniolo et al. (1989)
Prospective studies								
	139			+				Hirayama (1978)
	186			(+)		(–)		Phillips et al. (1980)
	62			(+)		(–)		Kinlen (1982)
NA	99	(–)						Jones et al. (1987)
NA	601	NA						Willett et al. (1987)

[a] +, increased risk; –, decreased risk; NA, no association; *, association limited to subgroups; ( ), not statistically significant; blank, not studied
[b] P, population or neighbourhood controls; H, hospital controls; F, family controls

premenopausal women. A high fat diet in adolescence may be related to early age at menarche, which is associated with increased risk, although there are no strong data to support this relation.

Alternative hypotheses relate to the synthesis of different types of prostaglandins, as described on p. 203. The balance of different types of fatty acids might turn out to be more important than the total amount of fat or than the ratio of polyunsaturated:saturated fat.

Other cancers

It has been suggested that fat intake may be associated with the risk for cancers at other sites, in particular those occurring in endocrine organs. There is quite strong evidence that the risk for prostatic cancer is increased by a high-fat diet, measured either by indices of total fat intake (Graham *et al.*, 1983; Kolonel *et al.*, 1983) or as consumption of meat, eggs and dairy products (Rotkin, 1977; Lew & Garfinkel, 1979; Schuman *et al.*, 1982). Diet was estimated in most of these studies by brief, crude questionnaires, and the statistical analyses did not take account of total caloric intake. The associations observed may therefore be the nonspecific expression of other underlying dietary factors.

Limited data are available with regard to fat intake and cancers of the endometrium and the ovary. There is strong evidence that overweight increases the risk for endometrial cancer. The prospective study of the American Cancer Society on 419 060 women indicated that the risk rises steadily in relation to increase in body weight (Lew & Garfinkel, 1979). Taking as the reference women whose body weight (for any specific height) was below average, the relative risk increased to 1.36, 1.85, 2.30 and 5.42 for those weighing 10–19%, 20–29%, 30–39% and 40% or more, respectively, in excess of the average weight. Obesity is clearly related to diet; however, it is not specifically related to fat, but rather to excess caloric intake. Only one study provides some evidence that high intake of fatty foods increases the risk for endometrial cancer (La Vecchia *et al.*, 1986). The picture is even less clear for cancer of the ovary. The American Cancer Society prospective study (Lew & Garfinkel, 1979) showed an increased risk associated with overweight only for women whose weight was 40% greater than average.

Cholesterol

A diet rich in fat (and particularly in saturated fat) is usually also rich in cholesterol. There is therefore an intrinsic positive correlation between dietary intake of cholesterol and of total and saturated fat, both at the individual and at the population level. International studies of the correlation between mortality from colon cancer and average per-caput intake of cholesterol have indicated a positive correlation with high dietary cholesterol (Liu *et al.*, 1979). Two case–control studies on breast cancer (Miller *et al.*, 1978; Lubin *et al.*, 1981) and one on colorectal cancer (Jain *et al.*, 1980) showed slight increases in risk associated with high intake of cholesterol. High cholesterol intake was also found to be associated with increased risks for cancers of the prostate and lung in Hawaii (Kolonel *et al.*, 1983).

These findings are in contrast to those of certain studies designed to investigate the relationship between cardiovascular disease and cholesterol level. In one intervention trial in 1971, the Los Angeles Veterans Administration Hospital Study (Pearce & Dayton, 1971), the number of deaths observed in the group randomly allocated to a low-cholesterol/high-polyunsaturated fat diet was twice that observed in the control group. In three successive intervention trials, however – the Finnish Mental Hospital Study (Turpeinen, 1979), the United States Coronary Drug Project (Coronary Drug Project Research Group, 1975), and the WHO Cooperative Trial on clofibrate (Committee of Principal Investigators, 1980) – no difference in cancer mortality was found between the low- and high-cholesterol groups. Subsequently, a number of observational follow-up studies indicated that subjects with serum cholesterol levels below 180 mg/dl might have an increased risk for colorectal cancer compared with subjects with higher levels (McMichael *et al.*, 1984; Keys *et al.*, 1985; Salonen *et al.*, 1985).

Several hypotheses have been formulated to explain the biological significance of the increased risk for colon cancer in subjects with low blood cholesterol. It has been suggested that individuals who maintain low serum cholesterol in spite of a high-fat diet may secrete more bile (containing bile acids and cholesterol) or excrete more nonabsorbed cholesterol in faeces (Broitman, 1981). As described above (p. 206), biliary secretion of acid and neutral steroids may influence colon carcinogenesis. However, several studies in which cholesterol and neutral steroid concentrations were measured in faeces provided inconsistent results concerning the relationship between faecal cholesterol concentration and colon cancer risk.

Dietary protein

Epidemiological studies on the possible association between dietary protein and cancer have given contrasting results, depending on the cancer site investigated. On the one hand, some studies on colorectal cancer and, to a lesser extent, breast cancer suggest that high intake of protein is associated with an increased risk. On the other hand, studies of oesophageal cancer indicate that subjects with low protein intake may be those at highest risk.

The evidence for an increased risk for colorectal cancer associated with high protein intake comes from three case–control studies in which total protein intake was measured (see Table 23) and five case–control studies in which meat consumption was used as an indicator of animal protein intake. About half of the case–control studies on colorectal cancer and all three prospective studies found no increase in risk associated with either protein or meat intake.

The association between protein or meat intake and breast cancer has been investigated in ten case–control studies, five of which found some indication of increased risk (Miller *et al.*, 1978; Nomura *et al.*, 1978; Lubin *et al.*, 1981; Hislop *et al.*, 1986; Toniolo *et al.*, 1989). The results from five prospective studies were also contradictory: in Japan (Hirayama, 1978), high meat intake was associated with increased mortality from breast cancer, while in other studies the association was weak and not statistically significant (Phillips *et al.*, 1980; Kinlen, 1982; see Table 24).

The complexity of the relationship between dietary protein level and cancer risk is further exemplified by the results of several studies on oesophageal cancer. Two studies, conducted in the USA (Ziegler *et al.*, 1981) and in France (Tuyns *et al.*, 1987), showed that subjects with low intake of animal proteins, particularly in the form of fresh meat and fish, were at markedly increased risk for oesophageal cancer. The main risk factors, however, were consumption of alcohol and, to a lesser extent, tobacco. It has been postulated that insufficient consumption of fresh foods of animal origin may interact with the carcinogenic effect of alcoholic beverages, although little experimental evidence is available to support this hypothesis (IARC, 1988).

Carbohydrates

While fat intake has received most attention as the energy providing nutrient in relation to cancer of the colorectum and breast, complex carbohydrates (starch) have often been mentioned as a possible etiological factor in gastric cancer. The case–control studies that suggested a role for starches provide only limited support, however, for such a relationship. In 12 studies, data were presented that allowed some testing of the association (see Table 25). In ten of these there was some indication that foods rich in complex carbohydrates might increase stomach cancer risk. A minor drawback of most of them was that only a limited number of indicator foods, such as rice, pasta and potatoes, were studied, and no attempt was made to measure or calculate total intake of simple and total complex carbohydrates. In only one of these studies (Tuyns et al., 1990) were estimates obtained of whole diet in terms of nutrient intake. In this study, a positive association was found between intake of polysaccharides and gastric cancer risk, which, however, disappeared after adjustment for total caloric intake. Another interesting observation in this study was a highly significantly increased effect on risk of mono- and disaccharides. This finding was in agreement with that of Risch *et al.* (1985), who found an increasing risk with consumption of total carbohydrates; however, they also found that the starch component of carbohydrates did not appear to be associated with gastric cancer risk.

Energy

In experiments in rats, caloric restriction in early life reduced the yield of spontaneous tumours and increased longevity (Ross & Bras, 1965). In other experiments, caloric restriction resulted in inhibition of the development of spontaneous and chemically induced tumours such as, for example, sarcomas and lung tumours (Tannenbaum, 1942a,b). Kritchesky *et al.* (1984) reported that a low-fat, high-calorie diet led to more mammary tumours in rats who had received 7,12-dimethylbenz[*a*]anthracene than a high-fat, low-calorie diet. They suggested that in this model caloric intake might be a greater determinant of a tumour-enhancing regimen than dietary fat.

Epidemiological findings on energy intake and cancer have been the object of much controversy. Estimates of energy intake are based on separate estimates of the intake of protein, fat, carbohydrates and alcohol. In human epidemiology as well as in animal studies, one of the main conceptual and practical puzzles has been how to vary energy intake without modifying nutrient balance and, *vice versa*, how to investigate the effect of different levels of a nutrient, say fat, while keeping energy intake constant. This problem has been the object of recent methodological work (Howe, 1985; Willett & Stampfer, 1986) which has drawn attention to certain weaknesses in early epidemiological work on diet and cancer.

Table 25. Main results from case–control studies on diet and risk for gastric cancer

No. of cases	Controls[a]	Salt & salty foods[b]	Carbohydrates/starchy foods	Vegetables	Fruit	Fibre	Vitamin C	Vitamin A	Calcium and dairy products	Alcohol	Reference
100	H	NA	NA	NA	NA							Acheson & Doll (1964)
454	P	+			NA	NA						Hirayama (1963)
93	H			NA						NA		Higginson (1966)
276	H	(+)	(+)	+/-[c]							NA	Graham et al. (1967)
228	H		+	-							NA	Graham et al. (1972)
220	H	+	+	-	-					-	+	Haenszel et al. (1972)
166	H, P		+									Modan et al. (1974)
783	H	NA	+/NA[d]		-							Haenszel et al. (1976)
40	H			-	-						+	Hoey et al. (1981)
39	H		(+)	-	-			NA	NA		+	Correa et al. (1985)
246	P	+	+[e]	-	-	-	(-)	-/NA[f]	NA		+	Risch et al. (1985)
111	H					-		-				Stehr et al. (1985)
110	H		+	-	-	-	-				NA	Trichopoulos et al. (1983)
110	H, P	(+)	+	(-)	-						+	Jedrychowski et al. (1986)
206	H	+	+	-	-		-	-/NA[f]				LaVecchia et al. (1987)
241	H	+	+	-	-							Hu et al. (1988)
564	P	+	NA	-	-		-	-/NA[f]	-	+		You et al. (1988)
163	P	+									NA	Tuyns et al. (1983a)
293	P	+										Tuyns et al. (1988)
449	P		+/NA[g]		-	-	-	-/+[f]	+			Tuyns et al. (1990)

[a] H, hospital controls; P, population controls

[b] Salt and salty foods comprised, among others: salt added to dishes during meals; pickled vegetables; salted dried fish; fish and soya bean fermentation products.

[c] An increased risk was observed for higher levels of cabbage consumption; for lettuce the association was in the opposite direction.

[d] Effect of rice consumption: a positive association with gastric cancer was noted only for two of the three subgroups (Hawaiian Japanese and Issei and not for Nisei).

[e] An increased risk effect was observed for total carbohydrates, but the starch component did not appear to be associated with gastric cancer risk.

[f] Protective effects were due to β-carotene; for retinol, no association or increased risk was noted.

[g] The positive association between polysaccharides and gastric cancer risk disappeared after adjustment for total calorie intake.

+, increased risk; -, decreased risk; NA, no association; ( ), not statistically significant; blank, not studied

With regard to colorectal cancer, a positive association with caloric intake was found in five studies (Jain *et al.*, 1980; Bristol *et al*, 1985; Potter & McMichael, 1986; Graham *et al.*, 1988; Slattery *et al.*, 1988); no association was found in two (Macquart-Moulin *et al.*, 1986; Tuyns *et al.*, 1988); while in about 12 other studies, total caloric intake was not measured.

Very few case–control studies of breast cancer have included estimates of total energy intake. In one that did (Toniolo *et al.*, 1989), an increased risk for breast cancer was found with increasing levels of caloric intake. Adjustment for intake of saturated fat and animal protein made the association weaker and not statistically significant. In the study of US nurses (Willett *et al.*, 1987), total caloric intake was not associated with breast cancer risk.

Nitrosated products and *N*-nitroso compounds

Many components of the human diet, including drinking-water, contain nitrites and nitrates, either naturally (for example, in many vegetables) or as preservatives in meats and other cured products. Vegetables such as beetroot, celery, lettuce, radishes, spinach and endives are important sources of dietary nitrates (National Research Council, 1981). Nitrites present in foods or derived from nitrates in saliva can interact with other dietary substances, such as amines and amides (particularly in the acid pH of the stomach (Ohshima & Bartsch, 1981; Correa & Haenszel, 1982)), to produce *N*-nitroso compounds, most of which are carcinogens in experimental animals (see p. 134). Volatile *N*-nitrosamines may also be present in foods, mainly in those treated with nitrites, such as bacon and cheeses, and in beer.

Several correlation studies provide indirect evidence that exposure to high levels of nitrates and nitrites in food and drinking-water increases the risk for stomach and oesophageal cancer (Tannenbaum *et al.*, 1979; Armijo *et al.*, 1981). In a study in the UK, however, high nitrate levels were correlated with a lower risk for gastric cancer (Forman *et al.*, 1985). In this study, the nitrates were largely derived from vegetables, and the vitamin C they contained could have been protective. This was the explanation given for a similar effect seen in a case–control study in Canada, in which nitrate consumption appeared to be protective until vitamin C intake was taken into account. In the same study, nitrite consumption increased the risk for gastric cancer (Risch *et al.*, 1985). In cross-sectional studies in populations with different incidences of oesophageal and gastric cancers, levels of endogenous formation of nitrosamines were shown to be higher in population groups with a high incidence (Bartsch *et al.*, 1989).

Salt and salted foods

Salted fish is commonly consumed by southern Chinese and is one of the first solid foods given to babies after weaning. Although no significant difference in current use of salted fish has been found in several case–control studies, in Hong Kong (Geser *et al.*, 1978), Kuala Lumpur (Armstrong *et al.*, 1983) or California (Henderson *et al.*, 1976), positive associations have been found between nasopharyngeal carcinoma and the use of salted fish during and soon after weaning. A case–control study in Hong Kong on cases under 35 years of age found a positive association with consumption of salted fish at any time, but this was particularly strong for consumption during childhood, with a relative increase in risk of nearly 40 fold for consumption of salted fish one or more times a week at age 10 in comparison to rare consumption (Yu *et al.*, 1986). Subsequent studies in southern China (Guangxi and Guangzhou) have confirmed the association with salted fish intake, particularly during the weaning period, but the relative risks were much lower (between 2 and 3) (Yu *et al.*, 1988, 1989). All of these studies are, however, based on the recall of events occurring several decades previously, and relatively few observations were made.

Some experimental support for the association is provided by the study of Yu and Henderson (1987), in which rats fed salted fish developed tumours in the nasal cavity.

Salt and salty foods have also been incriminated as carcinogenic in relation to gastric cancer. In studies of You *et al.* (1980) and Tuyns (1983a, 1988), questions were asked about taste preferences and amounts of salt usually added to foods during meals. Persons who preferred salty foods had a higher risk of developing stomach cancer. In these studies, information was obtained about consumption of specific salt-rich foods, such as pickles and fish fermentation products, which were suspected of being related to gastric cancer risk. Positive associations were found in the studies of Hirayama (1963) and Haenszel *et al.* (1988). One hypothesis that might explain a relationship between salt intake and gastric cancer is that excess salt acts as an irritant on the stomach wall and may induce the synthesis of *N*-nitrosamines in the stomach.

Coffee and tea

Coffee and tea contain substances that are either direct mutagens (glyoxal) or which enhance the mutagenic effect produced by other chemicals (caffeine, theobromine) (Nasao *et al.*, 1979; Ames, 1983). Epidemiological studies on coffee drinking have been concerned largely with cancers of the bladder and pancreas. However, although increased risks for bladder cancer have been reported (Cole, 1971; Fraumeni *et al.*, 1971; Simon *et al.*, 1975; Howe *et al.*, 1980), dose–response relationships have not been seen, and other studies showed no association (Morrison *et al.*, 1982; Hartge *et al.*, 1983; Jensen *et al.*, 1986). With regard to pancreatic cancer, a dose–response relationship was found for women (MacMahon *et al.*, 1981), and an association with decaffeinated coffee was seen in another study (Lin & Kessler, 1981). A weak association was seen by Gold *et al.* (1985), with a suggestion of a dose–response relationship for women but inconsistent findings for men; in another study, uniformly negative results were seen for both men and women (Wynder *et al.*, 1983). In a further study, coffee intake seemed to be associated with increased risk (Mack *et al.*, 1986). In a repeat of an earlier study, MacMahon and his colleagues found an increased risk only for people who drank five or more cups of coffee daily, with no evidence of a dose–response relationship (Hsieh *et al.*, 1986).

An association between coffee drinking and ovarian cancer has been suggested (Trichopoulos *et al.*, 1981), but suggestions that coffee drinking may increase the risk for breast cancer were not supported by a large US case–control study (Rosenberg *et al.*, 1985). A cohort study of Seventh-day Adventists suggested that coffee drinking increases the risk for fatal large-bowel cancer (Phillips &

Snowdon, 1985); however, the dietary data were limited and did not permit a full evaluation of the possible confounding effects of other foods.

The drinking of hot beverages in general has been associated with increased risks for oesophageal cancer. Drinking hot tea is frequent in various populations with a high incidence of oesophageal cancer, such as Chinese in Singapore (De Jong *et al.*, 1974), Japanese (Hirayama, 1971; Segi, 1975), Turkomans in northern Iran (Iran–IARC Cancer Study Group, 1977; Cook-Mozaffari *et al.*, 1979), and Turkomans and Kazakhs in the USSR (Grishin, 1962; Kolicheva, 1980). In a study in Puerto Rico, more oesophageal cancer cases than controls claimed to drink their coffee hot rather than warm or cold (Martinez, 1969).

Pyrolysis products of proteins and amino acids

Grilling or broiling of foods (especially meat and fish) results in the production of mutagenic compounds (Sugimura *et al.*, 1981). Although there are no data on the degree of risk that these compounds, chemically identified as three-ring *N*-heterocyclic aromatic amines (Sugimura, 1982), pose for humans, several are carcinogenic in experimental animals (IARC, 1986).

Contaminants

Foods may contain residues of pesticides of various types, including herbicides and fumigants; the amounts vary according to the procedures used for treating crops and the method of harvesting. For the major pesticides, international regulations exist with regard to permissible amounts of residues in foods – the ADI, or acceptable daily intake; these are drawn up periodically by expert groups convened by the World Health Organization and the Food and Agricultural Organization of the United Nations and published as technical reports and in the *WHO Pesticide Residue Series*. The use of fertilizers may influence the level of nitrites in foods, which can lead to the formation of carcinogenic *N*-nitrosamines (see p. 134).

Dietary factors that may reduce the risk for cancer

The human diet contains components that may interfere in cancer development. These include vitamin A, provitamin A (β-carotene), vitamin C (ascorbic acid), vitamin E (α-tocopherol), vitamin B_2 (riboflavin), trace elements such as selenium and zinc, various inhibitors found in plants, and dietary fibre. Most of the putative protective micronutrients, such as vitamins C and E, β-carotene and selenium, are antioxidants and may inhibit carcinogenesis by quenching free radicals or singlet oxygen and blocking the endogenous formation of carcinogens (Peto *et al.*, 1981; Wattenberg, 1983).

Vitamin A and β-carotene

Vitamin A deficiency increases susceptibility to chemically induced neoplasia in laboratory animals, and, in some experimental models, an increased intake of this vitamin appears to protect against carcinogenesis (Sporn & Roberts, 1983). Experiments with synthetic retinoids suggest that they are protective against cancers of the breast, lung, urinary bladder and skin (Sporn & Newton, 1981). Retinoids can induce regression of papillomas of the skin in mice (Bollag, 1979;

Bollag & Hartmann, 1983). Carotenoids are precursors of vitamin A and are converted into vitamin A *in vivo*. A few experimental studies have suggested a protective effect of carotenoids against chemically induced neoplasia (Shamberger, 1971; Mathews-Roth, 1982).

Low intake of vitamin A and β-carotene, or low intake of foods rich in these vitamins, has been associated with increased risks for cancers at different sites, including cancers of the lung (Bjelke, 1975; MacLennan *et al.*, 1977; Mettlin *et al.*, 1979; Shekelle *et al.*, 1981; Kvåle *et al.*, 1983; Hinds *et al.*, 1984; Ziegler *et al.*, 1984), larynx (Graham *et al.*, 1981; Byers & Graham, 1984), mouth (Marshall *et al.*, 1982; Winn *et al.*, 1984), oesophagus (Wynder & Bross, 1961; Iran–IARC Cancer Study Group, 1977; Cook-Mozaffari *et al.*, 1979; Mettlin *et al.*, 1981), stomach (Graham *et al.*, 1972; Hirayama, 1977), large bowel (Bjelke, 1978) and urinary bladder (Mettlin & Graham, 1979). In one study of lung cancer, an inverse association was found between the risk for squamous-cell cancer and vitamin A intake, but no association for adenocarcinoma (Byers *et al.*, 1984). Although Schuman *et al.* (1977) suggested a protective effect of vitamin A against prostatic cancer, other studies have suggested increased risks (Graham *et al.*, 1983; Graham, 1984). In many of these studies, a negative association was found with vegetable intake, suggesting that β-carotene or some other inhibitor in the vegetables could be the responsible factor.

In two case–control studies, an inverse association was found between intake of preformed vitamin A and lung cancer (Smith & Jick, 1978; Gregor *et al.*, 1980). In a prospective study in which it was possible to differentiate between β-carotene and vitamin A intake, the protective effect against lung cancer was associated with β-carotene rather than vitamin A (Shekelle *et al.*, 1981).

Cohort studies in which blood samples were collected from healthy people, stored and subsequently analysed for vitamin A and in which information on development of cancer a few years later was available suggest that high risks for cancer, and especially lung cancer, are *not* associated with low blood levels of vitamin A (Stähelin *et al.*, 1984; Willett *et al.*, 1984; Friedman *et al.*, 1986). Wald *et al.* (1980) found that an association between low blood retinol levels and cancer risk was restricted to people who developed cancer within two years after their blood was sampled, suggesting that preclinical disease may already have been present. The relation between baseline retinol levels and subsequent cancer reported by Kark *et al.* (1981) was not confirmed after longer follow-up (Peleg *et al.*, 1984).

In cohort studies of serum β-carotene, lower levels than in controls were recorded in women who subsequently developed breast cancer although the differences were not statistically significant (Wald *et al.*, 1984), and in people who subsequently died of lung cancer (Stähelin *et al.*, 1984).

Vitamin C

Several experimental models suggest that vitamin C may prevent tumours by inhibiting the formation of carcinogens or by reducing the effect of exogenous carcinogens. It has been shown that vitamin C inhibits the formation of *N*-nitroso compounds from nitrites and amines or amides, both *in vitro* and *in vivo* (Mirvish *et al.*, 1972; Ivankovic *et al.*, 1974; Bartsch *et al.*, 1988) and also inhibits the formation of 1,2-dimethylhydrazine-induced carcinomas of the large bowel (Reddy & Hirohata, 1979; Logue & Frommer, 1980) and of sarcomas in rats given benzo[*a*]pyrene (Kallistratas & Faske, 1980). Vitamin C inhibits the malignant transformation of mouse embryo cells exposed to 3-methylcholanthrene in tissue culture (Benedict *et al.*, 1980), and low concentrations suppress the growth *in vitro* of cells taken from patients with acute nonlymphocytic leukaemia (Park *et al.*, 1980).

In an early epidemiological study on stomach cancer, Meinsma (1964) reported that patients with stomach cancer usually ate less citrus fruit than controls. An inverse correlation between intake of fresh fruits and vegetables and cancer of the stomach has since been observed in several studies (Higginson, 1966; Haenszel *et al.*, 1972; Haenszel & Correa, 1975; Bjelke, 1978; Kolonel *et al.*, 1981; Risch *et al.*, 1985), which may indicate an effect of vitamin C, although confounding by other micronutrients present in the same foods cannot be excluded. An inverse relationship has also been observed between the intake of foods rich in vitamins A and C and oesophageal cancer (Iran–IARC Cancer Study Group, 1977; Cook-Mozaffari *et al.*, 1979; Mettlin *et al.*, 1981; Ziegler *et al.*, 1981; Tuyns, 1983b; Tuyns *et al.*, 1987). Low intake of vitamin C also seemed to increase the risk for developing cancer of the larynx and dysplastic changes in the cervix uteri (Graham *et al.*, 1981; Wassertheil-Smoller *et al.*, 1981). Vitamin C supplements may decrease the frequency of relapses of adenomatous polyps of the large bowel.

Vitamin E

Vitamin E can also inhibit the production of carcinogenic *N*-nitroso compounds from nitrites and amines or amides and is one of the most important traps for oxygen radicals in lipid membranes (Newberne & Suphakarn, 1983). Some studies have suggested that it inhibits the development of chemically induced tumours in experimental animals, such as those of soft tissue (Haber & Wissler, 1962), mammary gland (Lee & Chen, 1979), skin (Wattenberg, 1972) and large bowel (Cook & McNamara, 1980).

Relevant epidemiological data are limited. In two cohort studies, no relationship was found between vitamin E levels and risk for cancers at all sites combined (Willett *et al.*, 1983), or for cancers at various sites (Salonen *et al.*, 1985). However, in another cohort study, significantly lower vitamin E levels were found among women who subsequently developed breast cancer than among controls (Wald *et al.*, 1984).

Vitamin B$_2$

Evidence from both laboratory experiments (Wynder & Klein, 1965; Foy & Kondi, 1984; Newberne, 1984) and studies of population groups with a high incidence of oesophageal cancer (Muñoz *et al.*, 1982; Thurnham *et al.*, 1982; Crespi *et al.*, 1984; Zaridze *et al.*, 1985) suggest that low intake and low blood levels of vitamin B$_2$ are associated with a high incidence of oesophageal cancer. In an intervention study in a high-risk area for oesophageal cancer in China, a dietary supplement including vitamin B$_2$ did not influence the prevalence of oesophagitis or dysplasia found at oesophagoscopy after one year of treatment (Muñoz *et al.*, 1985), but it significantly reduced the prevalence of micronuclei in oesophageal cells (Muñoz *et al.*, 1987). However, it is possible tht the vitamin was given for too short a period or that it influences other stages of the natural history of oesophageal cancer.

Selenium

Selenium is a trace element, which plays an important role in the metabolism of glutathione peroxidase, an enzyme that protects against oxidative damage (Willett & MacMahon, 1984), although at high doses it is toxic. Addition of selenium to the diet of laboratory animals reduces the yields of chemically induced tumours at several sites (Shamberger, 1970; Griffin & Jacobs, 1977; Greeder & Milner, 1980) and inhibits the mutagenic activity of a variety of chemicals (Jacobs *et al.*, 1977; Shamberger *et al.*, 1978).

An inverse correlation has been found between the selenium content of soil and human blood and the incidence of cancer, mostly of the gastrointestinal tract (Shamberger *et al.*, 1976; Schrauzer *et al.*, 1977). In one case–control study and two small cohort studies, low levels of selenium in the blood were associated with an increased risk for cancer (McConnell *et al.*, 1980; Willett *et al.*, 1983; Salonen *et al.*, 1985). In the study of Salonen *et al.*, blood samples were analysed for both selenium and vitamin E before individuals subsequently developed cancer. The risk for fatal cancer was greater among individuals with low selenium levels than among those with higher levels; however, subjects with low selenium and low vitamin E levels had an even greater risk.

Dietary fibre

Experimentally, dietary fibre can protect against large-bowel carcinogenesis. It may act on the metabolism of bacteria in the gut, resulting in less carcinogenic end products, or it may act simply by increasing faecal mass and thus decreasing the concentration of carcinogenic as well as other faecal constituents (Reddy *et al.*, 1978). The effect of fibre on colon carcinogenesis seems to depend on the type of fibre given (Watanabe *et al.*, 1979).

A study conducted in Copenhagen, Denmark, and Kuopio, Finland – areas with a four-fold difference in colon cancer incidence – revealed a significant inverse relationship between dietary fibre intake and the frequency of this cancer (IARC Intestinal Microecology Group, 1977). In a second study in Denmark (Jensen *et al.*, 1982), a significant inverse trend with large-bowel cancer incidence was observed for cereal consumption and total dietary fibre; and, in a Japanese cohort study, the higher the daily intake of rice and wheat, the lower the standardized mortality ratio for colon and rectal cancer (Hirayama, 1981).

Two case–control studies also support the hypothesis of a protective effect of high fibre intake. Modan *et al.* (1975) found a significantly lower fibre consumption frequency among patients with colon cancer but not in those with rectal cancer, compared to controls. Dales *et al.* (1979) found a consistent dose–response gradient for fibrous foods: significantly more colon cancer patients than controls reported eating diets high in fat-containing foods, and low in fibre-containing foods, and fewer patients ate low fat-containing foods and high fibre-containing foods. However, in two further case–control studies of colorectal cancer, no protective effect of dietary fibre could be demonstrated (Miller *et al.*, 1983; Potter & McMichael, 1986).

Vegetables and fruit

Vegetables and fruits are important components of the diet in most parts of the world, but individual intake varies substantially due to personal taste, local tradition and availability of fresh produce. Vegetables and fruit are usually the main source of vitamin C and carotenoids as well as of fibre and several mineral salts; their consumption is therefore highly correlated with the intake of several of the micronutrients that are suspected to reduce cancer risk. In epidemiological studies based on self-reported diet, it is often difficult to separate possible effect of vegetables and fruits from those of specific nutrients. A growing number of studies have reported lower risks for cancers of the oropharynx and larynx, oesophagus, stomach, colon, rectum, lung and breast in association with high consumption of vegetables and fruit. The evidence for a protective effect of a diet rich in vegetables and fruit is not in contradiction with the results on specific micronutrients; on the contrary, it adds support to the hypothesis that several components of vegetables and fruits may have inhibiting effects on carcinogenesis.

References

Acheson, E.D. & Doll, R. (1964) Dietary factors in carcinoma of the stomach: a study of 100 cases and 200 controls. *Gut*, *5*, 126-131

Ames, B.N. (1983) Dietary carcinogens and anticarcinogens. *Science*, *221*, 1256-1266

Armijo, R., Gonzales, A., Orellana, M., Coulson, A.H., Sayre, J.W. & Detel, R. (1981) The epidemiology of gastric cancer in Chile: II. Nitrate exposures and stomach cancer frequency. *Int. J. Epidemiol.*, *10*, 57-62

Armstrong, R.W., Armstrong, M.J., Yu, M.C. & Henderson, B.E. (1983) Salted fish and inhalants as risk factors for nasopharyngeal carcinoma in Malaysian Chinese. *Cancer Res.*, *43*, 2967-2970

Bartsch, H., Ohshima, H., Pignatelli, B. & Calmels, S. (1989) Human exposure to endogenous *N*-nitroso compounds: quantitative estimates in subjects at high risk for cancer of the oral cavity, oesophagus, stomach and urinary bladder. *Cancer Surv.*, *8*, 335-362

Benedict, W.F., Wheatley, W.L. & Jones, P.A. (1980) Inhibition of chemically induced morphological transformation and reversion of the transformed phenotype by ascorbic acid in C3H/10T1/2 cells. *Cancer Res.*, *40*, 2796-2801

Berrino, F. & Panico, G. (1989) Dietary fat, nutritional status and endocrine associated cancers. In: Miller, A.B., ed., *Diet and the Aetiology of Cancers* (Monograph Series of the European School of Oncology), Berlin (West), Springer, pp. 3-12

Bjelke, E. (1975) Dietary vitamin A and human lung cancer. *Int. J. Cancer*, *15*, 561-565

Bjelke, E. (1978) Dietary factors and the epidemiology of cancer of the stomach and large bowel. In: Kasper, H., ed., *Aktuelle Probleme der Klinischen Diatetik*, Stuttgart, Georg Thieme, pp. 10-17

Bollag, W. (1979) Retinoids and cancer. *Cancer Chemother. Pharmacol.*, *3*, 307-315

Bollag, W. & Hartmann, H.R. (1983) Prevention and therapy of cancer with retinoids in animals and man. *Cancer Surv.*, *2*, 315-326

Bristol, J.B., Emmett, P.M., Heaton, K.W. & Williamson, R.C.N. (1985) Sugar, fat, and the risk of colorectal cancer. *Br. Med. J.*, *291*, 1467-1470

Broitman, S.A. (1981) Cholesterol excretion and colon cancer. *Cancer Res.*, *41*, 3738-3740

Byers, T. & Graham, S. (1984) The epidemiology of diet and cancer. *Adv. Cancer Res.*, *41*, 1-69

Byers, T., Vena, J., Mettlin, C., Swanson, M. & Graham, S. (1984) Dietary vitamin A and lung cancer risk. An analysis by histological subtypes. *Am. J. Epidemiol.*, *120*, 769-776

Cole, P. (1971) Coffee drinking and cancer of the lower urinary tract. *Lancet*, *i*, 1335-1337

Committee of Principal Investigators (1980) WHO cooperative trial on primary prevention of ischaemic heart disease using clofibrate to lower serum cholesterol: mortality follow-up. *Lancet*, *ii*, 379-385

Cook, M.G. & McNamara, P. (1980) Effect of dietary vitamin E on dimethylhydrazine-induced colonic tumors in mice. *Cancer Res.*, *40*, 1329-1331

Cook-Mozaffari, P.J., Azordegan, F., Day, N.E., Ressicaud, A., Sabai, C. & Aramesh, B. (1979) Oesophageal cancer studies in the Caspian littoral of Iran: results of a case–control study. *Br. J. Cancer*, *39*, 293-309

Coronary Drug Project Research Group (1975) Clofibrate and niacin in coronary heart disease. *J. Am. Med. Assoc.*, *231*, 360-381

Correa, P. & Haenszel, W. (1982) Epidemiology of gastric cancer. In: Correa, P. & Haenszel, W., eds, *Epidemiology of Cancer of the Digestive Tract (Developments in Oncology 6)*, The Hague, Martinus Nijhoff, pp. 59-84

Correa, P., Fontham, E., Pickle, L.W., Chen, V., Lin, Y. & Haenszel, W. (1985) Dietary determinants of gastric cancer in south Louisiana inhabitants, *J. Natl Cancer Inst.*, *75*, 645-654

Crespi, M., Muñoz, N., Grassi, A., Shen, Q., Wang, K.J. & Lin, J.J. (1984) Precursor lesions of esophageal cancer in a low-risk population in China: comparison with high-risk populations. *Int. J. Cancer*, *34*, 599-602

Dales, L.O., Friedman, G.D., Ury, H.K., Grossman, S. & Williams, S.R. (1979) A case–control study of relationships of diet and other traits to colorectal cancer in American blacks. *Am. J. Epidemiol.*, *109*, 132-144

De Jong, J.U.W., Breslow, N., Goh Eve Hong, J., Sridharan, M. & Shanmugaratnam, K. (1974) Aetiological factors in oesophageal cancer in Singapore Chinese. *Int. J. Cancer*, *13*, 291-301

Forman, D., Al-Dabbagh, S. & Doll, R. (1985) Nitrates, nitrites and gastric cancer in Great Britain. *Nature*, *313*, 620-625

Foy, H. & Kondi, A. (1984) The vulnerable esophagus: riboflavin deficiency and squamous cell dysplasia of the skin and the esophagus. *J. Natl Cancer Inst.*, *72*, 941-948

Fraumeni, J.F., Scotto, J. & Dunham, L.J. (1971) Coffee drinking and bladder cancer. *Lancet*, *ii*, 1204

Friedman, G.D., Blaner, W.S., Goodman, D.S., Vogelman, J.H., Brind, J.L., Hoover, R., Fireman, B.H. & Orentreich, N. (1986) Serum retinol and retinol-binding protein levels do not predict subsequent lung cancer. *Am. J. Epidemiol.*, *123*, 781-789

Geser, A., Charnay, N., Day, N.E., de-Thé, G. & Ho, H.C. (1978) Environmental factors in the etiology of nasopharyngeal carcinoma: report on a case–control study in Hong Kong. In: de-Thé, G. & Ito, Y., eds, *Nasopharyngeal Carcinoma: Etiology and Control* (IARC Scientific Publications No. 20), Lyon, IARC, pp. 213-229

Gold, E.B., Gordis, L., Diener, M.D., Seltser, R., Boinott, J.K., Bynum, T.E. & Hutcheon, D.F. (1985) Diet and other risk factors for cancer of the pancreas. *Cancer*, *55*, 460-467

Goodwin, P.J. & Boyd, W.F. (1987) Critical appraisal of the evidence that dietary fat intake is related to breast cancer risk in humans. *J. Natl Cancer Inst.*, *79*, 473-485

Graham, S. (1984) Epidemiology of retinoids and cancer. *J. Natl Cancer Inst.*, *73*, 1423-1428

Graham, S., Lilienfeld, A.M. & Tidings, J.E. (1967) Dietary and purgation factors in the epidemiology of gastric cancer. *Cancer*, *20*, 2224-2234

Graham, S., Scholz, W. & Martino, P. (1972) Alimentary factors in the epidemiology of gastric cancer. *Cancer*, *30*, 927-928

Graham, S., Dayal, H., Swanson, M., Mittleman, A. & Wilkinson, G. (1978) Diet in the epidemiology of cancer of the colon and rectum. *J. Natl Cancer Inst.*, *61*, 709-714

Graham, S., Mettlin, C., Marshall, J., Priore, R., Rzepka, T. & Shedd, D. (1981) Dietary factors in the epidemiology of cancer of the larynx. *Am. J. Epidemiol.*, *113*, 675-680

Graham, S., Marshall, J., Mettlin, C., Rzepka, T., Nemoto, T. & Byers, T. (1982) Diet in the epidemiology of breast cancer. *Am. J. Epidemiol.*, *116*, 68-75

Graham, S., Haughey, B., Marshall, J., Priore, R., Byers, T., Rzepka, T., Mettlin, C. & Pontes, J.E. (1983) Diet in the epidemiology of carcinoma of the prostate gland. *J. Natl Cancer Inst.*, *70*, 687-692

Graham, S., Marshall, J., Haughey, B., Mittelman, A., Swanson, M., Zielezny, M., Byers, T., Wilkinson, G. & West, D. (1988) Dietary epidemiology of cancer of the colon in western New York. *Am. J. Epidemiol.*, *128*, 490-503

Greeder, G.A. & Milner, J.A. (1980) Factors influencing the inhibitory effect of selenium on mice inoculated with Ehrlich ascites tumour cells. *Science*, *209*, 825-827

Gregor, A., Lee, P.N., Roe, F.J.C., Wilson, M.J. & Melton, A. (1980) Comparison of dietary histories in lung cancer cases and controls with special reference to vitamin A. *Nutr. Cancer, 2*, 93-97

Griffin, A.C. & Jacobs, M.M. (1977) Effects of selenium on azo dye hepatocarcinogenesis. *Cancer Lett., 3*, 177-181

Grishin, E.N. (1962) Etiology and incidence of cancer of the oesophagus in Aktinbinsk oblast. *Tz. Inst. Klin. Eksp. Khiz. Acad. Nauk. Kaz. SSR, 8*, 23-27

Haber, S.L. & Wissler, R.W. (1962) Effect of vitamin E on carcinogenicity of methylcholanthrene. *Proc. Soc. Exp. Biol. Med., 111*, 774-775

Haenszel, W. & Correa, P. (1975) Developments in the epidemiology of stomach cancer over the past decade. *Cancer Res., 35*, 3452-3459

Haenszel, W., Kurihara, M., Segi, M. & Lee, R.K.C. (1972) Stomach cancer among Japanese in Hawaii. *J. Natl Cancer Inst., 49*, 969-988

Haenszel, W., Berg, J.W., Segi, M., Kurihara, M. & Locke, F.B. (1973) Large-bowel cancer in Hawaiian Japanese. *J. Natl Cancer Inst., 51*, 1765-1779

Haenszel, W., Kurihara, M., Locke, F.B., Shimizu, K. & Segi, M. (1976) Stomach cancer in Japan. *J. Natl Cancer Inst., 56*, 265-278

Haenszel, W., Locke, F.B. & Segi, M. (1980) A case-control study of large-bowel cancer in Japan. *J. Natl Cancer Inst., 64*, 17-22

Hartge, P., Hoover, R., West, D.W. & Lyon, J.L. (1983) Coffee drinking and risk of bladder cancer. *J. Natl Cancer Inst., 70*, 1021-1026

Henderson, B.E., Louie, E., Jing, S.H., Buell, P. & Gardner, M.B. (1976) Risk factors associated with nasopharyngeal carcinoma. *New Engl. J. Med., 295*, 1101-1106

Higginson, J. (1966) Etiological factors in gastrointestinal cancer in man. *J. Natl Cancer Inst., 37*, 527-545

Hill, M.J. (1981) Dietary fat and human cancer. *Proc. Nutr. Soc., 40*, 15-19

Hill, M.J. (1985) Mechanisms of colorectal carcinogenesis. In: Joossens, J.V., Hill, M.J. & Geboers, J., eds, *Diet and Human Carcinogenesis*, Amsterdam, Elsevier, pp. 149-163

Hill, M.J. (1989) Experimental studies of fat, fibre and calories in carcinogenesis: In: Miller, A.B., ed., *Diet and the Aetiology of Cancers* (Monograph Series of the European School of Oncology), Berlin (West), Springer

Hill, M.J., Drasar, B.S., Aries, V., Crowther, J.S., Hawksworth, G. & Williams, R.E.O. (1971) Bacteria and aetiology of cancer of the large bowel. *Lancet, i*, 95-100

Hinds, M.W., Kolonel, L.N., Hankin, J.H. & Lee, J. (1984) Dietary vitamin A, carotene, vitamin C and risk of lung cancer in Hawaii. *Am. J. Epidemiol., 119*, 227-237

Hirayama, T. (1963) A study of the epidemiology of stomach cancer, with special reference to the effect of the diet factor. *Bull. Inst. Public Health, 12*, 85-96

Hirayama, T. (1971) An epidemiological study of cancer of the oesophagus in Japan, with special reference to the combined effect of selected environmental factors. In: *International Seminar on Epidemiology of Oesophageal Cancer, Bangalore, 4 November 1971*, p. 45-60

Hirayama, T. (1977) Changing patterns of cancer in Japan with special reference to the decrease of stomach cancer mortality. In: Hiatt, H.H., Watson, J.D. & Winston, J.D., eds, *Origins of Human Cancer*, Book C, *Human Risk Assessment*, Cold Spring Harbor, NY, CSH Press, pp. 55-75

Hirayama, T. (1978) Epidemiology of breast cancer with special reference to diet. *Prev. Med., 7*, 173-195

Hirayama, T. (1981) A large-scale cohort study on the relationship between diet and selected cancers of digestive organs. In: Bruce, W.R., Correa, P., Lipkin, M., Tannenbaum, S.R. & Wilkins, T.D., eds, *Gastrointestinal Cancer, Endogenous Factors* (Banbury Report 7), Cold Spring Harbor, NY, CSH Press, pp. 409-429

Hirohata, T., Shigematsu, T., Nomura, A.M.Y., Nomura, Y., Horie, A. & Hirohata, I (1985) Occurrence of breast cancer in relation to diet and reproductive history: a case-control study in Fukuoka, Japan. *Natl Cancer Inst. Monogr., 69*, 187-190

Hirohata, T., Nomura, A.M., Hankin, J.H., Kolonel, L. & Lee, J. (1987) An epidemiologic study on the association between diet and breast cancer. *J. Natl Cancer Inst., 78*, 595-600

Hislop, T.G., Coldman, A.J., Elwood, J.M., Brauer, G. & Kan, L. (1986) Childhood and recent eating patterns and risk of breast cancer. *Cancer Detect. Prev., 9*, 47-58

Hoey, J., Montvernay, C. & Lambert, R. (1981) Wine and tobacco: risk factors for gastric cancer in France. *Am. J. Epidemiol.*, *113*, 668-674

Hoff, G., Moen, I.E., Trygg, K., Frolich, W., Sauar, J., Vatn, M., Gjone, E. & Larsen, S. (1986) Epidemiology of polyps of the rectum and sigmoid colon: evaluation of nutritional factors. *Scand. J. Gastroenterol.*, *21*, 199-204

Howe, G.R. (1985) The use of polytomous dual response data to increase power in case-control studies: an application to the association between dietary fat and breast cancer. *J. Chronic Dis.*, *38*, 663-670

Howe, G.R., Burch, J.D., Miller, A.B., Cook, G.M., Estève, J., Morrison, B., Gordon, P., Chambers, L.W., Fodor, G. & Winsor, G.M. (1980) Tobacco use, occupation, coffee, various nutrients, and bladder cancer. *J. Natl Cancer Inst.*, *64*, 701-713

Hsieh, C.C., MacMahon, B., Yen, S., Trichopoulos, D., Warren, K. & Nardi, G. (1986) Coffee and pancreatic cancer. *New Engl. J. Med.*, *315*, 587-589

Hu, J., Zhang, S., Jia, E., Wang, Q., Liu, S., Liu, Y., Wu, Y. & Cheng, Y. (1988) Diet and cancer of the stomach: a case-control study in China. *Int. J. Cancer*, *41*, 331-335

IARC (1986) *IARC Monographs on the Evaluation of the Carcinogenic Risk of Chemicals to Humans*, Vol. 40, *Some Naturally Occurring and Synthetic Food Components, Furocoumarins and Ultraviolet Radiation*, Lyon, pp. 223-288

IARC (1988) *IARC Monographs on the Evaluation of Carcinogenic Risks to Humans*, Vol. 44, *Alcohol Drinking*, Lyon

IARC Intestinal Microecology Group (1977) Dietary fibre, transit time, faecal bacteria, steroids, and colon cancer in two Scandinavian populations. *Lancet*, *ii*, 207-211

Iran-IARC Cancer Study Group (1977) Esophageal cancer studies in the Caspian littoral of Iran: results of population studies. A prodrome. *J. Natl Cancer Inst.*, *59*, 1127-1138

Ivankovic, S., Preussmann, R., Schmähl, D. & Zeller, J.W. (1974) Prevention by ascorbic acid of in vivo formation of *N*-nitroso compounds. In: Bogovski, P. & Walker, E.A., eds, *N-Nitroso Compounds in the Environment* (IARC Scientific Publications No. 9), Lyon, IARC, pp. 101-102

Jacobs, M.M., Matney, T.S. & Griffin, A.C. (1977) Inhibitory effects of selenium on the mutagenicity of 2-acetylaminofluorene (AAF) and AAF derivatives. *Cancer Lett.*, *2*, 19-22

Jain, M., Cook, G.M., Davis, F.G., Grace, M.G., Howe, G.R. & Miller, A.B. (1980b) A case-control study of diet and colorectal cancer. *Int. J. Cancer*, *26*, 757-768

Jensen, O.M., MacLennan, R. & Wahrendorf, J. (1982) Diet, bowel function, fecal characteristics, and large-bowel cancer in Denmark and Finland. *Nutr. Cancer*, *4*, 5-19

Jensen, O.M., Wahrendorf, J., Knudsen, J.B. & Sørensen, B.L. (1986) The Copenhagen case-control study of bladder cancer. II. Effect of coffee and other beverages. *Int. J. Cancer*, *37*, 651-657

Jones, D.Y., Schatzkin, A., Green, S.B., Block, G., Brinton, L.A., Ziegler, R.G., Hoover, R. & Taylor, P.R. (1987) Dietary fat and breast cancer in the National Health and Nutrition Examination Survey. I. Epidemiologic follow-up study. *J. Natl Cancer Inst.*, *79*, 465-471

Kallistratas, G. & Faske, E. (1980) Inhibition of benz[*a*]pyrene carcinogenesis in rats with vitamin C. *J. Cancer Res. Clin. Oncol.*, *97*, 91-96

Kark, J.D., Smith, A.H., Switzer, B.R. & Hames, C.G. (1981) Serum vitamin A (retinol) and cancer incidence in Evans County, Georgia. *J. Natl Cancer Inst.*, *66*, 7-16

Katsouyanni, K., Trichopoulos, D., Boyle, P., Xirouchaki, E., Trichopoulou, A., Lisseos, B., Vasilaros, S. & MacMahon, B. (1986) Diet and breast cancer: a case-control study in Greece. *Int. J. Cancer*, *38*, 815-820

Keys, A., Aravanis, C., Blackburn, H., Buzina, R., Dontas, A.S., Fidanza, F., Karvonen, M.J., Menotti, A., Nedelkovic, S., Punsar, S. & Toshima, H. (1985) Serum cholesterol and cancer mortality in the Seven Countries Study. *Am. J. Epidemiol.*, *121*, 870-873

Kinlen, L.J. (1982) Meat and fat consumption and cancer mortality: a study of strict religious orders in Britain. *Lancet*, *i*, 946-949

Kolicheva, N.I. (1980) Epidemiology of esophagus cancer in the USSR. In: Levin, D., ed., *Joint USA/USSR Monograph on Cancer Epidemiology in the USA and USSR*

Kolonel, L.N., Nomura, A.M.Y., Hirohata, T., Hankin, J.H. & Hinds, M.W. (1981) Association of diet and place of birth with stomach cancer incidence in Hawaii Japanese and Caucasians. *Am. J. Clin. Nutr.*, *34*, 2478-2485

Kolonel, L.N., Nomura, A.M.Y., Hinds, M.W., Hirohata, T., Hankin, J.H. & Lee, J. (1983) Role of diet in cancer incidence in Hawaii. *Cancer Res.*, *43*, 2397s-2402s

Kritchesky, D., Weber, M.M. & Klurfeld, D.M. (1984) Dietary fat versus calorie content in initiation and promotion of 7,12-dimethylbenz(a)anthracene-induced mammary tumorigenesis in rats. *Cancer Res.*, *44*, 3174-3177

Kune, S., Kune, G.A. & Watson, L.F. (1987) case-control study of dietary etiological factors: the Melbourne colorectal cancer study. *Nutr. Cancer*, *9*, 21-42

Kvåle, G., Bjelke, E. & Gart, J.J. (1983) Dietary habits and lung cancer risk. *Int. J. Cancer*, *31*, 397-405

La Vecchia, C., De Carli, A., Fasoli, M. & Gentile, A. (1986) Nutrition and diet in the etiology of endometrial cancer. *Cancer*, *57*, 1248-1253

La Vecchia, C., De Carli, A., Franceschi, S., Gentile, A., Negri, E. & Parazzini, F. (1987) Dietary factors and the risk of breast cancer. *Nutr. Cancer*, *10*, 205-214

Lê, M.G., Moulton, L.H., Hill, C. & Kramer, A. (1986) Consumption of dairy produce and alcohol in a case-control study of breast cancer. *J. Natl Cancer Inst.*, *77*, 633-636

Lee, C. & Chen, C. (1979) Enhancement of mammary tumorigenesis in rats by vitamin E deficiency. *Proc. Am. Assoc. Cancer Res.*, *20*, 132

Lew, E.A. & Garfinkel, L. (1979) Variations in mortality by weight among 750,000 men and women. *J. Chronic Dis.*, *32*, 563-576

Lin, R.S. & Kessler, I.I. (1981) A multifactorial model for pancreatic cancr in man: epidemiologic evidence. *J. Am. Med. Assoc.*, *245*, 147-152

Liu, K., Moss, D., Persky, V., Stamler, J., Garside, D. & Soltero, I. (1979) Dietary cholesterol, fat and fibre, and colon cancer mortality: an analysis of international data. *Lancet*, *ii*, 782-785

Logue, T. & Frommer, D. (1980) The influence of oral vitamin C supplements on experimental colorectal tumour induction. *Aust. N.Z. J. Med.*, *10*, 588

Lubin, J.H., Burns, P.E., Blot, W.J., Ziegler, R.G., Lees, A.W. & Fraumeni, J.R. (1981) Dietary factors and breast cancer risk. *Int. J. Cancer*, *28*, 685-689

Lubin, F., Wax, Y. & Modan, B. (1986) Role of fat, animal protein, and dietary fiber in breast cancer etiology. A case-control study. *J. Natl Cancer Inst.*, *77*, 605-612

Mack, T.M., Yu, M.C., Hanisch, R. & Henderson, B.E. (1986) Pancreas cancer and smoking, beverage consumption and past medical history. *J. Natl Cancer Inst.*, *76*, 49-60

MacLennan, R., Da Costa, J., Day, N.E., Law, C.D., Ng, Y.K. & Shanmugaratnam, K. (1977) Risk factors for lung cancer in Singapore Chinese, a population with high female incidence rates. *Int. J. Cancer*, *20*, 854-860

MacMahon, B., Yen, S., Trichopoulos, D., Warren, K. & Nardi, G. (1981) Coffee and cancer of the pancreas. *New Engl. J. Med.*, *304*, 13-16

Macquart-Moulin, G., Riboli, E., Cornee, J., Charnay, B., Berthezene, P. & Day, N. (1986) case-control study on colorectal cancer and diet in Marseilles. *Int. J. Cancer*, *38*, 183-191

Macquart-Moulin, G., Riboli, E., Cornee, J., Kaaks, R. & Berthezene, P. (1987) Colorectal polyps and diet: a case-control study in Marseilles. *Int. J. Cancer*, *40*, 179-188

Manousos, O., Day, N.E., Trichopoulos, D., Gerovassilis, F., Tzonou, A. & Polychronopoulou, A. (1983) Diet and colorectal cancer: a case-control study in Greece. *Int. J. Cancer*, *32*, 1-5

Marshall, J., Graham, S., Mettler, C., Shedd, D. & Swanson, M. (1982) Diet in the epidemiology of oral cancer. *Nutr. Cancer*, *3*, 145-149

Martinez, I. (1969) Factors associated with cancer of the oesophagus, mouth and pharynx in Puerto Rico. *J. Natl Cancer Inst.*, *42*, 1069-1094

Martinez, I., Torres, R., Frias, Z., Colon, J.R. & Fernandez, M. (1979) Factors associated with adenocarcinomas of the large bowel. In: Birch, J.M., ed., *Advances in Medical Oncology, Research and Education*, Vol. 3, Oxford, Pergamon, pp. 45-52

Mathews-Roth, M.M. (1982) Antitumour activity of beta-carotene, canthaxanthin and phtoene. *Oncology*, *39*, 33-37

McConnell, K.P., Jager, R.M., Bland, K.I. & Blotcky, A.J. (1980) The relationship of dietary selenium and breast cancer. *J. Surg. Oncol.*, *15*, 67-70

McMichael, A.J., Jensen, O.M., Parkin, D.M. & Zaridze, D.G. (1984) Dietary and endogenous cholesterol and human cancer. *Epidemiol. Rev.*, *6*, 192-216

Meinsma, L. (1984) Voeding in Kanker. *Voeding*, *25*, 357-365

Mettlin, C. & Graham, S. (1979) Dietary risk factors in human bladder cancer. *Am. J. Epidemiol.*, *110*, 255-263

Mettlin, C., Graham, S. & Swanson, M. (1979) Vitamin A and lung cancer. *J. Natl Cancer Inst.*, *62*, 1435-1438

Mettlin, C., Graham, S., Priore, R., Marshall, J. & Swanson, M. (1981) Diet and cancer of the oesophagus. *Nutr. Cancer*, *2*, 143-147

Miller, A.B., Kelly, A., Choi, N.W., Matthews, V., Morgan, R.W., Munan, L., Burch, J.D., Feather, J., Howe, G.R. & Jain, M. (1978) A study of diet and breast cancer. *Am. J. Epidemiol.*, *107*, 499-509

Miller, A.B., Howe, G.R., Jain, M., Craib, K.J.P. & Harrison, L. (1983) Food items and food groups as risk factors in a case–control study of diet and colorectal cancer. *Int. J. Cancer*, *32*, 155-161

Mirvish, S.S., Wallcave, L., Eagen, M. & Shubik, P. (1972) Ascorbate-nitrite reaction: possible means of blocking the formation of carcinogenic N-nitroso compounds. *Science*, *177*, 65-68

Modan, B., Lubin, F., Barrell, V., Greenberg, R.A., Modan, M. & Graham, S. (1974) The role of starches in the etiology of gastric cancer. *Cancer*, *34*, 2087-2092

Modan, B., Barrell, V., Lubin, F., Modan, M., Greenberg, R.A. & Graham, S. (1975) Low-fiber intake as an etiologic factor in cancer of the colon. *J. Natl Cancer Inst.*, *55*, 15-18

Morrison, A.S., Buring, J.E., Verhoek, W.G., Aoki, K., Leck, I., Ohno, Y. & Obata, K. (1982) Coffee drinking and cancer of the lower urinary tract. *J. Natl Cancer Inst.*, *68*, 91-94

Muñoz, N., Crespi, M., Grassi, A., Qing, W.G., Qiong, S. & Cai, L.Z. (1982) Precursor lesions of esophageal cancer in high-risk populations in Iran and China. *Lancet*, *i*, 876-879

Muñoz, N., Wahrendorf, J., Lu, J.B., Crespi, M., Thurnham, D.I., Day, N.E., Zheng, H.J., Grassi, A., Li, W.Y., Lui, G.L., Lang, Y.G., Zhang, C.Y, Zheng, S.F., Li, J.Y., Correa, P., O'Conor, G.T. & Bosch, X. (1985) No effect of riboflavin, retinol and zinc on prevalence of precancerous lesions of the oesophagus. Randomized double-blind intervention study in high-risk population in China. *Lancet*, *ii*, 111-114

Muñoz, N., Hayashi, M., Lu, J.B., Wahrendorf, J., Crespi, M. & Bosch, F.X. (1987) Effect of riboflavin, retinol and zinc on micronuclei of buccal mucosa and of oesophagus: a randomized double-blind intervention study in China. *J. Natl Cancer Inst.*, *79*, 687-691

Nasao, M., Takahashi, Y., Yamanaka, H. & Sugimura, T. (1979) Mutagens in coffee and tea. *Mutat. Res.*, *68*, 101-106

National Research Council (1981) *The Health Effects of Nitrate, Nitrite and N-Nitroso Compounds*, Part 1, Washington DC, National Academy Press

Newberne, P.M. (1984) Enhanced esophageal carcinogenesis by riboflavin deficiency. In: *Proceedings of Society of Toxicology, 23 Annual Meeting, 12-16 March 1984, Atlanta, Georgia*

Newberne, P.M. & Suphakarn, V. (1983) Nutrition and cancer: a review with emphasis on the role of vitamins C, E and selenium. *Nutr. Cancer*, *5*, 107-119

Nomura, A., Hirohata, T., Rellahan, W., Burch, T., Harris, D. & Batten, G. (1978) Survivorship from large bowel cancer among Caucasians and Japanese in Hawaii. *Cancer*, *41*, 1571-1576

Ohgaki, H., Kusama, K., Matsukara, N., Morino, K., Hasegawa, H., Sato, S., Takayama, S. & Sugimura, T. (1984) Carcinogenicity in mice of a mutagenic compound, 2-amino-3-methyldimidazo(4,5-f)quinoline, from broiled sardine, cooked beef and beef extract. *Carcinogenesis*, *5*, 921-924

Ohshima, H. & Bartsch, H. (1981) Quantitative estimation of endogenous nitrosation in humans by monitoring *N*-nitrosoproline excreted in the urine. *Cancer Res.*, *41*, 3658-3662

Park, C.H., Amare, M., Savin, M.H. & Hoogstraten, B. (1980) Growth suppression of human leukemic cells *in vitro* by L-ascorbic acid, *Cancer Res.*, *40*, 1062-1065

Pearce, M.L. & Dayton, S. (1971) Incidence of cancer in men on a diet high in polyunsaturated fat. *Lancet*, *i*, 464-467

Peleg, I., Heyden, S., Knowles, M. & Hames, C.G. (1984) Serum retinol and risk of subsequent cancer. Extension of the Evans County, Georgia study. *J. Natl Cancer Inst.*, *73*, 1455-1462

Peto, R., Doll, R., Buckley, J.D. & Sporn, M.B. (1981) Can dietary beta-carotene materially reduce human cancer rates? *Nature*, *290*, 210-218

Phillips, R.L. (1975) Role of life-style and dietary habits in risk of cancer among Seventh-day Adventists. *Cancer Res.*, *35*, 3513-3522

Phillips, R.L. & Snowdon, D.A. (1985) Dietary relationships with fatal colorectal cancer among Seventh-day Adventists. *J. Natl Cancer Inst.*, *74*, 307-317

Phillips, R.L., Kuzma, J.W. & Lotz, T.M. (1980) Cancer mortality among comparable members versus non-members of the Seventh Day Adventist Church. In: Cairns, J., Lyon, L.J. & Skolnick, M., eds, *Cancer Incidence in Defined Populations* (Banbury Report No. 4), Cold Spring Harbor, NY, CSH Press, pp. 93-108

Potter, J.D. & McMichael, A.J. (1986) Diet and cancer of the colon and rectum: a case-control study. *J. Natl Cancer Inst.*, *76*, 557-569

Reddy, B.S. & Hirohata, T. (1979) Effect of dietary ascorbic acid on 1,2-dimethylhydrazine-induced colon cancer in rats. *Fed. Proc.*, *38*, 389-400

Reddy, B.S., Weisburger, J.M. & Wynder, E.L. (1975) Effects of high-risk and low-risk diets for colon carcinogenesis on fecal microflora and steroids in man. *J. Nutr.*, *105*, 287-290

Reddy, B.S., Hedges, A.R., Laakso, K. & Wynder, E.L. (1978) Metabolic epidemiology of large-bowel cancer: fecal bulk and constituents of high-risk North American and low-risk Finnish populations. *Cancer*, *42*, 2832-2838

Risch, H.A., Jain, M., Choi, N.W., Fodor, J.G., Pfeiffer, C.J., Howe, G.R., Harrison, L.W., Craib, K.J.P. & Miller, A.B. (1985) Dietary factors and the incidence of cancer of the stomach. *Am. J. Epidemiol.*, *122*, 947-959

Rosenberg, L., Miller, D.R., Helmrich, S.P., Kaufman, D.W., Schottenfeld, D., Stolley, P.D. & Shapiro, S. (1985) Breast cancer and the consumption of coffee. *Am. J. Epidemiol.*, *122*, 391-399

Ross, M.H. & Bras, G. (1965) Tumor incidence patterns and nutrition in the rat. *J. Nutr.*, *87*, 245-260

Rotkin, I.D. (1977) Studies on the epidemiology of prostate cancer: expanded sampling. *Cancer Treat. Rep.*, *61*, 173-180

Salonen, J.T., Salonen, R., Lappetelainen, R., Mäenpää, P.H., Alfthan, G. & Puska, P. (1985) Risk of cancer in relation to serum concentrations of selenium and vitamins A and E: matched case-control analysis of prospective data. *Br. Med. J.*, *290*, 417-420

Sarin, R., Tandon, R.K., Paul, S., Gandhi, B.M., Kapur, B.M. & Kapur, K. (1985) Diet, body fat and plasma lipids in breast cancer. *Indian J. Med. Res.*, *81*, 493-498

Schauzer, G.N., White, D.A. & Schneider, C.J. (1977) Cancer mortality correlation studies: II. Statistical associations with dietary selenium intakes. *Bioinorg. Chem.*, *7*, 23-31

Schuman, L.M., Mandel, J., Blackard, C., Bauer, H., Scarlett, J. & McHugh, R. (1977) Epidemiologic study of prostatic cancer: preliminary report. *Cancer Treat. Rep.*, *61*, 181-186

Schuman, L.M., Mandel, J.S., Radke, A., Saul, U. & Halberg, F. (1982) Some selected features of the epidemiology of prostatic cancer: Minneapolis-St Paul, Minnesota, case-control study, 1976-79. In: Magnus, K., ed., *Trends in Cancer Incidence: Causes and Practical Implications*, Washington DC, Hemisphere, pp. 345-354

Segi, M. (1975) Tea-gruel as a possible factor for cancer of the esophagus. *Gann*, *66*, 199-202

Shamberger, R.J. (1970) Relationship to cancer: I. Inhibitory effect of selenium on carcinogenesis. *J. Natl Cancer Inst.*, *44*, 931-936

Shamberger, R.J. (1971) Inhibitory effect of vitamin A on carcinogenesis. *J. Natl Cancer Inst.*, *47*, 667-673

Shamberger, R.J., Tytko, S.A. & Willis, C.E. (1976) Antioxidants and cancer. IV. Selenium and age-adjusted human cancer mortality. *Arch. Environ. Health*, *31*, 231-235

Shamberger, R.J., Beaman, K.D., Corlett, C.L. & Kasten, B.L. (1978) Effect of selenium and other antioxidants on the mutagenicity of malonaldehyde. *Fed. Proc.*, *37*, 261

Shekelle, R.B., Lui, S., Raynor, W.J., Lepper, M., Maliza, C. & Rossof, A.H. (1981) Dietary vitamin A and risk of cancer in the Western Electric study. *Lancet*, *ii*, 1185-1189

Simon, D., Yen, S. & Cole, P. (1975) Coffee drinking and cancer of the lower urinary tract. *J. Natl Cancer Inst.*, *54*, 587-591

Skegg, D.C.G. (1987) Alcohol, coffee, fat and breast cancer. *Br. Med. J.*, *295*, 1011-1012

Slattery, M.L., Schumacher, M.C., Smith, K.R., West, D.W., Abd-Elghany, N. (1988) Physical activity, diet and risk of colon cancer in Utah. *Am. J. Epidemiol.*, *128*, 989-999

Smith, P.G. & Jick, H. (1978) Cancers among users of preparations containing vitamin A. *Cancer, 42*, 808-811

Sporn, M.B. & Newton, D.L. (1981) Recent advances in the use of retinoids for cancer prevention. In: Buchenal, J.H. & Oettgen, H.F., eds, *Cancer Achievements, Challenges and Prospects for the 1980's*, Vol. 1, New York, Grune & Stratton, pp. 541-548

Sporn, M.B. & Roberts, A.B. (1983) Role of retinoids in differentiation and carcinogenesis. *Cancer Res., 43*, 3034-3040

Stähelin, H.B., Rosel, F., Buess, E. & Brubacher, G. (1984) Cancer, vitamins, and plasma lipids: prospective Basel study. *J. Natl Cancer Inst., 73*, 1463-1468

Stehr, P.A., Gloninger, M.F., Kuller, L.H., Marsh, G.M., Radford, E.P. & Weinberg, G.B. (1985) Dietary vitamin A deficiencies and stomach cancer. *Am. J. Epidemiol., 121*, 65-70

Stemmermann, G.N., Nomura, A.M.Y. & Heilbrun, L.K. (1984) Dietary fat and the risk of colorectal cancer. *Cancer Res., 44*, 4633-4637

Sugimura, T. (1982) Mutagens, carcinogens, and tumor promoters in our daily foods. *Cancer, 49*, 1970-1984

Sugimura, T. & Sato, S. (1983) Mutagens-carcinogens in foods. *Cancer Res., 43*, 2415s-2421s

Sugimura, T., Nagao, M. & Wakabayashi, K. (1981) Mutagenic heterocyclic amines in cooked food. In: Egan, H., Fishbein, L., Castegnaro, M., O'Neill, I.K. & Bartsch, H., eds, *Environmental Carcinogens - Selected Methods of Analysis*, Vol. 4, *Some Aromatic Amines and Azo Dyes in the General and Industrial Environment* (IARC Scientific Publications No. 40), Lyon, IARC, pp. 251-267

Talamini, R., La Vecchia, C., Decarli, A., Franceschi, S., Grattoni, E., Grigoletto, E., Liberati, A. & Tognoni, G. (1984) Social factors, diet and breast cancer in a northern Italian population. *Br. J. Cancer, 49*, 723-729

Tannenbaum, A. (1942a) The genesis and growth of tumors: II. Effects of caloric restriction *per se. Cancer Res., 2*, 460-467

Tannenbaum, A. (1942b) The genesis and growth of tumours: III. Effects of a high-fat diet. *Cancer Res., 2*, 468-474

Tannenbaum, S.R., Moran, D., Rand, W., Cuello, C. & Correa, P. (1979) Gastric cancer in Colombia: IV. Nitrite and other ions in gastric contents of residents from a high-risk region. *J. Natl Cancer Inst., 62*, 9-12

Thurnham, D.I., Rathakette, P., Hambidge, K.M., Muñoz, N. & Crespi, M. (1982) Riboflavin, vitamin A and zinc status in Chinese subjects in a high-risk area for oesophageal cancer in China. *Human Nutr. Clin. Nutr., 36C*, 337-349

Toniolo, P., Riboli, E., Protta, F., Charrel, M. & Cappa, A.P.M. (1989) Calorie-providing nutrients and risk of breast cancer. *J. Natl Cancer Inst., 81*, 278-286

Trichopoulos, D. & Polychronopoulou, A. (1986) Epidemiology, diet and colorectal cancer. *Eur. J. Clin. Oncol., 22*, 335-337

Trichopoulos, D., Papapostolou, M. & Polychronopoulou, A. (1981) Coffee and ovarian cancer. *Int. J. Cancer, 28*, 691-693

Trichopoulos, D., Ouranos, G., Day, N.E., Tzonou, A., Manousos, O., Papadimitriou, C. & Trichopoulou, A. (1985) Diet and cancer of the stomach: a case-control study in Greece. *Int. J. Cancer, 36*, 291-297

Turpeinen, O. (1979) Effect of cholesterol-lowering diet on mortality from coronary heart disease and other causes. *Circulation, 59*, 1-7

Tuyns, A.J. (1983a) Sodium chloride and cancer of the digestive tract. *Nutr. Cancer, 4*, 198-205

Tuyns, A.J. (1983b) Oesophageal cancer in non-smoking drinkers and in non-drinking smokers. *Int. J. Cancer, 32*, 443-444

Tuyns, A.J. (1988) Salt and gastrointestinal cancer. *Nutr. Cancer, 11*, 229-232

Tuyns, A.J., Riboli, E., Doornbos, G. & Pequignot, G. (1987) Diet and esophageal cancer in Calvados (France). *Nutr. Cancer, 9*, 81-92

Tuyns, A.J., Kaaks, R. & Haelterman, M. (1988) Colorectal cancer and the consumption of foods: a case-control study in Belgium. *Nutr. Cancer, 11*, 189-204

Tuyns, A.J., Kaaks, R. & Haelterman, M. (1990) Diet and gastric cancer in Belgium: a case-control study. *Nutr. Cancer* (in press)

Wald, N., Idle, M., Borchan, J. & Berkley, A. (1980) Low serum vitamin A and subsequent risk of cancer: preliminary results of a prospective study. *Lancet, ii*, 813-815

Wald, N.J., Boreham, J., Hayward, J.L. & Bulbrook, R.D. (1984) Plasma retinol, carotene and vitamin E levels in relation to the future risk of breast cancer. *Br. J. Cancer, 49*, 321-324

Wassertheil-Smoller, S., Romney, S.L., Wylie-Rosett, J., Slagle, S., Miller, G., Ludcido, D., Duttagupta, C. & Palan, P.R. (1981) Dietary vitamin C and uterine cervical dysplasia. *Am. J. Epidemiol., 114*, 714-724

Watanabe, K., Reddy, B.S., Weisburger, J.H. & Critchevsky, D. (1979) Effect of dietary alfalfa, pectin, and wheat bran on azoxymethane or methylnitrosourea-induced colon carcinogenesis in F344 rats. *J. Natl Cancer Inst., 63*, 141-145

Wattenberg, L.W. (1972) Inhibition of carcinogenic and toxic effects of polycyclic hydrocarbons by phenolic antioxidants and ethoxyquin. *J. Natl Cancer Inst., 48*, 1425-1430

Wattenberg, L.W. (1983) Inhibition of neoplasia by minor dietary constituents. *Cancer Res., 43*, 2448s-2453s

Willett, W.C. & MacMahon, B. (1984) Diet and cancer - an overview. *New Engl. J. Med., 310*, 633-638, 697-703

Willett, W.C. & Stampfer, M.J. (1986) Total energy intake: implications for epidemiologic analyses. *Am. J. Epidemiol., 124*, 17-27

Willett, W.C., Polk, B.P., Morris, J.S., Stampfer, M.J., Pressel, S., Rosner, B., Taylor, J.O., Schneider, K. & Hames, C.G. (1983) Prediagnostic serum selenium and risk of cancer. *Lancet, ii*, 130-134

Willett, W.C., Polk, B.F., Underwood, B.A., Stampfer, M.J., Pressel, S., Rosner, B., Taylor, J.O., Schneider, K. & Hames, C.G. (1984) Relation of serum vitamins A and E and carotenoids to the risk of cancer. *New Engl. J. Med., 310*, 430-434

Willett, W.C., Stampfer, M.J., Colditz, G.A., Rosner, B.A., Hennekens, C.M. & Speizer, F.E. (1987) Dietary fat and the risk of breast cancer. *New Engl. J. Med., 316*, 22-28

Williams, C.M. & Dickerson, J.W. (1987) Dietary fat, hormones and breast cancer: the cell membrane as a possible site of interaction of these two factors. *Eur. J. Surg. Oncol., 13*, 89-104

Winn, D.M., Ziegler, R.G., Pickle, L.W., Gridley, G., Blot, W.J. & Hoover, R.N. (1984) Diet in the etiology of oral and pharyngeal cancer among women from the southern United States. *Cancer Res., 44*, 1216-1222

Wynder, E.L. & Bross, I.J. (1961) A study of etiological factors in cancer of the oesophagus. *Cancer, 14*, 389-413

Wynder, E.L. & Klein, U.E. (1965) The possible role of riboflavin deficiency in epithelial neoplasia: 1. Epithelial changes in mice in simple deficiency. *Cancer, 18*, 167-180

Wynder, E.L., Kajatani, T., Ishikani, S., Dodo, H. & Takano, A. (1969) Environmental factors for cancer of the colon and rectum. II. Japanese epidemiological data. *Cancer, 23*, 1210-1220

Wynder, E.L., Hall, N.E.L. & Polansky, M. (1983) Epidemiology of coffee and pancreatic cancer. *Cancer Res., 43*, 3900-3906

You, M.-C., Blot, W.J., Chang, Y.-S., Ershow, A.G., Yang, Z.-T., An, Q., Henderson, B., Xu, G.-W., Fraumeni, J.F., Jr & Wang, T.-G. (1988) Diet and high risk of stomach cancer in Shandong, China. *Cancer Res., 48*, 3518-3523

Young, T.B. & Wolf, D.A. (1988) case-control study of proximal and distal colon cancer and diet in Wisconsin. *Int. J. Cancer, 42*, 167-175

Yu, M.C. & Henderson, B.E. (1987) Intake of Cantonese-style salted fish as a cause of nasopharyngeal carcinoma. In: Bartsch, H., O'Neill, I.K. & Schulte-Hermann, R., eds, *The Relevance of N-Nitroso Compounds to Human Cancer: Exposure and Mechanisms* (IARC Scientific Publications No. 84), Lyon, IARC, pp. 547-549

Yu, M.C., Ho, J.H.C., Lai, S.H. & Henderson, B.E. (1986) Cantonese-style salted fish as a cause of nasopharyngeal carcinoma: report of a case-control study in Hong Kong. *Cancer Res., 46*, 956-961

Yu, M.C., Mo, C.-C., Chong, W.-X., Yeh, F.-S. & Henderson, B.E. (1988) Preserved foods and nasopharyngeal carcinoma: a case-control study in Guangxi, China. *Cancer Res., 48*, 1954-1959

Yu, M.C., Huang, T.-B. & Henderson, B.E. (1989) Diet and nasopharyngeal carcinoma: a case-control study in Guangzhou, China. *Int. J. Cancer, 43*, 1077-1082

Zaridze, D.G., Blettner, M., Trapeznikov, N.N., Kuvshinov, J.P., Matiakin, E.G., Poljakov, B.P., Poddubni, B.K., Parshikova, S.M., Rottenberg, V.I., Chamrakulov, F.S., Chodjaeva, M.C., Stich, H.F., Rosin, M.P., Thurnham, D.I., Hoffmann, D. & Brunnemann, K.D. (1985) Survey of a population with a high incidence of oral and oesophageal cancer. *Int. J. Cancer*, *36*, 153-158   .

Zemla, B. (1984) The role of selected dietary elements in breast cancer risk among native and migrant populations in Poland. *Nutr. Cancer*, *6*, 187-195

Ziegler, R.G., Morris, L.E., Blot, W.J., Pottern, L.M., Hoover, R. & Fraumeni, J.F. (1981) Esophageal cancer among black men in Washington, DC. II. Role of nutrition. *J. Natl Cancer Inst.*, *67*, 1199-1206

Ziegler, R.G., Mason, T.J., Stemhagen, A., Hoover, R., Schoenberg, J.B., Gridley, G., Virgo, P.W., Altman, R. & Fraumeni, J.F. (1984) Dietary carotene and vitamin A and risk of lung cancer among white men in New Jersey. *J. Natl Cancer Inst.*, *73*, 1429-1435

Chapter 13. Pollution

Air pollution

The general population may be exposed to two major types of air pollution: (i) a 'reducing' form, known as 'London smog', the principal components of which are soots, sulfur dioxide and sulfuric acids resulting from the incomplete combustion of coal and oil; and (ii) an 'oxidizing' form, known as 'Los Angeles smog', which comprises carbon monoxide, hydrocarbons and photochemical decomposition products.

Some of the components of air pollution have been evaluated in the *IARC Monographs* programme on the evaluation of carcinogenic risks to humans (IARC, 1987); these are listed in Table 26. The presence among these components of several carcinogens and the carcinogenicity and mutagenicity of extracts of material from polluted urban air (Nisbet *et al.*, 1983) support the hypothesis that air pollution might increase the risk for cancer in exposed populations.

This chapter is restricted largely to consideration of the association between air pollution and lung cancer, since relevant studies are not available with regard to cancers at other sites. The major obstacle to a clear evaluation of the role of air pollution in inducing lung cancer is the importance of other exposures, such as active and passive smoking, occupational exposures and exposure to indoor air pollutants like radon gas and polycyclic aromatic hydrocarbons, which are associated with the occurrence of this tumour. Furthermore, since the carcinogenic effect of tobacco smoke can be enhanced by exposures to other carcinogens, such as asbestos and radon (see pp. 158,175), a similar enhancement by air pollution is plausible.

Most of the epidemiological investigations on air pollution and lung cancer are studies on the correlation between mortality from lung cancer with time or in geographical areas with known gradients of air pollution. Stocks (1936, 1947) observed that the mortality rate from lung cancer was higher in large towns than in small ones and was correlated with the density of population. This 'urban factor' was confirmed in a number of other studies (e.g., Mancuso *et al.*, 1955; Levin *et al.*, 1960). Stocks and Campbell (1955) found that lung cancer is about twice as common in urban smokers as in those in rural areas. The fact that migrants from the UK to South Africa, Australia and New Zealand appear to carry with them an excess incidence of lung cancer (Eastcott, 1956; Dean, 1961, 1962) has been attributed at least partly to exposure to carcinogenic factors in the urban environment. Rates of lung cancer in various urban and rural areas are shown in Table 27. The highest urban:rural ratio in males and one of the highest in females is seen in an area where there was formerly a major air pollution problem (north-western UK).

Table 26. Evidence of carcinogenicity for components of air pollution as evaluated by the *IARC Monographs* programme in volumes 1-42[a]

Substance	Evidence in humans	Evidence in animals	Overall evaluation
Inorganic			
Arsenic and arsenic compounds	Sufficient	Limited	1
Beryllium	Limited	Sufficient	2A
Cadmium and cadmium compounds	Limited	Sufficient	2A
Chromium and chromium compounds	Inadequate	Inadequate	3
Chromium metal	Inadequate	Inadequate	3
Hexavalent chromium compounds	Sufficient	Sufficient	1
Lead and lead compounds	Inadequate	Sufficient	2B
Nickel and nickel compounds	Sufficient	Sufficient	1
Silica: Crystalline silica	Limited	Sufficient	2A
Amorphous silica	Inadequate	Inadequate	3
Polynuclear compounds			
Anthracene	No data	Inadequate	3
Benzo[a]anthracene	No data	Sufficient	3
Benzo[b]fluoranthene	No data	Sufficient	2B
Benzo[j]fluoranthene	No data	Sufficient	2B
Benzo[k]fluoranthene	No data	Sufficient	2B
Benzo[ghi]fluoranthene	No data	Inadequate	3
Benzo[a]pyrene	No data	Sufficient	2A
Benzo[e]pyrene	No data	Inadequate	3
Chrysene	No data	Limited	3
Fluoranthene	No data	Inadequate	3
Fluorene	No data	Inadequate	3
Perylene	No data	Inadequate	3
Phenanthrene	No data	Inadequate	3
Pyrene	No data	Inadequate	3
Triphenylene	No data	Inadequate	3
Polynuclear nitroaromatic compounds			
3-Nitrofluoranthene	No data	Inadequate	3
1-Nitropyrene	No data	Limited	3
Others			
Formaldehyde	Limited	Sufficient	2A
Soots	Sufficient	Inadequate	1

[a] For definitions of the degrees of evidence and of groups 1, 2A, 2B and 3, see IARC (1987), pp. 29-32

Attempts have been made to assess trends in lung cancer mortality in relation to reductions in air pollution, such as occurred in England and Wales in the 1920s (Royal College of Physicians, 1970) and after the Clean Air Act of 1956 (Lawther & Waller, 1978). Interpretation of these trends is difficult, however, because changes in cigarette usage and 'tar' delivery were occurring during the same period (see p. 174). Stevens and Moolgavkar (1984), using a statistical model, suggested that the rate of lung cancer among male nonsmokers in the UK increased from 15 per 100 000 in 1941–45 to 19.3 per 100 000 in 1951–55 and then declined to 8.6 per 100 000 in 1971–75, implying a reduction in the effect of air pollution. However, the latent period appears to be too short to explain fully the decreasing pattern of lung cancer.

Table 27. Age-standardized rates per 100 000 population for mortality from carcinoma of the bronchus and trachea in urban and rural areas[a]

Registry	Males			Females		
	Urban	Rural	Ratio	Urban	Rural	Ratio
Japan, Miyagi	30.9	28.4	1.1	9.2	8.1	1.1
Czechoslovakia, Slovakia	68.2	70.5	1.0	9.4	6.5	1.4
FRG, Saarland	77.7	63.0	1.2	7.7	6.0	1.3
France, Calvados	46.1	39.6	1.2	3.4	2.9	1.2
France, Doubs	56.9	40.1	1.4	3.3	2.0	1.7
Hungary, Szabolcs	61.8	50.9	1.2	10.3	6.2	1.7
Norway	39.4	24.5	1.6	9.6	5.2	1.9
Romania, Cluj County	35.2	35.3	1.0	6.7	4.7	1.4
Switzerland, Vaud	63.8	56.6	1.1	8.7	5.6	1.6
UK, England and Wales	74.8	56.2	1.3	19.7	15.1	1.3
Australia, New South Wales	55.5	46.8	1.2	12.2	8.3	1.5

[a] From Muir *et al.* (1987)

Dean *et al.* (1978) studied mortality from lung cancer in urban and rural areas of the north of England in relation to cigarette smoking habits. The risk for lung cancer in urban areas was approximately twice that of the rural areas; however, in one of the heavily polluted urban areas, significantly more lung cancer deaths occurred among men (but not among women) living in urban rather than in rural areas, suggesting occupational exposure to the sources of pollution. Pike *et al.* (1979) showed that the excess of lung cancer seen among men in a highly polluted area of Los Angeles was attributable to their occupations and their smoking habits. Trichopoulos *et al.* (1987), comparing mortality from lung cancer during 1961-80 in heavily polluted Athens to that in other towns in Greece (after adjusting for tobacco consumption), found no evidence for an increased risk associated with air pollution in the population residing in Athens.

Some investigators have attempted to determine whether atmospheric pollution affects the incidence of lung cancer in nonsmokers. Doll (1953) estimated that lung cancer death rates among nonsmokers were very similar in Greater London, other urban areas and rural districts. Friberg and Cederlöf (1978) also found no indication that an urban factor caused lung cancer in nonsmokers. Only Hammond and Horn (1958) found that the rates of death from lung cancer among nonsmokers decreased from those in large towns, to medium-sized towns to small towns to no deaths in rural areas; however, few deaths were studied and it was not possible to exclude a possible confounding effect of occupation.

Small populations suspected of being exposed to emissions from specific industrial sources have been investigated in several studies. Pershagen (1985) carried out a case–control study of lung cancer in an area of northern Sweden where a copper smelting facility emitting arsenic was located and found a two-fold increase in relative risk among men living near the plant, after adjusting for age, smoking habits and occupation. Lloyd *et al.* (1985) and Smith *et al.* (1987) found an association between mortality from lung cancer and localized air pollution from iron and steel foundries in some areas in Scotland. Kaldor *et al.* (1984), evaluating residential exposure to air emissions from petroleum and chemical plants, considered that the higher risk in men suggested an occupational exposure.

In only a few studies has information been collected at the individual level on exposure and on potential confounding variables. Haenszel *et al.* (1962) recorded histories of smoking habits and of life-time residence from the families of a 10% sample of US men who had died of cancer and directly from a sample of the general population. Within each residence category there was a major gradient in risk according to smoking habits; within each smoking category there was a much smaller gradient from urban to rural and from large to small population units. The authors commented that some of the apparent differences by residence may have been due to incomplete control for differences in smoking habits.

Hitosugi (1968) asked about smoking habits and place of residence by administering a questionnaire to lung cancer patients residing in three areas with different levels of air pollution. A clear association was seen between lung cancer and smoking, but level of air pollution also appeared to be related to lung cancer among male workers who smoked. No effect was seen in men who did not smoke, and the results for women are unclear. Wicken (1966), studying the smoking and residential patterns of lung cancer patients in Northern Ireland in comparison to those of people who had died from other causes, found an association with degree of urbanization. Subsequently, Hammond and Garfinkel (1980), in an analysis of the American Cancer Society's cohort study of 1 000 000 US men and women, found no relationship with urban residence, after standardization for smoking and occupational hazards. In a hospital-based case–control study of lung cancer, investigating the potential effects of tobacco smoking, occupation and air pollution, Vena (1982) found an increased risk due to air pollution, which was limited to heavy smokers.

It is not possible, on the basis of the available epidemiological evidence, to make quantitative statements about the possible contribution of air pollution to the risk for lung cancer in humans. Although greatly overshadowed by the effects of cigarette smoking, it seems probable that, in heavily polluted areas, air pollution may contribute to mortality from lung cancer. In industrialized countries, concentrations of some pollutants derived from heating systems may have decreased, but those of others have increased, as has the size of exposed urban populations. In developing countries, both urban populations and air pollution have increased dramatically.

A consistent body of evidence has associated air pollution with mortality and morbidity from nonmalignant respiratory diseases. Several epidemics of deaths from acute respiratory diseases in Europe and the USA before 1960 were shown to be caused by heavy air pollution. One of the most serious occurred in London on 5–9 December 1952, when heavy pollution from industrial and domestic sources, together with unfavourable atmospheric conditions, were estimated to have caused some 4000 deaths (Wilkins, 1954). Several longitudinal studies have shown a decrease in chronic respiratory impairment associated with diminishing levels of air pollution (Van der Lende *et al.*, 1973; Ferris *et al.*, 1976; Fletcher *et al.*, 1976). Epidemiological investigations have also associated higher levels of air pollution with increased respiratory morbidity in children (Douglas & Waller, 1966; Lunn *et al.*, 1967; Colley *et al.*, 1973; Kiernan *et al.*, 1976).

Water pollution

The general population is widely exposed to a number of carcinogenic organic and inorganic contaminants of water supplies, including asbestos, halogenated hydrocarbons and other pesticides, heavy metals and radioactive isotopes. Evaluations of whether there is a carcinogenic risk for the general population from this source have usually been based on correlation studies, in which the relationship between cancer rates and contamination levels is examined across regions. This kind of study is vulnerable to a number of problems of interpretation (see p. 104).

Various types of asbestiform fibres have been detected in drinking-water supplies. The deposition of wastes from an iron ore processing plant into Lake Superior in North America resulted in 1–30 million amphibole-like fibres per litre of tap-water in Duluth, Minnesota (Cook *et al.*, 1974; Nicholson, 1974). Chrysotile fibres have been detected in drinking-water in villages in asbestos mining areas in Québec, Canada (Wigle, 1977) and in California (Kanarek *et al.*, 1980) and Washington (Polissar *et al.*, 1982), USA, from drinking-water sources passing through serpentine rock, the parent rock form of chrysotile asbestos. In several locations in the USA, including Connecticut (Harrington *et al.*, 1978) and Florida (Millette *et al.*, 1983), chrysotile fibres have been introduced into drinking-water supplies from the asbestos cement pipes in which the water was transported.

A number of epidemiological evaluations have been made of cancer incidence and mortality in relation to the asbestos content of drinking-water (Marsh, 1983; National Research Council, 1983; Levine, 1985; Working Group for the DHSS Committee to Coordinate Environmental and Related Programs, Subcommittee on Risk Assessment, 1987; Kanarek, 1989). Even though there is some consistency in the finding of an association with cancers of the pancreas and stomach (Table 28), the results for other sites are variable and generally negative.

Trihalomethanes, such as chloroform, which is carcinogenic to experimental animals (IARC, 1987) and other halogenated hydrocarbons (like trichloroethylene and tetrachloroethylene) and pesticides (Rook, 1974), occur as contaminants of drinking-water supplies, and some are suspected or well-known animal carcinogens (National Research Council, 1987). There have been few systematic studies to evaluate the effect of low levels of contamination with such substances on cancer incidence or mortality. The results of five case–control studies on trihalomethanes, utilizing death certificates, which are summarized in Table 29, suggest associations between the level of contamination and cancers of the urinary bladder, rectum and colon.

Table 28. Relative risks for cancers of the stomach and pancreas associated with ingestion of asbestos in drinking-water, as estimated from seven studies in North America

Stomach cancer		Pancreatic cancer		Reference
Males	Females	Males	Females	
1.51	1.37	1.28	1.27	Mason *et al.* (1974)
1.22	0.92	1.21	1.41	Levy *et al.* (1976)
1.08	1.07			Harrington *et al.* (1978)
1.40	1.20	1.00	1.70	Wigle (1977)
1.70	1.17	0.95	0.79	Toft *et al.* (1981)
1.15	0.65	1.00	1.33	Polissar *et al.* (1982)
1.18	1.06	1.11	1.14	Kanarek *et al.* (1980)

Three large studies have been reported in which information on residence history, consumption of drinking-water, other exposure to water (such as showering) and potential confounding factors, was elicited from individuals by interview or questionnaire. Wilkins and Comstock (1981) interviewed persons exposed to chlorinated surface water and unchlorinated well-water and observed increased mortality from breast cancer and an increased incidence of bladder cancer among the exposed persons over 12 years. Cantor *et al.* (1987) reported on a case–control study of bladder cancer covering ten areas in the USA and involving 2982 cases and 5782 controls. Relative risks increased with duration of exposure to chlorinated surface water in nonsmokers, reaching three fold after 60 years of exposure; increases in risk for bladder cancer were also seen with level of intake of beverages made with tap water. Young *et al.* (1987) questioned 347 patients with newly diagnosed colon cancer and two groups of matched controls for potential exposure to trihalomethanes and many other potential risk and confounding factors. Even though an association with colon cancer was seen for ingestion of chlorinated water, no association was seen between trihalomethane level and risk for colon cancer.

The levels of nitrate in surface and ground waters have markedly increased over the last 20 years, due to increased use of artificial fertilizers and the disposal of wastes from intensive animal farming (World Health Organization, 1985). In the human stomach, ingested nitrates contribute to the formation of

N-nitrosamines, which are potentially carcinogenic to humans (see p. 134; National Research Council, Committee on Nitrate and Alternative Curing Agents in Food, 1981); however, attempts to correlate the occurrence of gastric cancer and levels of nitrate in drinking-water have yielded inconsistent results (Fraser, 1985).

Table 29. Odds ratios obtained in case–control studies on mortality from cancer according to exposure to trihalomethanes in water

Cancer site	Alavanja et al. (1978)[a]		Brenniman et al. (1980)[b]		Young et al. (1981)[c]	Wilkins & Comstock (1981)[c]
	Males	Females	Males	Females	(Females)	(Males and females)
Oesophagus	2.39*	1.28	0.99	1.06	1.03	1.76
Stomach	1.67*	2.23*	0.91	1.07	1.81	0.61
Colon	1.99*	1.30	1.04	1.17	1.51*	0.89
Rectum	2.33*	1.25	1.14	1.35	1.39	1.42
Liver	2.76[d]*	1.55[d]	0.91	1.09	1.09	2.98
Pancreas	2.62*	1.26	1.03	1.02	1.06	0.80
Kidney	-	-	-	-	1.04	2.76
Bladder	2.02*	0.82	0.99	0.95	1.04	2.20
Lung	1.83*	1.55	-	-	0.85	0.96
Brain	-	-	-	-	2.48	1.10
Breast	-	-	-	-	1.36	2.27*

[a] Chlorinated *versus* unchlorinated water at death
[b] Chlorinated *versus* unchlorinated ground-water at death
[c] High level of chlorination *versus* no chlorination
[d] And kidney
* Significant difference between the two groups

High levels of radioactivity have been observed in drinking-water in Sweden and Finland and in several areas of the USA (National Research Council, 1977). Bean *et al.* (1982) compared cancer mortality of residents of Iowa municipalities who consumed well-water containing different levels of radium-226 and found associations for lung cancer in males and for breast cancer in females. Hess *et al.* (1983) found a correlation between levels of radon-222 in drinking-water and mortality from all cancers, from lung cancers and from cancers of the reproductive tract in 16 counties in Maine, USA.

A variety of metals occur at trace levels in drinking-water. They may be leached from the soil and decaying plant material; they may occur as a result of mining of coal or mineral ore; they may be discharged into industrial waste-water, such as that generated by plating and metal-finishing operations; and they may be corroded from metal parts of the water distribution system (National Research Council, 1977). Evaluations of the possible effects of elevated concentrations of trace metals have focused mainly on arsenic. Tseng *et al.* (1968) and Tseng (1977) showed dose–response relationships between levels of arsenic in the drinking-water and the prevalence of skin cancer in Taiwan. Although studies in various areas of the USA have not corroborated these results (Morton *et al.*, 1976; Harrington *et al.*, 1978), the levels of arsenic in Taiwan are considerably higher than those in the areas of USA that were studied. In a case–control study in Taiwan, Chen *et al.* (1986) found a dose–response relationship with arsenic levels in water and the frequency of cancers of the lung and bladder. Several other associations have been found between levels of metals and cancer mortality in the USA (Berg & Burbank, 1972; Isacson *et al.*, 1985).

Thus, a number of studies have been carried out to investigate the carcinogenicity of drinking-water, and several indicate the possibility of an increase in risk associated with contamination of water by specific carcinogens. Methodological difficulties, however, render the results of these studies generally inconclusive.

References

Alavanja, M., Goldstein, I. & Suuser, M. (1978) Case control study of gastrointestinal and urinary cancer mortality and drinking water chlorination. In: Jolley, R.J., Gorchev, H. & Hamilton, D.H., Jr, eds, *Water Chlorination: Environmental Impact and Health Effects*, Vol. 1, Ann Arbor, MI, Ann Arbor Science, pp. 395-409

Bean, J.A., Isacson, P., Hahne, R.M.A. & Kohler, J. (1982) Drinking water and cancer incidence in Iowa. II. Radioactivity in drinking water. *Am. J. Epidemiol.*, *116*, 924-932

Berg, J.W. & Burbank, F. (1972) Correlations between carcinogenic trace metals in water supplies and cancer mortality. *Ann. N.Y. Acad. Sci.*, *199*, 249-264

Brenniman, G.R., Vasilomanolakis-Lagos, J., Amsel, J., Namekata, T. & Wolff, A.H. (1980) case–control study of cancer deaths in Illinois communities served by chlorinated or non-chlorinated water. In: Jolley, R.L., Brungs, W.A., Cumming, R.B. & Jacobs, V.A., eds, *Water Chlorination: Environmental Impact and Health Effects*, Vol. 3, Ann Arbor, MI, Ann Arbor Science, pp. 1043-1057

Cantor, K.P., Hoover, R., Hartge, P., Mason, T.J., Silverman, D.T., Altman, R., Austin, D.F., Child, M.A., Key, C.R., Marrett, L.D., Myers, M.H., Narayana, A.S., Levin, L.I., Sullivan, J.W., Swanson, G.M., Thomas, D.B. & West, D.W. (1987) Bladder cancer, drinking water source, and tap water consumption: a case–control study. *J. Natl Cancer Inst.*, *79*, 1269-1278

Chen, C.J., Chuang, C.Y., Lin, M.T. & Wu, Y.H. (1986) Malignant neoplasma among residents of a blackfoot disease-endemic area in Taiwan: high-arsenic artesian well water and cancers. *Cancer Res.*, *45*, 5895-5899

Colley, J.R.T., Douglas, J.W.B. & Reid, D.D. (1973) Respiratory disease in young adults: influence of early childhood lower respiratory tract illness, social class, air pollution and smoking. *Br. Med. J.*, *iii*, 195-198

Cook, P.M., Glass, G.E. & Tucker, J.G. (1974) Asbestiform amphibole mineral: detection and measurement of high concentration in municipal water supplies. *Science*, *185*, 853-855

Dean, G. (1961) Lung cancer in white South Africans. *Br. Med. J.*, *ii*, 1599-1605

Dean, G. (1962) Lung cancer in Australia. *Med. J. Aust.*, *i*, 1003-1011

Dean, G., Leem P.N., Todd, G.F. & Wicken, A.J. (1978) *Report on a Second Retrospective Mortality Study in North-east England. Part II. Changes in Lung Cancer and Bronchitis Mortality and in Other Relevant Factors Occurring in Areas of North-east England 1963-72* (Research Paper 14), London, Tobacco Research Council

Doll, R. (1953) Mortality from lung cancer among non-smokers. *Br. J. Cancer*, *7*, 303-312

Douglas, J.W.B. & Waller, R.E. (1966) Air pollution and respiratory infection in children. *Br. J. Prev. Soc. Med.*, *20*, 1-8

Eastcott, D.F. (1956) The epidemiology of lung cancer in New Zealand. *Lancet*, *i*, 37-39

Ferris, B.G., Jr, Chen, H., Puleo, S. & Murphy, R.L. (1976) Chronic non-specific respiratory disease in Berlin, New Hampshire, 1967-1973. A further follow-up study. *Am. Rev. Respir. Dis.*, *113*, 475-485

Fletcher, C.M., Peto, R. & Tinker, C.M. (1976) *The Natural History of Chronic Bronchitis and Emphysema*, Oxford, Oxford University Press

Fraser, P. (1985) Nitrates: epidemiological evidence. In: Wald, N. & Doll, R., eds, *Interpretation of Negative Epidemiological Evidence for Carcinogenicity* (IARC Scientific Publications No. 65), Lyon, IARC, pp. 183-194

Friberg, L. & Cederlöf, R. (1978) Late effects of air pollution with special reference to lung cancer. *Environ. Health Perspect.*, 22, 45-66

Haenszel, W., Loveland, D.B. & Sirken, M.G. (1962) Lung cancer mortality as related to residence and smoking histories. I. White males. *J. Natl Cancer Inst.*, 28, 947-1001

Hammond, E.C. & Garfinkel, L. (1980) General air pollution and cancer in the United States. *Prev. Med.*, 9, 206-211

Hammond, E.C. & Horn, D. (1958) Smoking and death rates: report on forty four months of follow-up of 187,783 men. *J. Am. Med. Assoc.*, 166, 1159-1172, 1294-1308

Harrington, J.M., Craun, G., Meigs, J.W., Landrigan, P.J., Flannery, J.T. & Woodhull, R.S. (1978) An investigation of the use of asbestos cement pipe for public water supply and the incidence of gastrointestinal cancer in Connecticut, 1953-1973. *Am. J. Epidemiol.*, 107, 96-103

Hess, C.T., Weiffenback, C.W. & Norton, S.A. (1983) Environmental radon and cancer correlations in Maine. *Health Phys.*, 45, 339-348

Hitosugi, M. (1968) Epidemiological study of lung cancer with special reference to the effect of air pollution and smoking habit. *Bull. Inst. Public Health*, 17, 237-256

IARC (1987) *IARC Monographs on the Evaluation of Carcinogenic Risks to Humans*, Suppl. 7, *Overall Evaluations of Carcinogenicity: An Updating of* IARC Monographs *Volumes 1 to 42*, Lyon

Isacson, P., Bean, J.A., Splinter, R., Olson, D.B. & Kohler, J. (1985) Drinking water and cancer incidence in Iowa. III. Association of cancer with indices of contamination. *Am. J. Epidemiol.*, 121, 856-869

Kaldor, J., Harris, J.A., Glazer, E., Glaser, S., Neutra, R., Mayberry, R., Nelson, V., Robinson, L. & Reeds, D. (1984) Statistical association between cancer incidence and major-cause mortality, and estimated residential exposure to air emissions from petroleum and chemical plants. *Environ. Health Perspect.*, 54, 319-332

Kanarek, M.S. (1989) Epidemiological studies on ingested mineral fibres: gastric and other cancers. In: Bignon, J., Peto, J. & Saracci, R., eds, *Non-occupational Exposure to Mineral Fibres* (IARC Scientific Publications No. 90), Lyon, IARC, pp. 428-437

Kanarek, M.S., Conforti, P.M., Jackson, L.A., Cooper, R.C. & Murchio, J.C. (1980) Asbestos in drinking water and cancer incidence in the San Francisco Bay Area. *Am. J. Epidemiol.*, 112, 54-72

Kiernan, K.E., Colley, J.R.T., Douglas, J.B.W. & Reid, D.D. (1976) Chronic cough in young adults in relation to smoking habits, childhood environment and chest illness. *Respiration*, 33, 236-244

Lawther, P.J. & Waller, R.E. (1978) Trends in urban air pollution in th United Kingdom in relation to lung cancer mortality. *Environ. Health Perspect.*, 22, 71-73

Levin, M.L., Haenszel, W., Carroll, B.E., Gerhardt, P.R., Handy, V.H. & Ingraham, S.C. (1960) Cancer incidence in urban and rural areas of New York State. *J. Natl Cancer Inst.*, 24, 1243-1257

Levine, D.S. (1985) Does asbestos exposure cause gastrointestinal cancer? *Dig. Dis. Sci.*, 30, 1189-1198

Levy, B.S., Sigurdson, E., Mandel, J., Laudon, E. & Pearson, J. (1976) Investigating possible effects of asbestos in city water: surveillance of gastrointestinal cancer incidence in Duluth, Minnesota. *Am. J. Epidemiol.*, 104, 523-526

Lloyd, O.L.L., Williams, F.L.R. & Gailey, F.A.Y. (1985) Is the Armedale epidemic over? Air pollution and mortality from lung cancer and other diseases, 1961-82. *Br. J. Ind. Med.*, 42, 815-823

Lunn, J.E., Knowelden, J. & Handyside, A.J. (1967) Patterns of respiratory illness in Sheffield infant school-children. *Br. J. Prev. Soc. Med.*, 21, 7-16

Mancuso, T.F., MacFarlane, E.M. & Porterfield, J.D. (1955) Distribution of cancer mortality in Ohio. *Am. J. Public Health*, 45, 58-70

Marsh, G.M. (1983) Critical review of epidemiologic studies related to ingested asbestos. *Environ. Health Perspect.*, *53*, 49-56

Mason, T.J., McKay, F.W. & Miller, R.W. (1974) Asbestos-like fibers in Duluth water supply. *J. Am. Med. Assoc.*, *228*, 1019-1020

Millette, J.R., Clark, P.F., Stober, J. & Rosenthal, M. (1983) Asbestos in water supplies of the United States. *Environ. Health Perspect.*, *53*, 45-48

Morton, W., Starr, G., Pohl, D., Stoner, J., Wagner, S. & Weswig, P. (1976) Skin cancer and water arsenic in Lane County, Oregon. *Cancer*, *37*, 2523-2532

Muir, C., Waterhouse, J., Mack, T., Powell, J. & Whelan, S., eds (1987) *Cancer Incidence in Five Continents, Vol. V* (IARC Scientific Publications No. 88), Lyon, IARC

National Research Council (1977) *Drinking Water and Health*, Vol. 1, *A Report of the Safe Drinking Water Committee, Commission of Life Sciences*, Washington DC, National Academy Press, pp. 123-144

National Research Council (1983) *Drinking Water and Health*, Vol. 5, *A Report of the Safe Drinking Water Committee, Commission of Life Sciences*, Washington DC, National Academy Press, pp. 123-144

National Research Council, Committee on Nitrate and Alternative Curing Agents in Food (1981) *The Health Effects of Nitrate, Nitrite and N-Nitroso Compounds*, Washington DC, National Academy Press

Nicholson, W.J. (1974) Analysis of amphibole asbestiform fibers in municipal water supplies. *Environ. Health Perspect.*, *9*, 165-172

Nisbet, I.C.T., Schneiderman, M.A., Karch, N.S. & Sieger, D.M. (1983) *Review and Evaluation of the Evidence for Cancer Associated with Air Pollution* (Publication No. EPA-450/5-83006), Research Triangle Park, NC, US Environmental Protection Agency

Pershagen, G. (1985) Lung cancer mortality among men living near an arsenic emitting smelter. *Am. J. Epidemiol.*, *122*, 684-694

Pike, M.C., Jing, J.S., Rosario, I.P., Henderson, B.E. & Menck, H.R. (1979) Occupation: 'explanation' of an apparent air pollution related localized excess of lung cancer in Los Angeles County. In: Breslow, N. & Whittemore, A., eds, *Energy and Health*, Philadelphia, PA, SIAM, pp. 3-16

Polissar, L., Severson, R.K., Boatman, E.S. & Thomas, D.B. (1982) Cancer incidence in relation to asbestos in drinking water in the Puget Sound region. *Am. J. Epidemiol.*, *116*, 314-328

Rook, J.J. (1974) Formation of haloforms during chlorination of natural waters. *J. Soc. Water Treat. Exam.*, *23*, 234-243

Royal College of Physicians (1970) *Air Pollution and Health*, London, Putnam Medical

Smith, G.H., Williams, F.L. & Lloyd, O.L. (1987) Respiratory cancer and air pollution from iron foundries in a Scottish town: an epidemiological and environmental study. *Br. J. Ind. Med.*, *44*, 795-802

Stevens, R.G. & Moolgavkar, S. (1984) A cohort analysis of lung cancer and smoking in British males. *Am. J. Epidemiol.*, *119*, 624-641

Stocks, P. (1936) *Report of the British Empire Cancer Campaign*, London

Stocks, P. (1947) *Regional and Social Differences in Cancer Death Rates*, London, Her Majesty's Stationery Office

Stocks, P. & Campbell, J.M. (1955) Lung cancer death rates among non-smokers and pipe and cigarette smokers: evaluation in relation to air pollution by benzpyrene and other substances. *Br. Med. J.*, *ii*, 923-929

Toft, P., Wigle, D.T., Meranger, J.C. & Mao, Y. (1981) Asbestos and drinking water in Canada. *Sci. Total Environ.*, *18*, 77-89

Trichopoulos, D., Hatzakis, A., Wynder, E., Katsouyanni, K. & Kalandidi, A. (1987) Time trends of tobacco smoking, air pollution, and lung cancer in Athens. *Environ. Res.*, *44*, 169-178

Tseng, W.P. (1977) Effects and dose-response relationships of skin cancer and blackfoot disease with arsenic. *Environ. Health Perspect.*, *19*, 109-119

Tseng, W.P., Chu, H.M., How, S.W., Fong, J.M., Lin, C.S. & Yeh, S. (1968) Prevalence of skin cancer in an endemic area of chronic arsenicism in Taiwan. *J. Natl Cancer Inst.*, *40*, 353-363

Van der Lende, R., Tammeling, G.J. & Visser, B.F. (1973) Epidemiological investigations in the Netherlands into the influence of smoking and atmospheric pollution on respiratory symptoms and lung function disturbances. *Pneumologie*, *149*, 119-126

Vena, J.E. (1982) Air pollution as a risk factor in lung cancer. *Am. J. Epidemiol.*, *116*, 42-56

Wicken (1966) *Environmental and Personal Factors in Lung Cancer and Bronchitis Mortality in Northern Ireland 1960-62* (Tobacco Research Council Research Paper No. 9), London, Tobacco Research Council

Wigle, D.T. (1977) Cancer mortality in relation to asbestos in municipal water supplies. *Arch. Environ. Health*, *32*, 185-190

Wilkins, E.T. (1954) Air pollution and the London fog of December 1952. *J. R. Sanit. Inst.*, *74*, 1-21

Wilkins, J.R. & Comstock, G.W. (1981) Source of drinking water at home and site-specific cancer incidence in Washington County, Maryland. *Am. J. Epidemiol.*, *114*, 178-190

Working Group for the DHSS Committee to Coordinate Environmental and Related Programs, Subcommittee on Risk Assessment (1987) Report on cancer risks associated with the ingestion of asbestos. *Environ. Health Perspect.*, *72*, 253-265

World Health Organization (1985) *Environmental Health Criteria 5: Nitrates, Nitrites and N-Nitroso Compounds*, Geneva

Young, T.B., Kanarek, M.S. & Tsiatis, A.A. (1981) Epidemiologic study of drinking water chlorination and Wisconsin female cancer mortality. *J. Natl Cancer Inst.*, *67*, 1191-1198

Young, T.B., Wolf, D.A. & Kanarek, M.S. (1987) case-control study of colon cancer and drinking water trihalomethanes in Wisconsin. *Int. J. Epidemiol.*, *16*, 190-207

Chapter 14. Endogenous hormones, reproductive factors and sexual behaviour

Various aspects of sexual and reproductive behaviour influence cancer risk. Thus, the frequencies of cancers of the breast, ovary and endometrium are influenced by reproductive factors associated with ovarian activity; the frequency of cancer of the cervix, which is often inversely associated with the incidence of breast, endometrial and ovarian cancer, is more closely associated with factors relating to sexual activity. In addition, cancer of the colon in women is associated with low parity. Fewer associations have been noted between sexual and reproductive behaviour and cancers in males, yet it is necessary to consider such factors in relation to cancers of the prostate, penis and testis.

Although there is a certain similarity in the etiology of some of these cancers, it is more appropriate to consider individual cancer sites. Some of the cancers considered in this section are also associated with the exogenous use of hormones, and experiments in animals indicate a carcinogenic effect of various naturally occurring and synthetic hormones. These associations are discussed on pp. 151–153.

Cancer of the breast

Reproductive and hormonal factors that influence the incidence of breast cancer have been studied thoroughly for many years, but our understanding of their etiological role is far from complete, and a comprehensive model in which to accommodate these factors together with all the other epidemiological features of breast cancer is still lacking.

The age-specific incidence curve of breast cancer is quite different from that of the other epithelial cancers (see Figure 5, p. 40): instead of a steady increase with age, it rises sharply from early adulthood to about the time of menopause; after that, the rise occurs at a much lower rate. The basic shape of the incidence curve is quite similar in all populations, whatever the overall incidence rates, emphasizing the effect of ovarian activity on the susceptibility of breast epithelium to neoplastic transformation (Henderson *et al.*, 1988). Moolgavkar *et al.* (1980) and Pike (1987) described the age pattern of the incidence rates of breast cancer using mathematical models that provide a logical explanation of the increased risk associated with menopause, early age at menarche and late age at first full-term pregnancy, which are generally considered to be the most important risk factors for breast cancer.

At menopause, after a variable period of irregular cycles, the hormonal milieu changes dramatically, the main alteration being that the ovaries stop producing oestrogens. These changes also bring about a decrease in the turnover rate of breast epithelial cells; and early menopause, either natural or induced by ovariectomy, has been shown consistently to reduce the risk for breast cancer (Trichopoulos *et al.*, 1972): women whose menopause occurs before the age of 45 have 50% less risk for breast cancer than women whose menopause occurs after the age of 55. There is some epidemiological evidence that exogenous sources of oestrogens, such as menopausal replacement therapy (IARC, 1987; see p. 152) and increased peripheral conversion of adrenal androgens into oestrogens in obese women (Henderson *et al.*, 1988), may increase the risk. Adipose tissue is the major source of oestrogens in postmenopausal women, and it has been found consistently in a number of studies that obese menopausal women are at higher risk for breast cancer than menopausal women who are not obese. Studies in which oestrogen levels have been measured in blood and urine of breast cancer cases and of controls have given inconsistent, and mostly negative, results (Zumoff, 1981).

Another commonly recognized risk factor for breast cancer is early menarche. Several studies have shown an approximately 20% decrease in risk resulting from each year that menarche is delayed (Henderson *et al.*, 1988), but inconsistent findings have been reported (Paymaster & Gangadharan, 1972; Soini, 1977; Choi *et al.*, 1978; Adami *et al.*, 1980; La Vecchia *et al.*, 1987).

Low parity has been suspected of being a major risk factor for breast cancer for more than 200 years, and this is one of the most reproducible features of the epidemiology of breast cancer (Kvåle *et al.*, 1987). In the early studies, however, the effect of parity was not separated from the effects of related variables, and it was not until the large international study of MacMahon *et al.* (1970a) that it was recognized that a major factor was the age of a woman at the time of her first full-term pregnancy. Those women with a first birth occurring before the age of 20 had about one-half the risk of nulliparous women or of women who delayed their first birth until the age of 30 or later. It was also apparent that women whose first birth occurred after the age of 35 had a higher risk than nulliparous women; in between, there appears to be a smooth increase in risk with increasing age at first birth. The effect of age at first birth remains after controlling for parity; after controlling for age at first birth, however, subsequent births appeared to confer little or no further protection.

The protective effect of an early first birth was confirmed in most subsequent studies. A few population-based studies, however, showed no such association (Choi *et al.*, 1978; Adami *et al.*, 1980), and a prospective study carried out in Sweden (Kvåle & Heuch, 1987) showed an effect which disappeared after allowing for parity and age at last birth. Other studies have demonstrated a protective effect of high parity that is independent of the effect of age at first birth (Soini, 1977; Thein-Hlaing & Thein-Maung-Myint, 1978; Tulinius *et al.*, 1978; Brinton *et al.*, 1983; Wang & Fentiman, 1985). A reanalysis of the study of MacMahon *et al.* (1970a) by Trichopoulos *et al.* (1983) confirmed the effect of age at first birth but showed also that age at any birth after the first was associated with a small increase in relative risk for every year of increase in age. Trichopoulos *et al.* also found that any full-term pregnancy before the age of 35 confers some protection, whereas a pregnancy afterwards increases the risk. This finding is consistent with the results of the prospective study of Kvåle and Heuch (1987), in which age at last birth was significantly associated with the incidence of breast cancer: parous women whose last birth occurred after 35 years of age had a higher risk than nulliparous women, even if their first birth had occurred early.

These observations suggest that any pregnancy may have a dual effect – cause a transient increase, followed by a subsequent strong, long-lasting decrease in risk for breast cancer. A recent meta-analysis of several Italian case–control studies on breast cancer in premenopausal women (Bruzzi *et al.*, 1988) suggests that a critical time may be the few years immediately following a pregnancy. It is clear that the association between events related to pregnancy and breast cancer incidence requires further clarification. Social class and cultural differences, as well as trends in use of oral contraceptives, may affect the associations, especially in populations undergoing transition from a low to a high incidence (like Singapore) or with large internal differences according to these factors (Kvåle *et al.*, 1987).

The protective effect of early age at first birth appears to be restricted to completed pregnancies. Indeed, in some studies, suggestive evidence has been found for an increase in risk in relation to abortion (Choi *et al.*, 1978), particularly among women who had a first-trimester abortion before their first full-term pregnancy (Pike *et al.*, 1981; Hadjimichael *et al.*, 1986); but this was not observed in other studies (Paymaster & Gangadharan, 1972; Brinton *et al.*, 1983; La Vecchia *et al.*, 1987). In studies by Pike *et al.* (1981), the association was observed both for miscarriages and for induced abortions. Apparently, the early part of pregnancy has a negative effect which can be overridden by the beneficial effect of a completed pregnancy. This finding is in line with the dual effect of pregnancies at different ages that makes the interpretation of epidemiological data so complicated.

It has not yet been clearly demonstrated whether lactation protects against the development of breast cancer or not. Following the large international study of MacMahon *et al.* (1970b), which showed that the association between breast cancer and lactation was explained almost totally by the effect of early age at first birth, the possibility that breast feeding was protective appeared to be remote. New results, however, suggest that dismissal of the old theory originated by Rigoni-Stern in 1850 may have been premature. Two case–control studies (Byers *et al.*, 1985; McTiernan & Thomas, 1986) show that, after controlling for age at first birth and other potential confounders, breast feeding may still have a protective effect of about 50% in premenopausal, but not in postmenopausal, women. The study of Byers *et al.* (1985) suggested that failure of lactating mothers to produce sufficient milk, rather than absence of lactation *per se*, may be the relevant risk factor. Clearly, this could be an indicator of some underlying hormonal imbalance which deserves further investigation.

Experimental, physiological and clinical findings point to the existence of some hormonal determinant of breast cancer, and the search for a common endogenous hormonal pattern among breast cancer patients has produced a wide variety of theories (Kirschner, 1977; Zumoff, 1982; Moore *et al.*, 1986). Notwithstanding the large body of indirect evidence supporting the role of oestrogens, case–control studies based on biological measurements have been inconclusive. Studies on progesterone and on its urinary metabolite, pregnanediol, have also been largely inconsistent. Progesterone levels, however, vary so widely in normal women that gross misclassification is likely to occur in studies based on single measurements. More consistent results have been found in case–control studies on urinary or serum levels of testosterone, but the possibility that this is a consequence, rather than a cause, of breast cancer or of the stress associated with its diagnosis, has not been ruled out.

An association with parity was suspected at one time, but subsequent studies dismissed it because of the presumed correlation of pregnancy with the key sexual risk factors. However, in several recent studies in which adequate control for the confounding effects of sexual and reproductive factors has been made, a persistent association with multiparity has been found (Brinton *et al.*, 1989; Cuzick *et al.*, 1989; Parazzini *et al.*, 1989). In one of these studies, carried out in Latin America, a five-fold excess was seen in women with 14 or more pregnancies (after adjustment for age at first intercourse, number of sexual partners, interval since last Pap smear and years of education), and the association appears to be related to the numbers of live births rather than to total number of pregnancies (Brinton *et al.*, 1989).

The prevailing opinion today seems to be that the total amounts of hormones in the urine and peripheral blood are related only marginally to the risk for breast cancer (Moore *et al.*, 1986). Other theories are therefore focused on the concentration of hormones within breast tissues, or, alternatively, on the susceptibility of breast epithelium and on its capacity to utilize plasma hormones. These are based mainly on the observation that the intramammary concentration of several hormones, mainly oestrogens, is much higher (up to 20 times) than the concentration in blood (Vermeulen *et al.*, 1986). Until these new hypotheses are defined more clearly, it would be unwise to reject all past results as confused and obscure. None of the theories can be considered proven or disproven, and most of them maintain a core of biological plausibility, even in the absence of much empirical support.

Cancer of the uterine cervix

Many of the risk factors for cancer of the cervix appear to be the inverse of those for cancer of the breast. The disease is more frequent in married than in single women (Ernster *et al.*, 1979), particularly in those who first married at an early age, and increases in frequency with parity. The two major risk factors appear to be young age at first coitus and multiple sexual partners (Rotkin, 1973); however, more recent studies have suggested that the number of sexual partners is the more important determinant (Harris *et al.*, 1980; Reeves *et al.*, 1985; Brinton *et al.*, 1987), the association with age at first coitus disappearing or substantially decreasing after adjustment for number of sexual partners. Several studies indicate that the behavioural risk factors for carcinoma *in situ* of the uterine cervix are similar to those for invasive cancer (Thomas, 1973; Harris *et al.*, 1980).

The virtual absence of squamous-cell cancer of the cervix among nuns (Gagnon, 1950) and the absence of case reports indicating the presence of the disease in women who have never been sexually active, together with the association with multiple sexual partners, suggest that the disease is transmitted venereally. Although until fairly recently herpes simplex virus-type 2 was regarded as the possible etiological agent, attention has now shifted to the human papilloma virus, particularly but not exclusively subtypes 16 and 18 (see p. 188).

The disease can also occur in women who have had only one sexual partner. Kessler (1977) reported that cancer of the cervix tended to occur more frequently in the second wives of men whose first wife had died of the disease. Buckley *et al.* (1981) found that the number of sexual partners reported by the husbands of women who claimed to have had only one sexual partner was a significant risk factor. This finding is fully compatible with venereal transmission of the essential etiological factor.

It was suggested that women whose partner is not circumcised are at greater risk than those with circumcised partners (Wynder *et al.*, 1954). However, Dunn and Buell (1959) found no association and suggested that women might not know whether their partners were circumcised. Terris *et al.* (1973) also found no association. It is possible that circumcision is of etiological importance only in cultural groups unaware of penile hygiene (Jayant *et al.*, 1987). In India, Muslim women are far less likely to develop cancer of the cervix than Hindu women (Wahi *et al.*, 1972), and this has been attributed to the circumcision status of their husbands. Parsis have a much lower risk than Muslims, which could be due to better hygiene.

Five to ten per cent of cervical cancers are adenocarcinomas and have a number of biological and epidemiological features that differentiate them from the more common squamous-cell carcinomas. The risk factors for adenocarcinomas are the same as those for the squamous-cell type, but these tumours are also associated with factors related to endometrial cancer, such as excess weight (Brinton *et al.*, 1987; Parazzini *et al.*, 1988).

Cancer of the endometrium

Endometrial cancer shares many epidemiological features and risk factors with breast cancer, yet the understanding of its hormonal biology is more advanced (Pike, 1987; Henderson *et al.*, 1988). Its incidence rises rapidly in women up to the age of 50 – more steeply than that of breast cancer – and thereafter increases at a much reduced rate. The suggestion of a strong protective effect of menopause is evident, and case–control studies have established late menopause as a risk factor. Earlier age at menarche has been observed among cases too, at least in premenopausal women. Nulliparous women are at increased risk, but there appears to be no association with age at first birth (Elwood *et al.*, 1977; Kelsey *et al.*, 1982; La Vecchia *et al.*, 1984). Increasing parity provides an increasing degree of protection, especially in young women (Henderson *et al.*, 1983; Centers for Disease Control Cancer and Steroid Hormone Study, 1987).

The above observations, together with the finding that combination-type oral contraceptives confer protection and sequential contraceptives increase the risk (see pp. 152–153), corroborate the validity of the 'unopposed' oestrogen hypothesis. This postulates that during the premenopausal period the rate of increase in risk with age depends on the accumulation of mitotic activity during the first half of the normal menstrual cycle when oestrogens are unopposed by progesterone (Henderson *et al.*, 1988). With loss of ovarian function at menopause, the slope of the age-specific incidence curve depends entirely on oestrogen formation in adipose tissue (MacDonald *et al.*, 1978) and on the use of oestrogen replacement therapy (see p. 152).

Obesity is a risk factor for endometrial cancer both after and before the menopause (Henderson *et al.*, 1983; La Vecchia *et al.*, 1984). As there is no evidence of a significant elevation of plasma oestrogens in obese women before the menopause (Zumoff, 1982), it has been suggested that the mechanism by which obesity increases the risk for endometrial cancer in young women is through the induction of anovulation and the ensuing progesterone deficiency (Henderson *et al.*, 1988).

Cancer of the ovary

Ovarian cancer shares some risk factors with breast cancer and with endometrial cancer. It has been shown relatively consistently that factors associated with suppression of ovulation, such as pregnancy, whether complete or incomplete, use of combined oral contraceptives and breast feeding are protective (Centers for Disease Control Cancer and Steroid Hormone Study, 1983, 1987; Risch *et al.*, 1983). A number of authors have shown that the risk increases with the number of 'ovulatory years', computed as the number of years between menarche and menopause (or diagnosis if premenopausal) minus the number of years in which the woman was either pregnant or taking oral contraceptives, even though a protective effect of late menarche has not been found consistently (Casagrande *et al.*, 1979; Hildreth *et al.*, 1981; Franceschi *et al.*, 1982; Cramer *et al.*, 1983). The age-specific curve for ovarian cancer, which rises up to the age at menopause and then tends to flatten off, as for endometrial cancer, can be described in mathematical models as a function of the number of years of regular cycles (Pike, 1987).

According to the 'incessant ovulation' hypothesis, each ovulation-induced trauma to the ovarian surface carries a certain risk that malignant cells will be created during ensuing repair. The theory implies that the amount of protection should be independent of the particular cause of anovulation and depend only on the total period of anovulation, but this has not yet been clearly demonstrated (Risch *et al.*, 1983). The hypothesis is consistent with the observation that ovarian cancer is associated with nulliparity but not with infertility (Cramer *et al.*, 1983).

Cancer of the colon

The risk for cancer of the colon has been seen to be increased in women with low parity (Bjelke, 1974; Dales *et al.*, 1979; Weiss *et al.*, 1981; Potter & McMichael, 1983; Howe *et al.*, 1985); a sixth study did not show the association (Byers *et al.*, 1982). In two of the studies, age at first birth was shown to be a more important risk factor than low parity (Potter & McMichael, 1983; Howe *et al.*, 1985). The mechanism by which these associations come about is unclear, although McMichael and Potter (1980) suggested there may be some hormonal basis for cancer of the colon.

Cancer of the prostate

Although it has been suspected that prostatic cancer is related to sexual and reproductive factors, much of the available information does not confirm this theory. Greenwald *et al.* (1974) followed a cohort of men who had been examined while at university: a lower proportion of married men who later died from prostatic cancer had had no children at the time they were examined than married controls, but the difference did not attain statistical significance. No difference was found in the proportion never married, in age at first marriage, in age at birth of the first child or in age at birth of the last child. Neither detailed anthropometric measurements nor an index of baldness (based on photographs taken at a 25th graduation anniversary) showed any difference between cases and controls.

In a small case–control study, Steele *et al.* (1971) noted that cases had had more sexual relationships with multiple partners, both before and after marriage, and a more frequent past history of venereal disease. Krain (1974) also found that patients with prostatic cancer more frequently gave histories of past venereal disease, increased coital frequency and more sexual partners. Rotkin (1977) found no difference in the number of sexual partners; he found, instead, features suggesting delayed development of secondary sexual characteristics, including delayed interest in females during adolescence and a deficit of sexual activity in patients over 50 years of age. He postulated that limitation of sexual activity at any time of life may increase the risk. Schuman *et al.* (1977) and Mandel and Schuman (1987) found that prostatic cancer patients used prostitutes to a greater extent and had had more venereal disease than controls but had had slightly fewer partners.

Part of the difficulty in interpreting the results of these studies may be imprecision in information on sexual factors for relatively old patients and the possibility that there is some response bias in those studies which indicate increased sexual activity. Therefore, it would be premature to indicate that the associations noted are real.

Cancer of the testis

Testicular cancer is primarily a disease of young adult males. Although it is included here for the sake of completeness, there is no evidence that it is associated with marital status, sexual activity or fertility (Morrison, 1976; Ross *et al.*, 1979).

Cancer of the penis

Incidence rates in different countries and among different religious groups indicate that circumcision is a major protective factor for penile cancer (see Part I, p. 77). For full protection, circumcision must be performed in infancy (Hoppmann & Fraley, 1978). The wives of men with cancer of the penis appear to be more likely to have cancer of the cervix (Martinez, 1969; Graham *et al.*, 1979; Smith *et al.*, 1980). This observation suggests that one of the etiologic factors common to these two diseases may be sexually transmitted viral infections (see pp. 185–189).

References

Adami, H.O., Hanse, J., Jung, B. & Runsten, A. (1980) Age at first birth, parity and risk of breast cancer in a Swedish population. *Br. J. Cancer, 42*, 651-658

Bjelke, E. (1974) Colorectal cancer: clues from epidemiology. In: Bucalossi, P., Veronesi, U. & Cascinelli, N, eds, *Proceedings of the Eleventh International Cancer Congress* (Excerpta Medica Congress Series No. 354), Vol. 6, Amsterdam, Elsevier, pp. 324-330

Brinton, L.A., Hoover, R. & Fraumeni, J.F. (1983) Reproductive factors in the aetiology of breast cancer. *Br. J. Cancer, 47*, 757-762

Brinton, L.A., Hamman, R.F., Huggins, G.R., Lehman, H.F., Levine, R.S., Mallin, K. & Fraumeni, J.F., Jr (1987) Sexual and reproductive risk factors for invasive squamous cell cervical cancer. *J. Natl Cancer Inst., 79*, 23-30

Brinton, L.A., Reeves, W.C., Brenes, M.M., Herrero, R., de Britton, R.C., Gaitan, E., Tenorio, F., Garcia, M. & Rawls, W.E. (1989) Parity as a risk factor for cervical cancer. *Am. J. Epidemiol., 130*, 486-496

Bruzzi, P., Negri, E., La Vecchia, C., De Carli, A., Palli, D., Parazzini, F. & del Turco, M.R. (1988) Short term increase in risk of breast cancer after full term pregnancy. *Br. Med. J., 297*, 1096-1098

Buckley, J.D., Harris, R.W.C., Doll, R., Vessey, M.P. & Williams, P.T. (1981) case-control study of the husbands of women with dysplasia or carcinoma of the cervix uteri. *Lancet, ii*, 1010-1015

Byers, T., Graham, S. & Swanson, M. (1982) Parity and colorectal cancer in women. *J. Natl Cancer Inst., 69*, 1059-1062

Byers, T., Graham, S., Rzepka, T. & Marshall, J. (1985) Lactation and breast cancer. Evidence for a negative association in premenopausal women. *Am. J. Epidemiol., 121*, 664-674

Casagrande, J.T., Louie, E.W., Pike, M.C., Roy, S., Ross, R.K. & Henderson, B.E. (1979) 'Incessant ovulation' and ovarian cancer. *Lancet, ii*, 170-173

Centers for Disease Control Cancer and Steroid Hormone Study (1983) Oral contraceptive use and the risk of ovarian cancer. *J. Am. Med. Assoc., 249*, 1596-1599

Centers for Disease Control Cancer and Steroid Hormone Study (1987) Combination oral contraceptives use and the risk of endometrial cancer. *J. Am. Med. Assoc., 257*, 796-800

Choi, N.W., Howe, G.R., Miller, A.B., Matthews, V., Morgan, R.W., Munan, L., Burch, J.D., Feather, J., Jain, M. & Kelly, A. (1978) An epidemiologic study of breast cancer. *Am. J. Epidemiol., 107*, 510-521

Cramer, D.W., Hutchinson, G.B., Welch, W.R., Scully, R.E. & Ryan, K.J. (1983) Determinants of ovarian cancer risk. I. Reproductive experiences and family history. *J. Natl Cancer Inst., 71*, 711-716

Cuzick, J., De Stavola, B., McCance, D., Ho, T.H., Tan, G., Cheng, H., Chew, S.Y. & Salmon, Y.M. (1989) A case-control study of cervix cancer in Singapore. *Br. J. Cancer, 60*, 238-243

Dales, L.G., Friedman, G.D., Ury, H.K., Grossman, S. & Williams, S.R. (1979) A case-control study of relationships of diet and other traits to colorectal cancer in American blacks. *Am. J. Epidemiol., 109*, 132-144

Dunn, J.E. & Buell, P. (1959) Association of cervical cancer with circumcision of sexual partner. *J. Natl Cancer Inst., 22*, 749-764

Elwood, J.M., Cole, P., Rothman, K.J. & Kaplan, S.D. (1977) Epidemiology of endometrial cancer. *J. Natl Cancer Inst., 59*, 1055-1060

Ernster, V.L., Sacks, S.T., Selvin, S. & Petrakis, N.L. (1979) Cancer incidence by marital status. US Third National Cancer Survey. *J. Natl Cancer Inst., 63*, 567-585

Franceshi, S., La Vecchia, C., Helmrich, S.P., Mangioni, C. & Tognoni, G. (1982) Risk factors for epithelial ovarian cancer in Italy. *Am. J. Epidemiol., 115*, 714-719

Gagnon, F. (1950) Contribution to the study of the etiology and prevention of cancer of the cervix of the uterus. *Am. J. Obstet. Gynecol., 60*, 516-522

Graham, S., Priore, R., Graham, M., Browne, R., Burnett, W. & West, D. (1979) Genital cancer in wives of penile cancer patients. *Cancer, 44*, 1870-1874

Greenwald, P., Damon, A., Kirmiss, V. & Polan, A.K. (1974) Physical and demographic features of men before developing cancer of the prostate. *J. Natl Cancer Inst., 53*, 341-346

Hadjimichael, O.C., Boyle, C.A. & Meigs, J.W. (1986) Abortion before first livebirth and risk of breast cancer. Br. J. Cancer, 53, 281-284

Harris, R.W.C., Brinton, L.A., Cowdell, R.H., Skegg, D.C.G., Smith, P.G., Vessey, M.P. & Doll, R. (1980) Characteristics of women with dysplasia or carcinoma in situ of the cervix uteri. Br. J. Cancer, 42, 359-369

Henderson, B.E., Casagrande, J.T., Pike, M.C., Mack, T., Rosario, I. & Duke, A. (1983) The epidemiology of endometrial cancer in young women. Br. J. Cancer, 47, 749-756

Henderson, B.E., Ross, R. & Bernstein, L. (1988) Estrogens as a cause of human cancer: the Richard and Hinda Rosenthal Foundation Award lecture. Cancer Res., 48, 246-253

Hildreth, N.G., Kelsey, J.L., LiVolsi, V.A., Fischer, D.B., Holford, T.R., Mostow, E.D., Schwartz, P.E. & White, C. (1981) An epidemiologic study of epithelial carcinoma of the ovary. Am. J. Epidemiol., 114, 398-405

Hoppmann, H.J. & Fraley, E.E. (1978) Squamous cell carcinoma of the penis. J. Urol., 120, 393-398

Howe, G.R., Craib, K.J.P. & Miller, A.B. (1985) Age at first pregnancy and risk of colo-rectal cancer: a case-control study. J. Natl Cancer Inst., 74, 1155-1159

IARC (1987) IARC Monographs on the Evaluation of Carcinogenic Risks to Humans, Suppl. 7, Overall Evaluations of Carcinogenicity: An Updating of IARC Monographs Volumes 1 to 42, Lyon

Jayant, K., Notani, P.N., Gadre, V.V., Gulatti, S.S. & Shah, P.R. (1987) Personal hygiene in groups with varied cervical cancer rates: a study in Bombay. Indian J. Cancer, 24, 47-52

Kelsey, J.L., LiVolsi, V.A., Holford, T.R., Fischer, D.B., Mostow, E.D., Schwartz, P.E., O'Connor, T. & White, C. (1982) A case-control study of cancer of the endometrium. Am. J. Epidemiol., 116, 333-342

Kessler, I.I. (1977) Venereal factors in human cervical cancer. Cancer, 39, 1912-1919

Kirschner, M. (1977) The role of hormones in the etiology of human breast cancer. Cancer, 39, 2716-2726

Krain, L.S. (1974) Some epidemiologic variables in prostatic carcinoma in California. Prev. Med., 3, 154-159

Kvåle, G. & Heuch, I. (1987) A prospective study of reproductive factors and breast cancer. II. Age at first and last birth. Am. J. Epidemiol., 126, 842-850

Kvåle, G. Heuch, I. & Eide, G.E. (1987) A prospective study of reproductive factors and breast cancer. I. Parity. Am. J. Epidemiol., 126, 831-841

La Vecchia, C., Franceschi, S., De Carli, A., Gallus, G. & Tognoni, G. (1984) Risk factors for endometrial cancer at different ages. J. Natl Cancer Inst., 73, 667-671

La Vecchia, De Carli, A., Franceschi, S., Gentile, A., Negri, E. & Parazzini, F. (1987) Dietary factors and the risk of breast cancer. Nutr. Cancer, 10, 205-214

MacDonald, P.C., Edman, C.D., Hemsell, D.L., Porter, J.C. & Siiteri, P.K. (1978) Effect of obesity on conversion of plasma androstenedione to estrone in postmenopausal women with and without endometrial cancer. Am. J. Obstet. Gynecol., 130, 448-455

MacMahon, B., Cole, P., Lin, T.M., Lowe, C.R., Mirra, A.P., Ravnihar, B., Salber, E.J., Valaoras, V.G. & Yuasa, S. (1970a) Age at first birth and cancer of the breast. A summary of an international study. Bull. World Health Organ., 43, 209-221

MacMahon, B., Lin, T.M., Lowe, C.R., Mirra, A.P., Ravnihar, B., Salber, E.J., Trichopoulos, D., Valaoras, V.G. & Yuasa, S. (1970b) Lactation and cancer of the breast. A summary of an international study. Bull. World Health Organ., 42, 185-194

Mandel, J.S. & Schuman, L.M. (1987) Sexual factors and prostatic cancer: results from a case-control study. J. Gerontol., 42, 259-264

Martinez, I. (1969) Relationship of squamous cell carcinoma of the cervix uteri to squamous cell carcinoma of the penis among Puerto Rican women married to men with penile carcinoma. Cancer, 24, 777-780

McMichael, A.J. & Potter, J.D. (1980) Reproduction, endogenous and exogenous sex hormones, and colon cancer: a review and hypothesis. J. Natl Cancer Inst., 65, 1201-1207

McTiernan, A. & Thomas, D.B. (1986) Evidence for a protective effect of lactation on risk of breast cancer in young women. Results from a case-control study. Am. J. Epidemiol., 124, 353-358

Moolgavkar, S.H., Day, N.E. & Stevens, R.G. (1980) Two-stage model for carcinogenesis: epidemiology of breast cancer in females. J. Natl Cancer Inst., 65, 559-569

Moore, J.W., Clark, G.M.G., Hoare, S.A., Millis, R.R., Hayward, J.L., Quinlan, M.K., Wang, D.Y. & Bulbrook, R.D. (1986) The binding of oestradiol to blood proteins and the aetiology of breast cancer. *Int. J. Cancer*, *38*, 625-630

Morrison, A.S. (1976) Some social and medical characteritics of army men with testicular cancer. *Am. J. Epidemiol.*, *104*, 511-516

Parazzini, F., La Vecchia, C., Negri, E., Fasoli, M. & Cecchetti, G. (1988) Risk factors for adenocarcinoma of the cervix: a case-control study. *Br. J. Cancer*, *57*, 201-204

Parazzini, F., La Vecchia, C., Negri, E., Cecchetti, G. & Fedele, L. (1989) Reproductive factors and the risk of invasive and intraepithelial cervical neoplasia. *Br. J. Cancer*, *59*, 805-809

Paymaster, J.C. & Gangadharan, P. (1972) Some observations on the epidemiology of cancer of the breast in women in western India. *Int. J. Cancer*, *10*, 443-450

Pike, M.C. (1987) Age-related factors in cancers of the breast, ovary, and endometrium. *J. Chronic Dis.*, *40*, 59s-69s

Pike, M.C., Henderson, B.E., Casagrande, J.T., Rosario, I. & Gray, G.E. (1981) Oral contraceptive use and early abortion as risk factors for breast cancer in young women. *Br. J. Cancer*, *43*, 72-76

Potter, J.D. & McMichael, A.J. (1983) Large bowel cancer in women in relation to reproductive and hormonal factors: a case-control study. *J. Natl Cancer Inst.*, *71*, 703-709

Reeves, W.C., Brinton, L.A., Brenes, M.M., Guiroz, E., Rawls, W.E. & de Britton, R.C. (1985) case-control study of cervical cancer in Herrera Province, Republic of Panama. *Int. J. Cancer*, *36*, 55-60

Risch, H.A., Weiss, N.S., Lyon, J.L., Daling, J.R. & Luff, J.M. (1983) Events of reproductive life and the incidence of epithelial ovarian cancer. *Am. J. Epidemiol.*, *117*, 128-139

Ross, R.K., McCurtis, J.W., Henderson, B.E., Menck, H.R., Mack, T.M. & Martin, S.P. (1979) Descriptive epidemiology of testicular and prostate cancer in Los Angeles. *Br. J. Cancer*, *39*, 284-292

Rotkin, I.D. (1973) A comparison review of key epidemiological studies in cervical cancer related to current searches for transmissible agents. *Cancer Res.*, *33*, 1353-1367

Rotkin, I.D. (1977) Studies on the epidemiology of prostatic cancer: expanded sampling. *Cancer Treat. Rep.*, *61*, 173-180

Schuman, L.M., Mandel, J., Blackard, C., Bauer, H., Scarlett, J. & McHugh, R. (1977) Epidemiologic study of prostatic cancer: preliminary report. *Cancer Treat. Rep.*, *61*, 181-186

Smith, P.G., Kinlen, L.J., White, G.C., Adelstein, A.M. & Fox, A.J. (1980) Mortality of wives of men dying with cancer of the penis. *Br. J. Cancer*, *41*, 422-428

Soini, I. (1977) Risk factors of breast cancer in Finland. *Int. J. Epidemiol.*, *6*, 365-373

Steele, R., Lees, R.E., Kraus, A.S. & Rao, C. (1971) Sexual factors in the epidemiology of cancer of the prostate. *J. Chronic Dis.*, *24*, 29-37

Terris, M., Wilson, F. & Nelson, J.H. (1973) Relation of circumcision to cancer of the cervix. *Am. J. Obstet. Gynecol.*, *117*, 1056-1066

Thein Hlaing & Thein-Maung-Myint (1978) Risk factors of breast cancer in Burma. *Int. J. Cancer*, *21*, 432-437

Thomas, D.B. (1973) An epidemiologic study of carcinoma in situ and squamous dysplasia of the uterine cervix. *Am. J. Epidemiol.*, *98*, 10-28

Trichopoulos, D., MacMahon, B. & Cole, P. (1972) Menopause and breast cancer risk. *J. Natl Cancer Inst.*, *48*, 605-613

Trichopoulos, D., Hsieh, C., MacMahon, B., Lui, T., Lowe, C.R., Mirra, A.P., Ravnihar, B., Salber, E.J., Valaoras, V.G. & Yuasa, S. (1983) Age at any birth and breast cancer risk. *Int. J. Cancer*, *31*, 701-704

Tulinius, H., Day, N.E., Johannesson, G., Bjarnason, O. & Gonzales, M. (1978) Reproductive factors and risk for breast cancer in Iceland. *Int. J. Cancer*, *21*, 724-730

Vermeulen, A., Deslypere, J.P., Paridaens, R., Leclerq, G., Roy, F. & Heuson, J.C. (1986) Aromatase, 17-beta-hydroxysteroid dehydrogenase and intratissular sex hormone concentrations in cancerous and normal glandular breast tissue in postmenopausal women. *Eur. J. Cancer Clin. Oncol.*, *22*, 515-525

Wahi, P.M., Luthra, U.K., Mali, S. & Shimkin, M.B. (1972) Prevalence and distribution of cancer of the uterine cervix in Agra District, India. *Cancer, 30,* 720-725

Wang, D.Y. & Fentiman, I.S. (1985) Epidemiology and endocrinology of benign breast disease. *Breast Cancer Res. Treat., 6,* 5-36

Weiss, N.S., Daeing, J.R. & Woang, H.C. (1981) Incidence of cancer of the large bowel in women in relation to reproductive and hormonal factors. *J. Natl Cancer Inst., 67,* 57-60

Wynder, E.L., Cornfield, J. & Schroff, P.D. (1954) A study of environmental factors in carcinoma of the cervix. *Am. J. Obstet. Gynecol., 68,* 1016-1047

Zumoff, B. (1981) Influence of obesity and malnutrition on the metabolism of some cancer-related hormones. *Cancer Res., 41,* 3805-3807

Zumoff, B. (1982) Relationship of obesity and blood estrogens. *Cancer Res., 42,* 3289s-3294s

Chapter 15. Psychological factors

The possibility that certain personality types are more prone to cancer was first noted in the eighteenth century (Bahnson, 1980), and in 1893 Herbert Snow reported that patients with cancer of the breast and uterine cervix had often undergone a stressful life event, such as the loss of a close relative, in the recent past (Le Shan, 1959). However, during most of the present century, the possible role of psychological factors in the etiology of cancer has not been considered seriously by the scientific community (Angell, 1985). The low level of commitment in this area undoubtedly owes something to prejudice against the 'softer' social sciences; however, it can also be traced to the preeminence of the cellular theories of carcinogenesis, which leaves little theoretical place for organic phenomena such as mental states, and to certain major methodological problems which confront the epidemiological investigation of psychological factors, so that existing studies have not adequately confronted them.

There have been two distinct threads in the etiological studies carried out so far in this area. One is the role of personality type, as defined by psychological testing questionnaires such as the Minnesota Multiphasic Personality Inventory (MMPI) and Eysenck's Personality Inventory, which are used to assess various stable personality characteristics. Temoshok (1987) provides an extensive review of this work. In early studies, cancer patients were compared with controls who were either healthy or suffering from nonmalignant disease, and it was found that the cancer patients had a lower ability to express anger (Bacon *et al.*, 1952; Kissen, 1966; Bahnson & Bahnson, 1969). These studies are open to the obvious criticism that a patient's psychological state could well be influenced by the diagnosis of cancer or by the disease itself.

In order to circumvent this problem, several prospective studies have been carried out in which personality was assessed well before diagnosis of disease, or at the time of biopsy for disease before the diagnosis was known. The results of these studies have been somewhat varied. Shekelle *et al.* (1981) found that middle-aged men evaluated as having a depressive personality profile on one of the scales used had twice the risk of developing cancer in the 17 years subsequent to evaluation than non-depressive subjects, after adjusting for a number of important confounding variables, including age, alcohol and tobacco consumption and social class. In contrast, Dattore *et al.* (1980) reported that, after adjustment for age, patients with *lower* depression scores had a higher risk for cancer. Schmale and Iker (1971) found that women who were assessed as having an attitude of hopelessness at the time of cervical cancer biopsy were more likely to develop cancer than a reference group of patients. In similarly designed studies of women who underwent breast biopsies, inability to express anger (Greer *et al.*, 1979; Morris *et al.*, 1981; Jansen & Muenz, 1984) and emotional suppression (Wirsching *et al.*, 1982) predicted an unfavourable diagnosis. Other personality types characterized as being at an increased risk for cancer are those exhibiting 'rational and anti-emotional behaviour' (Grossarth-Maticek *et al.*, 1983) and 'loners' (Shaffer *et al.*, 1987). Although generally more convincing than the case–control studies, many of these prospective studies involved epidemiological designs that are somewhat different from those employed in studies of other risk factors for cancer. Furthermore, comparison across studies is hampered by the multiplicity of scales that have been used to evaluate personality.

The other major type of etiological study of psychological factors has involved investigation of the role of stressful life events, particularly in the period preceding the cancer diagnosis. A comprehensive review is given by Burgess (1987). Perhaps because they involve a more concrete risk factor than the personality studies, namely external events, the results of these studies have been somewhat easier to interpret. The conclusion from a number of investigations (Muslin *et al.*, 1966; Snell & Graham, 1971; Greer & Morris, 1975; Schonfield, 1975; Jones *et al.*, 1984; Ewertz, 1986) was that recent stressful events, most often the loss of a close relative, spouse or friend, were unrelated to the risk for breast cancer, but that for some other cancers, including lung cancer (Horne & Picard, 1979), stomach cancer (Lehrer, 1980) and childhood cancer (Jacobs & Charles, 1980), there was an association between recent life events and risk. It will be important to confirm these observations in future studies.

One of the main arguments against the role of psychological factors in cancer etiology has been the relative lack of plausible mechanisms. The relationship between psychological factors and hormonal and immune function has been investigated in several studies. There is evidence that the anger-suppressing personality type is associated with a specific antibody profile (Pettingale *et al.*, 1977) and that lymphocyte levels are depressed in subjects who have recently suffered the loss of a spouse (Bartrop *et al.*, 1977). The effect of stress on the immune system has also been tested in experiments in animals (Keller *et al.*, 1981). While the role of the immune system in cancer induction remains controversial, it could mediate a relationship between stress and cancer risk.

If psychological factors are to play a more prominent role in future epidemiological studies, it will be essential that instruments be standardized and that data on potential confounding variables be obtained and analysed systematically. It is not clear whether personality type is amenable to intervention; however, major life events, such as the loss of a loved one, are known to have a heavy impact on health (Kraus & Lilienfeld, 1959; Young *et al.*, 1963), which could be softened by supportive care. Whether cancer can also be prevented in this way remains to be demonstrated.

References

Angell, M. (1985) Disease as a reflection of the psyche. *New Engl. J. Med.*, *312*, 1570-1572

Bacon, C.L., Renneker, R. & Cutler, M. (1952) A psychosomatic survey of cancer of the breast. *Psychosom. Med.*, *14*, 453-460

Bahnson, C.B. (1980) Stress and cancer: the state of the art. Part 1. *Psychosomatics, 21*, 975-981

Bahnson, C.B. & Bahnson, M.B. (1969) Ego defences in cancer patients. *Ann. N.Y. Acad. Sci.*, *164*, 546-559

Bartrop, R.W., Luckhurst, E., Lazaris, L., Kiloh, L.G. & Penny, R. (1977) Depressed lymphocyte function after bereavement. *Lancet*, *i*, 834-836

Burgess, C. (1987) Stress and cancer. *Cancer Surv.*, *6*, 403-416

Dattore, P.J., Shontz, R.C. & Coyne, L. (1980) Premorbid personality differentiation of cancer and non cancer groups: a test of the hypothesis of cancer proneness. *J. Consult. Clin. Psychol.*, *48*, 388-394

Ewertz, M. (1986) Bereavement and breast cancer. *Br. J. Cancer, 53*, 701-703

Greer, S. & Morris, T. (1975) Psychological attributes of women who develop breast cancer: a controlled study. *J. Psychosom. Res.*, *19*, 147-153

Greer, S., Morris, T. & Pettingale, K.W. (1979) Psychological response to breast cancer: effect on outcome. *Lancet, ii*, 785-787

Grossarth-Maticek, R., Kanazir, D.T., Vetter, H. & Schmidt, P. (1983) Psychosomatic factors involved in the process of cancerogenesis: preliminary results of the Yugoslav prospective study. *Psychother. Psychosom.*, *40*, 191-210

Horne, R.L. & Picard, R.S. (1979) Psychosocial risk factors for lung cancer. *Psychosom. Med.*, *41*, 503-514

Jacobs, T.J. & Charles, E. (1980) Life events and the occurrence of cancer in children. *Psychosom. Med.*, *42*, 11-24

Jansen, M.A. & Muenz, L.R. (1984) A retrospective study of personality variables associated with fibrocystic disease and breast cancer. *J. Psychosom. Res.*, *28*, 35-42

Jones, D.R., Goldblatt, P.O. & Leon, D.A. (1984) Bereavement and cancer. Some data on deaths of spouses from the longitudinal study of Office of Population Censuses and Surveys. *Br. Med. J.*, *289*, 461-464

Keller, S.E., Weiss, J.M., Schleifer, S.J., Miller, N.E. & Stein, M. (1981) Suppression of immunity by stress: effect of a graded series of stressors on lymphocyte stimulation in the rat. *Science, 213*, 1397-1400

Kissen, D.M. (1966) The significance of personality in lung cancer in men. *Ann. N.Y. Acad. Sci.*, *125*, 820-826

Kraus, A.S. & Lilienfeld, A.M. (1959) Some epidemiologic aspects of the high mortality in a young widowed group. *J. Chronic Dis.*, *10*, 207-217

Lehrer, S. (1980) Life change and gastric cancer. *Psychosom. Med.*, *42*, 499-502

Le Shan, L. (1959) Psychological states as factors in the development of malignant disease: a critical review. *J. Natl Cancer Inst.*, *22*, 1-18

Morris, T., Greer, S., Pettingale, K.W. & Watson, M. (1981) Patterns of expressing anger and their psychological correlates in women with breast cancer. *J. Psychosom. Res.*, *25*, 111-117

Muslin, H.L., Gyarfas, K. & Pieper, W.J. (1966) Separation experience and cancer of the breast. *Ann. N.Y. Acad. Sci.*, *125*, 802-806

Pettingale, K.W., Greer, S. & Tee, D.E.H. (1977) Serum IgA and emotional expression in breast cancer patients. *J. Psychosom. Res.*, *21*, 395-399

Schmale, A.H. & Iker, H. (1971) Hopelessness as a predictor of cervical cancer. *Soc. Sci. Med.*, *5*, 95-100

Schonfield, J. (1979) Psychological and life-experience differences between Isareli women with benign and cancerous breast lesions. *J. Psychosom. Res.*, *19*, 229-234

Schaffer, J.W., Graves, P.L., Swank, R.T. & Pearson, T.A. (1987) Clustering of personality traits in youth and the subsequent development of cancer among physicians. *J. Behav. Med.*, *10*, 441-447

Shekelle, R.B., Raynor, W.J., Jr, Ostfeld, A.M., Garron, D.C., Bieliauskas, L.A., Liu, S.C., Maliza, C. & Paul, O. (1981) Psychological depression and 17 year risk of death from cancer. *Psychosom. Med.*, *43*, 117-125

Snell, L. & Graham, S. (1971) Social trauma as related to cancer of the breast. *Br. J. Cancer, 25*, 721-734

Temoshok, L. (1987) Personality, coping style, emotion and cancer: towards an integrative model. *Cancer Surv.*, *6*, 545-567

Wirsching, M., Stierlin, H., Hoffmann, F., Weber, G. & Wirsching, B. (1982) Psychological identification of breast cancer patients before biopsy. *J. Psychosom. Res.*, *26*, 1-10

Young, M., Benjamin, B. & Wallis, C. (1963) The mortality of widowers. *Lancet, ii*, 454-456

Chapter 16. Socioeconomic factors

Socioeconomic differences in the frequency of cancer may be attributable to differences in the circumstances of life of different sections of society. Societies are not homogeneous, and variations between people of different social classes in many aspects of life style, culture and behaviour have clear repercussions on health. In most studies of socioeconomic differences in cancer occurrence, measures have been used that are constructed on the basis of occupation, education, income and wealth or area of residence (Liberatos et al., 1988). Classifications involving such measures have been criticized as providing imprecise definitions and having an uncertain relation to sociological concepts of class. They persist in epidemiological research because data on morbidity and mortality and on health behaviour reveal clear social divisions.

Three types of reasons for studying social class can be identified (Marmot et al., 1987):

(i)   Public health action: Socio-economic differences in cancer frequency are often wide and some have become steeper recently. Elimination of social inequalities between and within countries is one of the major targets of the WHO programme, 'Health for all by the year 2000'.

(ii) Understanding the etiology of diseases: Wide differences between social classes may help in understanding disease causation, although the aspects of lifestyle or circumstances that are correlated with socioeconomic factors are very diverse.

(iii) Theory: Analysis of social class should allow an examination of how the organization of society affects health and disease.

Differentials and environmental causes of cancer mortality

Early studies of deaths from cancer in the USA (Maynard, 1910) and in England and Wales (Brown & Lal, 1914; Stevenson, 1923) were not concerned with individual cancer sites. Stevenson's (1923) occupational/industrial classification was the forerunner of what is known as the Registrar General's Social Classes. The decennial supplements of occupational mortality are based on deaths allocated to a social class according to the occupation specified on death certificates. While this provides the numerator for the mortality rates, the denominator is provided by information on the occupational distribution of the population collected by the census.

Using the supplements, Young (1926) provided the first systematic data on site-specific differentials in cancer mortality: 11 of the 16 individual sites examined showed evidence of a 'negative' gradient with class, i.e., the mortality rates in the lower socioeconomic groups (less advantaged) are greater than those in the higher socioeconomic groups (more advantaged). Stomach cancer, the numerically most important single site at the time, showed a particularly strong negative gradient. Cancer of the bowel was one of the few sites that showed a positive class gradient, with the highest mortality among the higher social classes.

In subsequent decennial supplements, the social class schema was refined (Registrar General, 1927), and social class differentials in mortality among women were analysed by husband's social class. By showing that the differences for men and women were similar for a number of cancer sites, Stocks (Registrar General, 1938) concluded that life style rather than occupational factors must be the dominant environmental influence behind the observed differences.

An important finding of the 1951 *Decennial Supplement on Occupational Mortality* (Stocks, 1952; Registrar General, 1954) was the identification of a distinct negative social class gradient in mortality from lung cancer, rates in Social Class I (professional) being lower than those in Social Class V (unskilled, manual). Earlier supplements had shown no evidence of an effect of social class on mortality from lung cancer.

Outside the UK, the same methodology has produced similar results. Clemmesen (1941) analysed occupational mortality in Denmark and found results broadly similar to those of the decennial supplements for England and Wales. Buell *et al.* (1960) analysed male cancer mortality in California, USA, around the time of the 1950 US census, according to an occupationally based social class schema similar to that of the Registrar General.

Logan (1982) produced a consolidated analysis of cancer mortality in the UK by occupation and social class on the basis of data from the decennial supplements. His findings are summarized in Table 30.

In the 1971 *Decennial Supplement* (Office of Population Censuses and Surveys, 1978), the concept of standardization within a social class was introduced. Instead of comparing the mortality rates for a group, such as an occupation order, with the rates for all men, comparison is made with men in the same social class or classes. This method takes into account many of the differences between occupations associated with social class, but permits concentration on those that remain, for which other explanations should be sought. Fox and Adelstein (1978), using this approach, showed that a correlation between smoking and risk for lung cancer for 25 occupational orders was reduced by three-quarters after standardization for social class.

In the Third National Cancer Survey in the USA, blacks had the highest incidence rate for all neoplasms among the major ethnic groups. In both black and white men, a decreasing risk for lung cancer was associated with increasing income, and the increased risk among blacks as compared to whites was totally explained by adjusting for income and education (Devesa & Diamond, 1983). No significant difference in lung cancer risk by ethnic group or socioeconomic status was apparent among women.

In an analysis of occupational and social class differences among New Zealand males, mortality from all neoplasms and from cancers of the liver, larynx, lung, buccal cavity and stomach were particularly high in people of low social classes, and mortality from multiple myeloma, malignant melanoma and lymphatic leukaemia particularly high among those of upper social classes. Smoking patterns explained much of the increased risk for smoking-related cancers among social classes III and IV, but not the very high mortality seen in class V (Pearce & Howard, 1986).

Table 30. Socioeconomic differentials for selected cancer sites[a]

Site	Sex	Differential type	Variation over time	Further details
Buccal cavity and pharynx	M	Negative, moderate	Narrowing of differentials	Salivary gland is only component of site aggregate to show a negative differential in most studies.
	F	? Negative	No systematic change	Few available data
Oesophagus	M	Negative, moderate	Negative gradient has become steeper and smoother	
	F	–		
Stomach	M	Negative, stronger	Constant	One of the strongest and most consistent relationships with socioeconomic position
	F	–	Sharp decline in mortality rate	
Colon	M	? Positive	Positive gradient apparent to and including 1951; subsequently no relationship with social class seen	Strong positive differentials observed in studies of colon cancer in Cali, Colombia, and in Hong Kong: no consistent relationship seen in other recent studies
	F	–		
Rectum		No evidence of consistent differential		
Liver	M	Negative, weak	In early period, non–linear relationship seen; negative gradient most apparent in 1971	Few available data
	F	? Negative	No systematic change	Few available data
Pancreas		No evidence of consistent differential		
Larynx	M	Negative, strong	Relatively constant negative gradient maintained	Negative differentials seen in earliest available data, in contrast to lung cancer
	F	–		
Lung	M	Negative, strong	Social class differentials first apparent in 1951 for males and 1961 for females; gradient steepest in 1971	Outside of England and Wales, negative differentials seen for males and females in 1940s
	F	–		In general, some evidence that male differentials wider than female differentials
Malignant melanoma	M	Positive, moderate	Differential slightly wider for females in 1971 than in 1961 or 1951	Few available data
	F	–		
Breast	F	Positive, weak	No earlier data available Sharp narrowing of differential 1931–61 Small positive differential remaining for married and single women in 1971	Small positive differentials found with great consistency
Site	Sex	Differential type	Variation over time	Further details

Site	Sex	Differential	Time trend	Notes
Cervix	F	Negative, strong	Slight widening of differentials for married and single women 1951–71; no earlier data available in disaggregated form	Earliest socioeconomic differential observed; almost always the largest differential reported in any study; found with complete consistency in every population investigated
Other uterus (principally corpus uteri)	F	No evidence of consistent differential		
Ovary	F	Positive, weak	Narrowing of differentials 1931–61; small positive differential remaining for married and single women in 1971	Similar pattern to breast, particularly with narrowing of differential over time; positive differential found in most studies
Prostate	M	Variable	Pronounced positive gradient in 1911 diminished with time to produce suggestion of weak negative gradient in 1971	Results of different studies contradictory
Testis	M	Positive, strong	Large positive differential remained relatively constant 1921–71	Positive differential shows consistency; however, few data available from decennial supplements
Bladder	M F	Variable –	Basic negative differential developed into smooth negative gradient between 1921 and 1971	Negative differential seen in decennial supplements is not confirmed in other studies, some of which indicate the existence of a positive differential, while others show no relationship with socio-economic position
Brain	M F	Positive, weak –	Early pronounced positive differential narrowed over time, leaving a small but perceptible positive differential in 1971	Positive differential found in most studies
Leukaemia	M F	? Positive –	Weak positive differential seen in most periods	Results of different studies are inconsistent; decennial supplements indicate that differentials may vary according to type of leukaemia
Hodgkin's disease	M F	Positive, weak –	Clear positive gradient in 1951 absent or only weakly present later	Some confirmation of positive differential from US data

a Adapted from Logan (1982)

Studies using area or grouped data

Clemmesen and Nielsen (1951) compared cancer incidence rates between groups of administrative districts in Copenhagen that had been aggregated according to mean annual house rents. The differentials observed between the five rental categories were in most respects similar to those reported in the decennial supplements for England and Wales.

In New Haven, Connecticut, USA, cancer registry data for 1935–49 were used to study the socioeconomic distribution of cancers of the stomach (Cohart, 1954), oesophagus, colon, rectum and pancreas (Cohart & Muller, 1955), lung (Cohart, 1955a), breast, ovary and uterus (Cohart, 1955b), using a composite index of socioeconomic levels that took into account a district's industrial composition and characteristics of its inhabitants. Men had a strong negative gradient for cancer of the oesophagus, and both men and women had negative gradients for cancers of the stomach and lung. An opposite effect was seen for cancers of the female breast and ovary, the highest rates occurring in the 'well-to-do' districts.

Pinkel and Nefzger (1959) used median house rentals recorded in the 1972 census tracts of Buffalo, NY, USA, as the basis for allocating cancer cases and members of the general population to one of a number of socioeconomic categories. The incidence of childhood leukaemia was greatest in those tracts with the highest rentals. In the same area, Graham *et al.* (1960) found a negative gradient for the incidences of cancers of the oesophagus, stomach, liver, lung and larynx in males, and for cancers of the stomach, liver and cervix in females. Breast cancer was the only site for which incidence increased sharply with increasing social status.

Dorn and Cutler (1959) collected data on cancer incidence in 1947 from ten major cities in the USA. A socioeconomic measure based on median family income was used. Steep negative gradients were found among white males for cancers of the lip, tongue and pharynx. For the major sites, such as stomach, the results for blacks were similar to those for whites.

Seidman (1970) used data from New York City to look at cancer mortality in religious groups according to a composite socioeconomic index. Mortality from cancers of the oesophagus, larynx and lung was considerably lower among Jewish men than that in other religious groups. However, for all of these sites, pronounced negative socioeconomic gradients were seen within each religious group. A similar situation prevailed among females for mortality from cervical cancer.

In the Third US National Cancer Survey (Devesa & Diamond, 1980, 1983), black and white males showed a strong negative socioeconomic gradient for lung cancer, while black and white females showed pronounced negative gradients for cervical cancer. Racial differences in mortality from cervical and breast cancer, although reduced by adjustment for socioeconomic factors, remained significant. Similar studies have been conducted in Sydney, Australia (Fisher, 1978), Finland (Teppo *et al.*, 1980) and Montréal, Canada (Thouez, 1984).

Data from the cancer registry of Cali, Colombia, and socioeconomic data by census tract (Haenszel *et al.*, 1975; Cuello *et al.*, 1982) provided results different from those found in the UK, Denmark and the USA for a number of sites. Among males, cancers of the buccal cavity, larynx, lung and bronchus and bladder all showed evidence of positive gradients, incidence rates being highest among men in the most affluent section of the community. Women in the top social class had a breast cancer rate that was double that of women in the lowest class, while males and females both showed a positive gradient for cancer of the colon. Both stomach and cervical cancer showed strong negative gradients.

Crowther *et al.* (1976) measured socioeconomic differences among groups in Hong Kong. Mortality from colorectal cancer in people of each sex showed a strong positive gradient with socioeconomic position, and assays of gut bacteria and bile acids in faecal samples from volunteers showed an increase in the concentration of bile acids with increasing income level.

A correlation study in 23 Brazilian states of the frequency of cancer in relation to various socioeconomic variables indicated that cancers of the colon, larynx and lung were positively related to measures of affluence, while a strong negative correlation was found for cancers of the cervix and penis (Franco *et al.*, 1988).

Record-linkage studies

The existence of socioeconomic differences at an individual level has been confirmed by studies in which the socioeconomic characteristics of individuals have been related to their subsequent risk of dying from or being diagnosed with cancer. Kitagawa and Hauser (1973) linked census records to a large random sample of all deaths throughout the USA that had occurred in the four months following the 1960 census. The differentials shown were similar to those seen in previous studies. Studies in France (Desplanques, 1976), Denmark (Lynge, 1979), Norway (Haldorsen & Glattre, 1976; Kristoffersen, 1979), Sweden (Vagero & Persson, 1986), Finland (Sauli, 1979; Hakama *et al.*, 1982; Teppo, 1984) and England and Wales (Fox & Goldblatt, 1982; Leon, 1988) have also used the linkage of routine data in analyses of socioeconomic differences in cancer incidence or mortality. Their results are largely consistent.

Increasing unemployment in industrialized countries has posed the need for investigating health problems among unemployed persons. Deterioration of mental health is well documented (Platt, 1984), but two record-linkage studies in the UK and Denmark have also shown that unemployed people have increased mortality from all cancers and particularly from lung cancer (Moser *et al.*, 1984; Iversen *et al.*, 1987). In both studies, the increased risk was attributed primarily to unemployment and not to a possible bias towards ill health in this population.

Differences in survival from cancer

Socioeconomic differences in survival have been examined mainly in the USA, but information is also available for a few other countries. In most studies, poorest survival is associated with low socioeconomic status. Recent interest in differences in survival is due partly to the observation of a large variation among different ethnic groups in the USA (Young *et al.*, 1984), which were shown to reflect, to some extent, socioeconomic differences. Variation in the length of time before a cancer is detected has been the cause most frequently incriminated for variations in survival. Differences in treatment, tumour characteristics, genetic factors and psychological influences have also been investigated as contributing causes, but there is little evidence for their importance.

Reasons for differences in cancer frequency by social class

A British government publication on health inequalities (Whitehead, 1987) heavily influenced thinking about the causes of social class differences in health. Four categories of explanation were considered: artefacts, natural and social selection, material or structural reasons and cultural or behavioural explanations.

It is sometimes argues that socioeconomic differences in mortality and morbidity are a consequence of selection, i.e., that it is health that determines social position rather than the opposite. People in poor health often experience downwards social mobility; however, this type of selection would appear to be an unimportant component of differences in deaths from all causes or from cancer specifically. Buell *et al.* (1960) pointed to the short clinical history of most cancers: if social mobility were important, it should have less effect on diseases that are rapidly fatal. Kitagawa and Hauser (1973) argued that there would be socioeconomic differences among persons of different educational levels; by its very nature, attained education provides a measure of socioeconomic status that is not susceptible to the effects of health selection.

Variations in cancer occurrence among social classes are associated with differences in life style and exposure, as is well illustrated by exposure to tobacco smoking, occupational exposures and reproductive history.

In 1972 in England and Wales, 31.5% of professional men and 57.7% of skilled manual workers were smokers. The corresponding percentages for women with husbands in these two social classes were 28.9% and 44.9%. In the USA in 1970, 'blue-collar' and service workers comprised the highest proportion of current smokers and professionals the lowest (Weinkam & Sterling, 1987). Ten years later, the prevalence of smoking was lower in both countries, but social class differences in smoking patterns remained or had become even steeper. Much of the variation between social classes in the incidence of and mortality from cancers related to smoking (cancers of the lung, oesophagus, larynx, bladder) can be attributed to smoking.

High cancer mortality has been observed in many non-manual occupations (Walrath *et al.*, 1985), and any list of occupational carcinogens reveals that the workers principally exposed are 'blue-collar' workers, such as those in the metal industry, asbestos insulators and dye manufacturers. It is difficult to determine, however, the degree to which this elevated cancer mortality is related to occupation and that to which it is related to general social circumstances. Both occupation and way of life have been shown to contribute to the variation in cancer mortality between occupational orders (Fox & Adelstein, 1978).

Breast cancer has been found consistently to be more frequent among women of higher socioeconomic status. This has been attributed to variations in reproductive factors, but childbearing history is probably not sufficient to explain the differences (Devesa & Diamond, 1980).

The identification of intervening variables (like smoking, reproductive history and occupation) that contribute to socioeconomic differences in cancer frequency may occasionally lead to important public health benefits. In order that an intervention be successful, however, the social causes of differences in exposure or life style must be kept in mind. For instance, it is not enough to identify smoking as a causal factor in the wide social class differences in the frequency of lung cancer, but it is also appropriate to identify the reasons why smoking is more prevalent among lower social classes.

Specific risk factors may not account for even the major part of the differences in cancer mortality (Syme & Berkman, 1976; Marmot *et al.*, 1984). Psychosocial factors may contribute to the general increase in physical illness among low socioeconomic groups, although studies on this topic (see p. 251) have not provided evidence as convincing as that from studies of mortality from cardiovascular diseases (Fox & Adelstein, 1978).

References

Brown, J.W. & Lal, M. (1914) An inquiry into the relation between social status and cancer mortality. *J. Hyg.*, *14*, 186-200

Buell, P., Dunn, J.E. & Breslow, C. (1960) The occupational-social class risks of cancer mortality in men. *J. Chronic Dis.*, *12*, 600-621

Clemmesen, J. (1941) *Cancer and Occupation in Denmark 1935-1939*, Copenhagen, Nyt Nordisk Forlag - Arnold Busck

Clemmesen, J. & Nielsen, A. (1951) The social distribution of cancer in Copenhagen, 1943-1947. *Br. J. Cancer*, *5*, 159-171

Cohart, E.M. (1954) Socio-economic distribution of stomach cancer in New Haven. *Cancer*, *7*, 455-461

Cohart, E.M. (1955a) Socio-economic distribution of cancer of the female sex organs in New Haven. *Cancer*, *8*, 34-41

Cohart, E.M. (1955b) Socio-economic distribution of cancer of the lung in New Haven. *Cancer*, *8*, 1126-1129

Cohart, E.M. & Muller, C. (1955) Socio-economic distribution of cancer of the gastrointestinal tract in New Haven. *Cancer*, *8*, 379-388

Crowther, J.S., Drasar. B.S., Hill, M.J., MacLennan, R., Magnin, D., Peach, S. & Teon-Chan, C.H. (1976) Faecal steroids and bacteria and bowel cancer in Hong Kong by socio-economic groups. *Br. J. Cancer*, *34*, 191-198

Cuello, C., Correa, P. & Haenszel, W. (1982) Socio-economic class differences in cancer incidence in Cali, Colombia. *Int. J. Cancer*, *29*, 637-643

Desplanques, G. (1976) *La Mortalité des Adultes suivant le Milieu Social 1955-71* (Collections de l'INSEE No. 195, Série D., No. 44), Paris, Institut National de Statistiques et Etudes Economiques

Devesa, S.S. & Diamond, E.L. (1980) Association of breast cancer and cervical cancer incidences with income and education among whites and blacks. *J. Natl Cancer Inst.*, *65*, 515-528

Devesa, S.S. & Diamond, E.L. (1983) Socio-economic and racial differences in lung cancer incidence. *Am. J. Epidemiol.*, *118*, 808-813

Dorn, H.F. & Cutler, S.J. (1959) *Morbidity from Cancer in the United States* (Public Health Monograph 56, Public Health Service Publication No. 590), Washington DC, US Government Printing Service

Fisher, S. (1978) Relationship of mortality to socio-economic status and some other factors in Sydney in 1971. *J. Epidemiol. Community Health*, *32*, 41-46

Fox, A.J. & Adelstein, A.M. (1978) Occupational mortality: work or way of life? *J. Epidemiol. Community Health*, *32*, 73-78

Fox, A.J. & Goldblatt, P.O. (1982) *Socio-economic Mortality Differentials 1971-1975* (OPCS Series LS1), London, Her Majesty's Stationery Office

Franco, E.L., Campos, F.N., Villa, L.L. & Torloni, H. (1988) Correlation patterns of cancer relative frequencies with some socioeconomic and demographic indicators in Brazil: an ecologic study. *Int. J. Cancer*, *41*, 24-29

Graham, S., Levin, M. & Lilienfeld, A.M. (1960) The socio-economic distribution of cancer of various sites in Buffalo NY, 1948-1952. *Cancer, 13*, 180-191

Haenszel, W., Correa, P. & Cuello, C. (1975) Social class differences among patients with large bowel cancer in Cali, Colombia. *J. Natl Cancer Inst., 54*, 1031-1035

Hakama, M., Hakulinen, T., Pukkala, E., Saxén, E. & Teppo, L. (1982) Risk indicators of breast and cervical cancer on ecologic and individual levels. *Am. J. Epidemiol., 16*, 990-1000

Haldorsen, T. & Glattre, E. (1976) *Occupational Mortality 1970-73* (Statistike Analyser No. 210), Oslo, Statistisk Sentralburo

Iversen, L., Andersen, O., Andersen, P.K., Christoffersen, K. & Keiding, N. (1987) Unemployment and mortality in Denmark 1970-1980. *Br. Med. J., 295*, 879-884

Kitagawa, E.M. & Hauser, P.M. (1973) *Differential Mortality in the United States: A Study in Socio-economic Epidemiology*, Cambridge, MA, Harvard University Press

Kristoffersen, L. (1979) *Occupational Mortality* (Rapporter fra Statistik Sentralbyro 79/19), Oslo, Statistik Sentralbyro

Leon, D.A. (1988) *Longitudinal Study 1971-75. The Social Distribution of Cancer* (Office of Population Censuses and Surveys, No. 3), London, Her Majesty's Stationery Office

Liberatos, P., Link, B.G. & Kelsey, J.L. (1988) The measurement of social class in epidemiology. *Epidemiol. Rev., 10*, 87-121

Logan, W.P.D. (1982) *Cancer Mortlaity by Occupation and Social Class 1851-1971* (IARC Scientific Publications No. 36), Lyon, IARC

Lynge, E. (1979) *Dødelighed og Erhverv, 1970-75* (Statistiske Undersøgelser No. 37), Copenhagen, Danmarks Statistik

Marmot, M.G. Shipley, M.J. & Rose, G. (1984) Inequalities in death-specific explanations of a general pattern. *Lancet, i*, 1003-1006

Marmot, M.G., Kogevinas, M. & Elston, M.A. (1987) Socio/economic status and disease. *Ann. Rev. Public Health, 8*, 111-135

Maynard, G.D. (1910) A statistical study in cancer death rates. *Biometrika, 7*, 276-304

Moser, K.A., Fox, A.J. & Jones, D.R. (1984) Unemployment and mortality in the OPCS longitudinal study. *Lancet, ii*, 1324-1329

Office of Population Censuses and Surveys (1978) *Occupational Mortality. The Registrar General's Decennial Supplement for England and Wales 1970-1972*, London, Her Majesty's Stationery Office

Pearce, N.E. & Howard, J.K. (1986) Occupation, social class and male cancer mortality in New Zealand, 1974-1978. *Int. J. Epidemiol., 15*, 456-462

Pinkel, D. & Nefzger, D. (1959) Some epidemiological features of childhood leukaemia in Buffalo, NY area. *Cancer, 12*, 351-358

Platt, S. (1984) Unemployment and suicidal behaviour: a review of the literature. *Soc. Sci. Med., 19*, 93-115

Registrar General (1927) *Decennial Supplement, England and Wales, 1921*, Part II, London, Her Majesty's Stationery Office

Registrar General (1938) *Decennial Supplement, England and Wales, 1931*, Part IIa, London, Her Majesty's Stationery Office

Registrar General (1954) *Decennial Supplement, England and Wales, 1951*, Part II, London, Her Majesty's Stationery Office

Sauli, H. (1979) *Occupational Mortality in 1971-75*, Helsinki, Central Statistical Office of Finland

Seidman, H. (1970) Cancer death rates by site and sex for religious and socio-economic groups in New-York City. *Environ. Res., 3*, 234-250

Stevenson, T.H.C. (1923) The social distribution of mortality from different causes in England and Wales, 1910-12. *Biometrika, 15*, 382-400

Stocks, P. (1952) Epidemiology of cancer of the lung in England and Wales. *Br. J. Cancer, 6*, 99-111

Syme, S.L. & Berkman, L.F. (1976) Social class susceptibility and sickness. *Am. J. Epidemiol., 104*, 1-8

Teppo, L. (1984) Cancer incidence by living area, social class and occupation. *Scand. J. Work Environ. Health, 10*, 361-366

Teppo, L., Pukkala, E., Hakama, M., Hakulinen, T., Herva, A. & Saxén, E. (1980) Way of life and cancer incidence in Finland. A municipality-based ecological analysis. *Scand. J. Soc. Med.*, *Suppl. 19*

Thouez, J.P. (1984) La mortalité differentielle par cancer suivant le milieu social: le cas de la région métropolitaine de Montréal, 1971. *Soc. Sci. Med.*, *18*, 73-81

Vagero, I. & Persson, G. (1986) Occurrence of cancer in socioeconomic groups in Sweden. An analysis based on the Swedish Cancer Environment Registry. *Scand. J. Soc. Med.*, *14*, 151-160

Walrath, J., Li, F.P., Hoar, S.K., Mead, M.W. & Fraumeni, J.F., Jr (1985) Causes of death among female chemists. *Am. J. Public Health*, *75*, 883-885

Weinkamm, J.J. & Sterling, T.D. (1987) Changes in smoking characteristics by type of employment from 1970 to 1979/80. *Am. J. Ind. Med.*, *11*, 539-561

Whitehead, M. (1987) *The Health Divide: Inequalities in Health in the 1980s*, London, Health Education Authority

Young, M. (1926) The variation in the mortality from cancer of different parts of the body in groups of men of different social status. *J. Hyg.*, *25*, 209-217

Young, J.L., Jr, Gloeckler-Ries, L. & Pollock, E.S. (1984) Cancer patient survival among ethnic groups in the United States. *J. Natl Cancer Inst.*, *73*, 341-352

PART III

EARLY DETECTION OF CANCER

Chapter 17. Description of screening measures

Introduction

Cancer may be detected earlier than usual in its natural history, either when a patient recognizes symptoms and refers then promptly to a medical practitioner or through the application of a screening test, aimed at diagnosing precancerous changes or cancer itself in asymptomatic individuals. It makes intuitive sense (but, as we shall see, is more difficult to demonstrate empirically) that cancers that are detected early can be treated more effectively.

The chance that a patient will recognize symptoms early on can be heightened substantially by public education programmes, but the usefulness of early detection in reducing mortality is not assured for all cancers. On the one hand is the example of melanoma in Australia, where very high incidence rates are accompanied by good survival rates (Lemish *et al.*, 1983), possibly due to campaigns aimed at helping people to recognize suspicious skin lesions. In contrast is cancer of the pancreas, which in 85% of cases is fatal within 12 months of its first symptoms (National Cancer Institute, Division of Cancer Prevention and Control, 1988). In many developing countries, greater awareness of the early signs of cervical cancer could result in a real reduction in mortality, provided adequate radiotherapy and surgical facilities were available.

Although there has been little systematic evaluation of the effects of education programmes on cancer mortality (Hakama *et al.*, 1989), there are strong ethical grounds for improving public knowledge of abnormal signs and symptoms.

The remainder of this chapter consists of a discussion of early detection methods that are applied to asymptomatic individuals and are known as 'population screening' or 'secondary prevention'. The aim of a screening test is to separate people who probably have the disease in question (or a very high likelihood of developing it) from those who probably do not. Individuals who are found to give positive results on screening must be subjected to conventional, more intensive diagnostic procedures. Since it is to be applied to a large number of apparently healthy individuals, a test must first of all be accurate, in the sense that the probability of a false result is limited. In addition, it must be relatively inexpensive, safe and convenient. Tests that achieve a reasonable degree of accuracy without overwhelming cost become candidates for large-scale implementation in an organized screening programme, and their capacity to reduce mortality or morbidity from the disease can then be evaluated. In the following sections, we discuss in more detail the benefits and costs of population screening and how a programme can be assessed, before going on to a site-by-site review of the value of currently available screening tests. A series of monographs published by the International Union Against Cancer (Miller, 1978; Prorok & Miller, 1984; Hakama *et al.*, 1986; Chamberlain & Miller, 1988; Day & Miller, 1988) gives a much fuller account of cancer screening.

Benefits and costs of a screening programme

In the simplest terms, the success of a screening programme is measured by the number of premature deaths prevented by its implementation. Expressed more precisely, a programme is beneficial if the mortality rate for the disease in question is lower in individuals who have been offered screening than in those who have not. An alternative to reduction of mortality as a measure of benefit is a reduction in number of years of life lost from the disease (see p. 21), which in some analyses has been assigned an economic value. Screening may not only reduce mortality but also decrease morbidity or the degree of therapeutic intervention required. These benefits are much harder to quantify than a reduction in mortality.

The benefits must be weighed against the costs of screening. The direct medical costs can be calculated as the cost of carrying out the testing, minus the amount saved by avoiding the more extensive therapeutic methods that are required when the disease is detected late. The cost of testing includes both the screening test itself and the follow-up evaluation that must be carried out when the screening test gives rise to a positive result.

The other costs of screening fall upon the individual patient and are not all financial. They include extension of the period of morbidity for those individuals whose disease does not benefit from early detection, unnecessary alarm raised by false-positive results, and delay in responding to true symptoms which may follow a false but reassuring negative result. The screening test may be unpleasant or time consuming and, in the case of some methods, such as the mammography procedures used in the 1960s, engender a risk in itself (Bailar, 1977).

Evaluation of screening

The costs of a screening test can be estimated fairly well as the technique is developed and its implementation begins. Evaluation of benefit is much more difficult, and the appropriate methodology is still being refined. Early attempts to prove the value of screening consisted simply of comparisons between the survival rate of cases detected by screening and those diagnosed clinically; these comparisons are unfortunately subject to several major biases. First of all, the screened population may not be a random sample of the population who gave rise to the clinical cases with regard to other prognostic factors for the disease such as social class. Secondly, an increase in the average time between diagnosis and death may simply be a result of advancing the date of diagnosis rather than retarding the date of death (Hutchison & Shapiro, 1968). Finally, a higher proportion of cases detected by screening are tumours that grow more slowly, which would in any case have a more favourable prognosis (Zelen & Feinleib, 1969). The effect of these biases on comparisons of case fatality can be estimated, but it is a complicated procedure dependent on assumptions about the natural history of the disease.

The rate of diagnosis of late-stage cancers (not the proportion of such cases, which will automatically fall if the number of early-stage cancers detected by screening is increased) can be used as an indication of whether a screening programme is likely to be of benefit, prior to any demonstration of a decrease in mortality, but is not proof of any benefit.

Ideally, screening should be evaluated by means of a randomized, controlled trial (Prorok *et al.*, 1984), such as that used in the Health Insurance Plan (HIP) study of breast cancer screening in New York, USA (Shapiro, 1977). When such a study is not feasible, a population-based study in which different geographical regions with and without screening programmes are compared, such as that in the UK (UK Trial of Early Detection of Breast Cancer, 1981), provides an alternative. To be interpretable, this approach requires that there be a high degree of compliance with the screening procedure in the screened areas and that any underlying geographical difference be taken account of in the statistical analyses.

Randomized trials have been carried out for only a few types of screening. Their use is limited by cost and organizational difficulties and the arguments about their ethics that arise when segments of the medical community are already convinced of the worth of a particular screening test. In the absence of controlled trials, evaluation of the benefits of screening must be made on the basis of observations of the results from implemented programmes.

Time trends in incidence and mortality, when examined in relation to the introduction of a screening programme or changes in an existing one, can provide convincing evidence of an effect of screening. The most noteworthy examples have been the decreases in rates of cervical cancer in Canada, Scandinavia and north-east Scotland following the implementation of screening programmes (Miller *et al.*, 1976; MacGregor *et al.*, 1985; Läärä *et al.*, 1987).

Cohort studies, in which disease rates among individuals with different screening histories are compared, can be viewed as the closest approximation to a randomized trial. Case–control studies of screening are a more recent development (Clarke & Anderson, 1979; Collette *et al.*, 1984; Prorok *et al.*, 1984; Verbeek *et al.*, 1984), offering the possibility of collecting data on many fewer individuals than in a cohort study but with little loss of information. A major problem with both designs is the non-representativeness of the screened population. For example, women who do not undergo regular cervical screening may be precisely those who are at highest risk of cervical cancer.

A single randomized trial or observational evaluation of a 'screening' method may be insufficient to estimate the potential benefit that might be achieved by screening at different ages and frequencies. Since it is impractical to conduct a new study to evaluate each different screening policy, the alternative is to use data from existing trials to formulate a model of the natural history of the disease (Day & Walter, 1984). The approach can be applied to data from a prospective trial, a cohort study or a case–control study (Brookmeyer *et al.*, 1986). Rates of disease incidence or mortality at different intervals after previous screens can be used to estimate the variation in relative risk associated with different screening intervals. (See section on cancer of the cervix, below.)

Emphasis on frequency of screening and other technical aspects should nevertheless not distract from the importance of the attendance or compliance rate of a programme. Improving compliance can increase the benefit more than shortening the screening interval. Degree of compliance cannot readily be inferred by comparing two populations, but it can readily be assessed in an uncontrolled demonstration project whenever screening is applied to a well-defined population (Prorok & Miller, 1984).

For certain types of cancer, the effectiveness of screening, and, indeed, of any method for preventing cancer (see p. 102), can be increased if it is restricted to subpopulations known to be at high risk. In fact, screening for all cancers is carried out in selected age groups in which the highest numbers of cases arise. Defining high-risk groups by criteria other than age is more difficult. There are some obvious examples, such as the familial syndromes in which a predisposition to certain cancers is inherited, or workers who are known to have been exposed for a long period to an occupational carcinogen before the hazard was known. In these situations, regular examinations of an appropriate kind may help in reducing mortality. For other, weaker risk factors, the benefit of selective screening is less clear, either because too many cases remain in the unselected part of the population, or the size of the selected group approaches that of the total population, rendering selection valueless (Hakama, 1984).

References

Bailar, J.C., III (1977) Screening for early breast cancer: pros and cons. *Cancer, 39 (Suppl. 6),* 2783-2795

Brookmayer, R., Day, N.E. & Moss, S. (1986) case-control studies for estimation of the natural history of preclinical disease from screening data. *Stat. Med., 5,* 127-138

Chamberlain, J. & Miller, A.B., eds (1988) *Screening for Gastrointestinal Cancer,* Bern, Hans Huber

Clarke, E.A. & Anderson, T.W. (1979) Does screening by 'Pap' smears help prevent cervical cancer? *Lancet, ii,* 1-4

Collette, H.J.A., Day, N.E., Rombach, J.J. & de Waard, F. (1984) Evaluation of screening for breast cancer in a non-randomized study (the Dom Project) by means of a case-control study. *Lancet, i,* 1224-1226

Day, N.E. & Miller, A.B., eds (1988) *Screening for Breast Cancer,* Bern, Hans Huber

Day, N.E. & Walter, S.D. (1984) Simplified models of screening for chronic disease: estimation procedures from mass screening programme. *Biometrics, 40,* 1-13

Hakama, M., Miller, A.B. & Day, N.E., eds (1986) *Screening for Cancer of the Uterine Cervix* (IARC Scientific Publications No. 76), Lyon, IARC

Hakama, M., Beral, V., Cullen, J. & Parkin, D.M. (1989) UICC workshop on evaluating interventions to reduce cancer risk. *Int. J. Cancer, 43,* 967-969

Hutchison, G.B. & Shapiro, S. (1968) Lead time gained by diagnostic screening for breast cancer. *J. Natl Cancer Inst., 41,* 665-673

Läärä, E., Day, N.E. & Hakama, M. (1987) Trends in mortality from cervical cancer in the Nordic countries: association with organized screening programmes. *Lancet, i,* 1247-1249

Lemish, W.M., Heenan, P.J., Holman, C.D.J. & Armstrong, B.K. (1983) Survival from preinvasive and invasive malignant melanome in Western Australia. *Cancer, 52,* 580-585

MacGregor, J.E., Moss, S.M., Parkin, D.M. & Day, N.E. (1985) A case-control study of cervical cancer screening in north-east Scotland. *Br. Med. J., 290,* 1543-1546

Miller, A.B., ed. (1978) *Screening in Cancer,* Geneva, International Union Against Cancer

Miller, A.B., Lindsay, J. & Hill, G.B. (1976) Mortality from cancer of the uterus in Canada and its relationship to screening for cancer of the cervix. *Int. J. Cancer, 17,* 602-612

National Cancer Institute, Division of Cancer Prevention and Control (1988) *1987 Annual Cancer Statistics Review Including Cancer Trends: 1950-1985* (NIH Publication No. 88-2789), Bethesda, MD, US Department of Health and Human Services, Public Health Service, National Institutes of Health, National Cancer Institute, p. VI-12

Prorok, P.C. & Miller, A.B., eds (1984) *Screening for Cancer. I. General Principles on Evaluation of Screening for Cancer and Screening for Lung, Bladder and Oral Cancer* (UICC Technical Report Series Vol. 78), Geneva, International Union Against Cancer

Prorok, P.C., Chamberlain, J., Day, N.E., Hakama, M. & Miller, A.B. (1984) UICC workshop on the evaluation of screening programmes for cancer. *Int. J. Cancer, 34*, 1-4

Shapiro, S. (1977) Evidence on screening for breast cancer from a randomized trial. *Cancer, 39*, 2772-2782

UK Trial of Early Detection of Breast Cancer (1981) Trial of early detection of breast cancer: description of method. *Br. J. Cancer, 44*, 618-627

Verbeek, A.L., Hendriks, J.H., Holland, R., Mravunac, M., Sturmans, F. & Day, N.E. (1984) Reduction of breast cancer mortality through mass screening with modern mammography. First results of the Nijmegen project, 1975-1981. *Lancet,* i, 1222-1224

Zelen, M. & Feinleib, M. (1969) On the theory of screening for chronic diseases. *Biometrika, 56*, 601-614

Chapter 18. Effects of population screening measures

In the following sections, arranged site by site, population screening measures are described, and studies in which their efficacy has been evaluated are reviewed. For those measures which appear to be beneficial, the effect of their introduction is quantified, when possible.

Screening tests are well established for cancer of the cervix (Hakama *et al.*, 1986) and for cancer of the breast (Day & Miller, 1988). Screening for colorectal cancer is a more recent development which is currently the subject of controlled trials (Chamberlain & Miller, 1988). Other sites for which potential screening tests have been identified but not yet demonstrated to be of value include bladder and oral cavity (Prorok & Miller, 1984), ovary and endometrium (Hakama *et al.*, 1986), liver and stomach (Chamberlain & Miller, 1988) and skin (malignant melanoma; Reynolds & Austin, 1984; Elwood *et al.*, , 1988).

Cancer of the oral cavity

The possibilities for preventing mortality from oral cancer through early detection would appear to be good, for a number of reasons. Firstly, the oral cavity is a comparatively accessible region of the body and one which is subject to routine examination for dental purposes. Secondly, a number of other oral lesions which are considered to be precursors of squamous-cell carcinoma can easily be detected morphologically by nonmedical personnel (Warnakulasuriya *et al.*, 1984). Finally, there are suggestions that precursor lesions can be induced to regress by reducing smoking and chewing habits (Mehta *et al.*, 1982). Although surgical excision of stage-I and early stage-II carcinomas results in a high survival rate (Binnie, 1975), there has not as yet been any systematically implemented programme, much less any adequate evaluation of their efficacy in reducing mortality (Prorok *et al.*, 1984).

Cancer of the nasopharynx

Serology for immunoglobulin A antibodies to Epstein-Barr virus has been proposed as the basis for screening tests for nasopharyngeal cancer (see p. 190). The only region in which a mass serological survey has been conducted is in the Guangxi autonomous region of China (Zeng *et al.*, 1982). Although cases were discovered at a higher level among seropositive individuals (de-Thé & Zeng, 1986), carefully designed studies will be necessary to evaluate the effect of screening on reducing morbidity and mortality from this cancer.

Cancer of the stomach

Extensive programmes of screening for stomach cancer have been introduced in Japan, using air contrast photofluorography examinations. It is clear that, when cancers are detected by screening, survival is much better than following symptomatic diagnosis. However, there has been no controlled trial of screening, so that it is impossible to know whether this is the result of the biases referred to above (p. 268) or is a real indication of success of the programme. The evidence has been reviewed by Oshima (1988) and Hisamichi (1989).

Geographic studies suggest that mortality rates from gastric cancer are lower in areas where screening has been most widely applied (Kuroichi *et al.*, 1983). Declines in gastric cancer mortality rates are more marked among people in age groups in which they are likely to undergo screening (Hirayama, 1985); however, temporal and geographic variations in risk factors in Japan may explain some of these observations.

Studies of the benefit that individuals obtain from participating in screening programmes are difficult to interpret, since it is likely that persons at low risk of developing or dying from gastric cancer are overrepresented in the screened population. This probably explains the favourable outcome for screened individuals that is usually observed in prospective studies, although in one (Hisamichi & Sugawara, 1984) there was no evidence for a difference in the incidence of gastric cancer between participants and nonparticipants in four towns in Miyagi prefecture. The same bias complicates interpretation of case–control studies. Two have been reported. Oshima *et al.* (1986) concluded that the mass screening programme in Osaka had been effective in reducing stomach cancer mortality by up to 50%, while Fukao *et al.* (1987) found that the relative risk for having an advanced cancer diagnosed in individuals screened within the last three years was 45% compared with that in those undergoing screening at a five-year interval or longer.

A major problem of gastric cancer screening is its cost. A large percentage of X-ray examinations must be followed by gastroscopy, with a very small final yield of early-stage cancers. Outside Japan, the relatively low incidence of stomach cancer, or the high costs of screening, argue against the implementation of such programmes (Chamberlain & Miller, 1988).

Cancers of the colon and rectum

Two techniques have been used for early detection of colorectal cancer. Testing for faecal occult blood by guaiac-impregnated paper slides is the method most frequently applied in large groups of people. Especially in the USA, regular sigmoidoscopy has been recommended as an important part of the physician's examination to detect early carcinomas (or their presumed precursors, adenomatous polyps) of the rectum and rectosigmoid colon (e.g., American Cancer Society, 1980). Flexible sigmoidoscopy has recently been introduced in place of rigid sigmoidoscopy; this method is more acceptable to patients and increases the area of the sigmoid colon that can be examined.

In a randomized study of multiphasic health testing which included sigmoidoscopy, the group undergoing regular examinations had fewer deaths from colorectal cancer than the control group, who were nonetheless free to request sigmoidoscopy at any time (Dales *et al.*, 1979). In a further follow-up, Friedman *et al.* (1986) observed a 50% reduction in mortality from colorectal cancer in the group assigned to annual sigmoidoscopy. Sigmoidoscopy is nevertheless an uncomfortable and expensive procedure and has not yet been shown to be feasible on a large scale. Studies of screening by determining occult blood and other methods have not yet indicated a clear reduction in mortality from colorectal cancer (Chamberlain *et al.*, 1986), although large trials are under way in Denmark (Klaaborg *et al.*, 1986), Sweden (Kewenter *et al.*, 1987), the UK (Hardcastle *et al.*, 1983) and the USA (Gilbertsen *et al.*, 1980; Winawer *et al.*, 1980).

Cancer of the liver

Attempts have been made to screen populations for liver cancer, particularly in China. The test is a serological assay for α-fetoprotein, raised titres of which suggest malignancy. For individuals with suspicious results, ultrasound examination is used to search for small cancers, which might be surgically resectable (Sun *et al.*, 1988). The value of this procedure in unknown, but it might be useful for screening chronic carriers of hepatitis B virus surface antigen, who, in high-risk areas for liver cancer, comprise only 10–15% of the population but give rise to 80% of cases.

Cancer of the lung

Because lung cancer is very common and reduction of incidence through programmes of primary prevention is likely to be a long-term undertaking, reduction of mortality by early detection has considerable appeal. Several trials have been reported. The Cooperative Early Lung Cancer Detection Program in the USA comprised three trials on men who were cigarette smokers and over 45 years of age. Two of these (Melamed *et al.*, 1984; Tockman *et al.*, 1985) examined the benefit of adding four-monthly sputum cytology to annual chest X ray; the third compared a screened group offered four-monthly chest X-ray and sputum examination with controls who were recommended an annual chest X-ray (Fontana, 1984). A further randomized trial of middle-aged male smokers in Czechoslovakia compared the outcome of six-monthly chest X-rays in the screened group with no intervention in the controls (Kubik *et al.*, 1990). Although cases detected by screening are less advanced and have better survival, in none of the trials was mortality from lung cancer lower in the group offered more extensive screening, and it cannot therefore be advocated as public health policy (Prorok *et al.*, 1984).

Melanoma

Relatively little is known about the natural history of melanoma and its putative precursor lesions (National Institutes of Health, 1984). It is clearly established that melanoma patients have many more benign naevi than controls (Holman & Armstrong, 1984; Green *et al.*, 1985; Elwood *et al.*, 1986). The relationship of these lesions to the development of melanoma is as yet unclear. They may be, like complexion and tanning ability, simply a further marker for constitutional factors that predispose to melanoma, or they may be early lesions which undergo malignant transformation, as suggested by the fact that a high proportion of patients report a pre-existing naevus at the site of the melanoma (Elder *et al.*, 1981). Careful prospective studies are required to determine whether melanoma can be prevented through early detection of transformed or transformation-prone naevi.

Syndromes have been described in which naevi that are clinically recognizable and histologically dysplastic seem to be markers of risk for the development of a melanoma (Elder *et al.*, 1982). They may be familial or sporadic (Greene *et al.*, 1985). It has been recommended that people with the dysplastic naevus syndrome should have their skin inspected regularly by a dermatologist to facilitate the early detection of melanoma (National Institutes of Health, 1984).

It is well established that rates of survival from melanoma differ widely depending on the stage at diagnosis. Education programmes aimed at professionals and the public appear to offer one means of reducing mortality (Doherty & MacKie, 1988). Another approach is to introduce screening for early detection of melanomas, although this is unlikely to be cost-effective if applied to an entire population because melanoma is relatively uncommon. Surveillance of people at high risk, however, may prove to be cost-effective: melanoma is one disease for which identification of people at high risk is simple; in addition, up to half of all melanomas may arise in less than 20% of the population at highest risk (English & Armstrong, 1988). High-risk individuals can be identified on the basis of numbers of naevi and other constitutional risk factors, like propensity to sunburn (Rhodes *et al.*, 1987; English & Armstrong, 1988; MacKie *et al.*, 1989).

Cancer of the breast

Breast cancer is the only malignancy for which randomized controlled trials have successfully demonstrated the benefits of early detection by mass screening. The lesions detected are principally early-stage invasive cancers rather than precancerous lesions, so that no reduction in the incidence of the disease can be expected. However, the results of two randomized trials of mammographic screening have demonstrated that mortality rates can be substantially reduced in groups allocated to screening.

The first randomized trial of breast cancer screening was initiated among HIP members in New York, USA, in 1963. Sixty-two thousand women aged 40–64 were randomized into two equal groups, one allocated to screening, the other to routine medical care. Four rounds of screening were planned at yearly intervals. Screening consisted of a clinical examination, usually by a surgeon, and two-view mammography. The results of 14 years of follow-up at both 14 years and 18 years of age have been reported by Shapiro *et al.* (1982, 1988); data on mortality are given in Table 31. In the first five years, the reduction in mortality was nearly 40%, slowly diminishing in proportionate but not in absolute terms to a value just greater than 20% after 14 years. The reduction in mortality in the first five years of the study was confined to women aged 50 years or more at date of entry to the study. By 14 years of follow-up, however, a similar reduction was seen in all age groups, and this was confirmed in the 18-year follow-up (Shapiro *et al.*, 1988). The numbers of deaths from breast cancer within each five-year age-at-entry group 18 years from entry are shown in Table 32. It should be noted, however, that the number of breast cancer deaths in each cell of Table 32 is too small for any firm conclusion on the age effect to be drawn.

Table 31. Cumulative numbers of deaths due to breast cancer by selected time intervals from date of entry into study of screening (from Shapiro *et al.*, 1982)

Interval to breast cancer diagnosis (years)	No. of breast cancers[a]	No. of deaths with breast cancer as underlying cause through year following entry			
		year 5	year 7	year 10	year 14
Within five					
Study	306	39	71	95	118
Control	300	63	106	133	153
Difference (%)		38.1	33.0	28.6	22.9
Within seven					
Study	425	39	81	123	165
Control	443	63	124	174	212
Difference (%)		38.1	34.7	29.3	22.2
Within ten					
Study	600	39	81	146	218
Control	604	63	124	192	262
Difference (%)		38.1	34.7	24.0	16.8

[a] Breast cancers histologically confirmed within a specified interval after entry plus deaths among women with breast cancer as the underlying cause but with no histologically confirmed diagnosis prior to death

Table 32. Cumulative numbers of deaths due to breast cancer[a] by age at entry into study of screening to five and 18 years after entry (from Shapiro *et al.*, 1988)

Age at entry (years)	Interval from entry (years)				Percent difference (1 - study control)	
	Five		Eighteen			
	Study	Control	Study	Control	5 years	18 years
40-45	9	11	18	28	18.2	35.6
45-49	10	9	31	37	-11.1	16.2
50-54	8	23	32	41	65.2	22.0
55-59	7	10	25	33	30.0	24.2
60-64	5	10	20	24	50.0	16.7
Total	39	63	126	163	38.1	22.7

[a] Deaths with breast cancer as the underlying cause among cases histologically confirmed within five years of entry plus deaths among women with breast cancer as the underlying cause but no histologically confirmed diagnosis before death

The second randomized controlled trial of breast cancer screening to have obtained results on mortality was performed on all women aged 40 or more resident in two counties of Sweden (a total of 162 981 women), randomly allocated into two groups – one to be screened, the other left to routine medical care. The only screening modality was mammography with a single view. Women aged less than 50 were to be screened every two years, the rest of the study cohort every 30–36 months (Tabar *et al.*, 1985). Results for mortality for the first eight years of follow-up have now been published (Tabar *et al.*, 1989) and are summarized in Table 33. As with the early results from the US study, no effect was seen among women aged less than 50 at date of entry; among women aged 50–69 years, breast cancer mortality in the screened group was 35–40% less than that in the control group.

Table 33. Deaths from breast cancer in screened and control populations: women aged 40–74 at entry (Tabar *et al.*, 1989)

Age group (years)	Group	No. of deaths	Population (at entry)	Relative risk[a] (95% confidence interval)
40-49	Screened	28	19 844	0.92 (0.52-1.60)
	Control	24	15 604	
50-59	Screened	45	23 485	0.60 (0.40-0.90)
	Control	54	16 805	
60-69	Screened	52	23 412	0.65 (0.44-0.95)
	Control	58	16 269	
70-74	Screened	35	10 339	0.77 (0.47-1.27)
	Control	31	7 307	
All ages	Screened	160	77 080	0.69[b] (0.55-0.88)
	Control	171	55 985	

[a] Adjusted for county
[b] Adjusted for age

The results of several case–control studies evaluating the effect on mortality from breast cancer of nonrandomized screening programmes have also been reported (Collette *et al.*, 1984; Verbeek *et al.*, 1984; Palli *et al.*, 1986). In Utrecht, The Netherlands, women aged 50–64 at the start of the programme in 1974, were invited to attend for screening by clinical examination and mammography at intervals of between one and two years. In a study of breast cancer deaths to the end of 1981, mortality among those who had presented at least once for screening was 70% less than those who had refused. In Nijmegen, all women aged 35 or over were invited for breast cancer screening every two years. The sole screening modality was single-view mammography. Overall, a 52% reduction in risk was seen (Verbeek *et al.*, 1984). In a further report (Verbeek *et al.*, 1985), including deaths up to the end of 1982, this reduction was examined by age. Women aged under 50 at first invitation showed no decrease in mortality from breast cancer, but the numbers were small.

In a rural area near Florence, Italy, a population-based programme was started in 1970, offering mammography to women aged 40–70 every 2.5 years (Palli *et al.*, 1986). In women over 50, the protective effect of screening was strong – a reduction in risk of about 50% for women screened only once and 75% for those screened at least twice; there was no significant benefit to women under the age of 50, however.

The results demonstrate unequivocally that mortality from breast cancer can be substantially reduced by regular screening. In particular, the results from Sweden, supported by those from Nijmegen, show that much of the reduction can be obtained by single-view mammography repeated every two to three years for women aged 50 years or more (Day *et al.*, 1984). For younger women, the situation is less clear: the Swedish, Nijmegen and Florence studies support the US finding that no reduction in mortality is seen in the first five years; it remains to be seen whether a reduction appears eventually.

Because of the costs involved in screening programmes based on mammography (with or without physical examination), there is a great appeal in programmes for breast-self examination (BSE), where the subject herself performs the screening test and can do so as frequently as is necessary to detect changes. A review of requirements for programmes of BSE and an evaluation of their known benefits has been published (Miller *et al.*, 1985); this report concludes that, at present, there is insufficient evidence that BSE has been effective in reducing mortality. Reviewing the results of 12 studies, Hill *et al.* (1988) concluded that there was evidence for reduced size and favourable stage distribution of lesions detected by BSE or reported by women who practise BSE, and two studies (Foster & Costanza, 1984; Huguley *et al.*, 1988) have found higher survival rates in self-examiners. However, the contributions of bias due to selection, lead time and the detection of slower growing tumours in the BSE group cannot be assessed, and no study has compared mortality reduction in a population practising BSE with that in a suitable control group. A randomized study in factories in the USSR has started, but it is unlikely that clear-cut results will emerge for many years. In the UK, mortality from breast cancer is being compared in six districts, in two of which all women aged 45–64 have been invited to BSE classes, while four districts act as 'controls'. After seven years' follow-up there has been no difference in mortality rates (UK Trial of Early Detection of Breast Cancer Group, 1988).

Cancer of the uterine cervix

It is now accepted that squamous-cell cancer of the cervix originates from intraepithelial precursors known as dysplasia and carcinoma *in situ* (or, collectively, cervical intraepithelial neoplasia, CIN). Several follow-up studies have indicated that the greater the degree of dysplasia, the greater the probability of progression to invasive cancer. These precancerous lesions of the cervix can be detected by cervical cytology, and a large body of observations demonstrates that cytological screening, if properly performed, can make a major reduction in both the incidence and the mortality rates from cervical cancer in the general female population, and that, for an individual woman, regular screening during adult life can greatly reduce her risk. The evidence that cervical cytology is an effective form of secondary prevention comes from three sources – geographical comparisons, studies of time trends and cohort and case–control analytical studies; randomized controlled trials have not been undertaken.

The most conclusive data on geographic comparisons and time trends come from the Nordic countries (Hakama, 1982; Läärä *et al.*, 1987) and from north-east Scotland (MacGregor *et al.*, 1985), together with earlier data from the USA (Cramer, 1974) and Canada (Miller *et al.*, 1976). Figure 21 displays the changing incidence in the Nordic countries. Nationwide mass screening was introduced in Iceland and Finland in the mid-1960s, rapidly achieving high coverage, and a sharp fall in incidence ensued in a few years; a fall of some 60% in national rates has been attributed to the mass screening. In Denmark and Sweden, mass screening was introduced county by county, and national coverage was achieved only slowly; the change in incidence is less marked. In Norway, no mass screening programme, apart from that in Østfold county set up as a trial in 1959 (Pedersen *et al.*, 1971), had been initiated by 1980, and cervical cancer rates rose steadily, if slowly, throughout the 1960s and 1970s. Changes in mortality were similar to those in incidence, as for example in Iceland (Figure 22; Johannesson *et al.*, 1982).

Figure 21. Incidence of cervical cancer in Nordic countries[a]

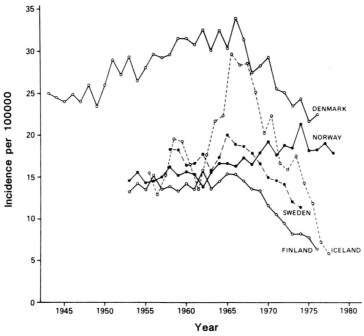

[a] From Hakama (1982)

A case–control study on the effects of screening was reported from Toronto, Canada (Clarke & Anderson, 1979). After adjusting for a number of risk factors for cervical cancer, women who had had a screening test in the previous five years had a risk that was 2.9-fold less than that of women who had not. A considerable number of case–control studies have been performed since (Aristizabal *et al.*,

1984; La Vecchia *et al.*, 1984; Raymond *et al.*, 1984; A MacGregor *et al.*, 1985). These studies have tended to define with more precision this reduction, called 'relative protection', by estimating it as a function of the time elapsed since the last test was performed. A collaborative study involving centres in Canada, Italy, Scandinavia, Scotland and Switzerland was undertaken to provide estimates of relative protection in terms of a woman's previous screening history (IARC Working Group, 1985; IARC, 1986).

Figure 22. Changes over time in mortality from and incidence (by stage of disease) of cervical cancer in Iceland[a]

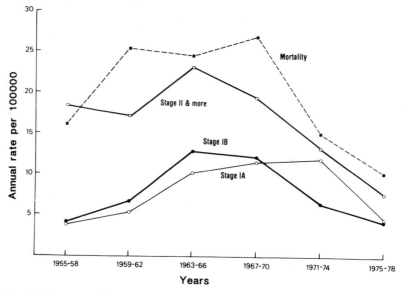

[a] Average annual age-specific rates, in the age range 20-75

A noteworthy feature of many screening programmes is that women whose socioeconomic condition and life style put them at high risk are less frequent attenders. Announcement of a screening policy, therefore, is no guarantee that it will work, and the experience in England and Wales is cautionary in this respect: despite a policy of screening all women over age 35 every five years, little change has occurred in the national rates for the disease. Although this is due partly to the fact that the risk for cervical cancer is increasing in generations of women born since 1931 (so that, without screening, incidence rates would have risen), it is probable that only about 25% of cancer cases have been prevented by the programme (Parkin *et al.*, 1985). Investigations into the relative lack of effect showed that the majority of invasive cases, particularly among women over 40, had never been screened; for the majority of the remainder, follow-up or treatment of abnormal cytological findings had been inadequate. Too infrequent screening and smears found on review to have been false negatives each contributed a further small proportion to the limited success of the programme (Chamberlain, 1984; Chisholm & Haran, 1984). These findings demonstrate that for screening to be effective at the population level, proper follow-up and referral systems, together with the necessary treatment facilities, must be in place, and active steps taken to ensure high participation among the target population. The requirements of an effective screening programme are best met by a centrally organized system of notification, follow-up, referral and treatment, as summarized by a working group of the International Union Against Cancer (Hakama *et al.*, 1986).

Cancer of the endometrium

Screening tests for endometrial cancer based on sampling of endometrial cells are available; however, they are expensive, and no data are available to assess their effect on mortality from the disease. Hence, screening for endometrial cancer cannot currently be recommended as a public health policy (Hakama *et al.*, 1986).

Cancer of the prostate

Three methods are available for detecting asymptomatic prostatic cancer – digital rectal examination (Chodak & Schoenberg, 1984), transrectal ultrasonography (Waterhouse & Resnick, 1989) and measurement of prostate-specific antigen (Scardino, 1989). None of these has high specificity, so that it would be necessary to use a combination of tests, e.g., digital examination followed by one of the more expensive methods. Since the appropriate treatment for early stages of this cancer is not yet known, it is unclear whether screening would confer any benefit, even if it were acceptable to the elderly males who are at highest risk.

Cancer of the ovary

Screening tests for ovarian cancer using ultrasound and monoclonal antibody techniques have been proposed (Hakama *et al.*, 1986). As yet, however, there is insufficient information to assess the sensitivity and specificity of these tests, and studies have not yet been carried out to evaluate their effectiveness in terms of reducing mortality from ovarian cancer. Screening for ovarian cancer, therefore, cannot currently be recommended as public health policy.

Cancer of the urinary bladder

Some pilot studies have been done of screening high-risk populations for bladder cancer in areas where schistosomiasis is endemic (see p. 193). El-Bolkainy *et al.* (1982) proposed methods for detecting bladder cancer by urinary cytology, which should be tested on a large scale.

In developed countries, most screening has involved urinary cytology of industrially exposed populations at risk. This approach is limited by doubt about what treatment to use when relatively wide in-situ changes are found, and the appropriate treatment for such conditions must first be evaluated. In the meantime, given the absence of any indication of reduction in mortality due to screening for bladder cancer, it cannot be advocated as a public health policy (Prorok *et al.* 1984).

Cancer of the thyroid

A small proportion of thyroid cancers occur as part of a hereditary condition, multiple endocrine neoplasia type 2a (see p. 100). Affected families can be investigated for the presence of the responsible genes (Sobol *et al.*, 1989), so that individuals with a high probability of inheriting the disease can be identified and the possibility of prophylactic thyroidectomy foreseen.

References

American Cancer Society (1980) Guidelines for the cancer-related checkup. Recommendations and rationale. *CA Cancer J. Phys.*, *30*, 193-240

Aristizabal, N., Cuello, C., Correa, P., Collazos, T. & Haenszel, W. (1984) The impact of vaginal cytology on cervical cancer risks in Cali, Colombia. *Int. J. Cancer*, *34*, 5-9

Binnie, W.H. (1975) Oral cancer. In: Dolby, A.E., ed., *Oral Mucosa in Health and Disease*, London, Blackwell Scientific, pp. 301-334

Chamberlain, J. (1984) Planning of screening programmes for evaluation and non-randomized approaches to evaluation. In: Prorok, P.C. & Miller, A.B., eds, *Screening for Cancer. I. General Principles on Evaluation of Screening for Cancer and Screening for Lung, Bladder and Oral Cancer* (UICC Technical Report Series Vol. 78), Geneva, International Union Against Cancer, pp. 5-17

Chamberlain, J. & Miller, A.B., eds (1988) *Screening for Gastrointestinal Cancer*, Bern, Hans Huber

Chamberlain, J., Day, N.E., Hakama, M., Miller, A.B. & Prorok, P.C. (1986) UICC workshop of the project on evaluation of screening programmes for gastrointestinal cancer. *Int. J. Cancer*, *37*, 329-334

Chisholm, D.K. & Haran, D. (1984) Cases of invasive cervical cancer in the north west in spite of screening. *Br. J. Fam. Planning*, *10*, 3-8

Chodak, G.W. & Schoenberg, H.W. (1984) Early detection of prostate cancer by routine screening. *J. Am. Med. Assoc.*, *252*, 3261-3264

Clarke, E.A. & Anderson, T.W. (1979) Does screening by 'Pap' smears help prevent cervical cancer? *Lancet*, *ii*, 1-4

Collette, H.J.A., Day, N.E., Rombach, J.J. & de Waard, F. (1984) Evaluation of screening for breast cancer in a non-randomized study (the Dom Project) by means of a case–control study. *Lancet*, *i*, 1224-1226

Cramer, D.W. (1974) The role of cervical cytology in the declining morbidity and mortality of cervical cancer. *Cancer*, *34*, 2018-2027

Dales, L.G., Friedman, G.D. & Collen, M.F. (1979) Evaluating periodic multiphasic health checkups - a controlled trial. *J. Chronic Dis.*, *32*, 385-404

Day, N.E. & Miller, A.B., eds (1988) *Screening for Breast Cancer*, Bern, Hans Huber

Day, N.E., Walter, S.D. & Collette, B. (1984) Statistical models of disease natural history: their use in the evaluation of screening programmes. In: Prorok, P.C. & Miller, A.B., eds, *Screening for Cancer. I. General Principles on Evaluation of Screening for Cancer and Screening for Lung, Bladder and Oral Cancer* (UICC Technical Report Series Vol. 78), Geneva, International Union Against Cancer, pp. 55-70

Doherty, U.R. & MacKie, R.M. (1988) Experience of a public education programme on early detection of cutaneous malignant melanoma. *Br. Med. J.*, *297*, 388-391

El-Bolkainy, M.N., Chu, E.W., Ghoneim, M.A. & Ibrahim, A.S. (1982) Cytologic detection of bladder cancer in a rural Egyptian population infected with schistosomiasis. *Acta Cytol.*, *26*, 303-310

Elder, D., Greene, M.H., Bondi, E.E. & Clark, W.H. (1981) Acquired melanocytic nevi and melanoma. The dysplastic nevus syndrome. In: Ackerman, A.B., ed., *Pathology of Malignant Melanoma*, New York, Masson, pp. 185-215

Elder, D.E., Greene, M.H., Guerry, D., IV, Kraemer, K.H. & Clark, W.H., Jr (1982) The dysplastic nevus syndrome: our definition. *Am. J. Dermatopathol.*, *4*, 455-560

Elwood, J.M., Williamson, C. & Stapleton, P.J. (1986) Malignant melanoma in relation to moles, pigmentation, and exposure to fluorescent and other lighting sources. *Br. J. Cancer*, *53*, 65-74

Elwood, J.M., Cooke, K.R., Coombs, B.D., Cox, B., Hand, J.E. & Skegg, D.C. (1988) A strategy for the control of malignant melanoma in New Zealand. *N.Z. Med. J.*, *101*, 602-604

English, D.R. & Armstrong, B.K. (1988) Identifying people at high risk of cutaneous malignant melanoma: results from a case-control study in Western Australia. *Br. Med. J.*, *296*, 1285-1288

Fontana, R.S., (1984) Early detection of lung cancer; the Mayo project. In: Prorok, P.C. & Miller, A.B., eds, *Screening for Cancer. I. General Principles on Evaluation of Screening for Cancer and Screening for Lung, Bladder and Oral Cancer* (UICC Technical Report Series Vol. 78), Geneva, International Union Against Cancer, pp. 107-122

Foster, R.S. & Costanza, M.C. (1984) Breast self-examination practices and breast cancer survival. *Cancer*, *53*, 999-1005

Friedman, G.D., Collen, M.F. & Fireman, B.H. (1986) Multiphasic health checkup evaluation: a 16-year follow-up. *J. Chronic Dis.*, *39*, 453-463

Fukao, A., Hisamichi, S. & Sugawara, N. (1987) A case-control study on evaluating the effect of mass screening in decreasing advanced stomach cancer (in Japanese). *J. Jpn. Soc. Gastroenterol. Mass Survey*, *75*, 112-118

Gilbertsen, V.A., McHugh, R.B., Schuman, L.M. & Williams, S.E. (1980) Colon cancer control study: an interim report. In: Winawer, S.J., Schottenfeld, D. & Sherlock, P., eds, *Colorectal Cancer: Prevention, Epidemiology, and Screening*, New York, Raven Press, pp. 261-266

Green, A., MacLennan, R. & Siskind, V. (1985) Common acquired naevi and the risk of malignant melanoma. *Int. J. Cancer*, *35*, 297-300

Greene, M.H., Clark, W.H., Tucker, M.A., Elder, D.E., Kraemer, K.H., Guerry, D., Witmer, W.K., Thompson, J., Matozzo, I. & Fraser, M.C. (1985) Acquired precursors of cutaneous malignant melanoma. The familial dysplastic nevus syndrome. *New Engl. J. Med.*, *312*, 91-97

Hakama, M. (1982) Trends in the incidence of cervical cancer in the Nordic countries. In: Magnus, K., ed., *Trends in Cancer Incidence. Causes and Practical Implications*, New York, Hemisphere, pp. 279-292

Hakama, M., Miller, A.B. & Day, N.E., eds (1986) *Screening for Cancer of the Uterine Cervix* (IARC Scientific Publications No. 76), Lyon, IARC

Hardcastle, J., Farrands, P.A., Balfour, T.W., Chamberlain, J., Amar, S.S. & Sheldon, M.G. (1983) Controlled trial of faecal occult blood testing in the detection of colorectal cancer. *Lancet*, *ii*, 1-4

Hill, D., White, V., Jolley, D. & Mapperson, K. (1988) Self examination of the breast: is it beneficial? Meta-analysis of studies investigating breast self examination and extent of disease in patients with breast cancer. *Br. Med. J.*, *297*, 271-275

Hirayama, T. (1985) Screening for gastric cancer. In: Miller, A.B., ed., *Screening for Cancer*, Geneva, International Union Against Cancer, pp. 367-377

Hisamichi, S. (1989) Screening for gastric cancer. *World J. Surg.*, *13*, 31-37

Hisamichi, S. & Sugawara, N. (1984) Mass screening for gastric cancer by X ray examination. *Jpn. J. Clin. Oncol.*, *14*, 211-223

Holman, C.D.J. & Armstrong, B.K. (1984) Pigmentary traits, ethnic origin, benign nevi, and family history as risk factors for cutaneous malignant melanoma. *J. Natl Cancer Inst.*, *72*, 257-266

Huguley, C.M., Brown, R.L., Greenberg, R.S. & Clark, W.S. (1988) Breast self-examination and survival from breast cancer. *Cancer*, *62*, 1389-1396

IARC (1986) Screening for squamous cervical cancer: duration of low risk after negative results of cervical cytology and its implications for screening policies. *Br. Med. J.*, *293*, 659-664

IARC Working Group (1985) Summary chapter. In: Hakama, M., Miller, A.B. & Day, N.E., eds, *Screening for Cancer of the Uterine Cervix* (IARC Scientific Publications No. 76), Lyon, IARC, pp. 133-144

Johannesson, G., Geirsson, G., Day, N. & Tulinius, H. (1982) Screening for cancer of the uterine cervix in Iceland 1965-1978. *Acta Obstet. Gynaecol. Scand.*, *61*, 199-203

Kewenter, J., Bjorck, S., Haglind, E., Jonsson, O., Svanvik, J. & Svensson, C. (1987) A controlled trial of occult blood screening for colorectal neoplasms: a comparison between rehydrated and nonrehydrated hemoccult II slides. In: Chamberlain, J. & Miller, A.B., eds, *Screening for Gastrointestinal Cancer*, Toronto, Hans Huber, pp. 33-39

Klaaborg, K., Madsen, M.S., Sondergaard, O. & Kronborg, O. (1986) Participation in mass screening for colorectal cancer with fecal occult blood test. *Scand. J. Gastroenterol., 21*, 1180-1184

Kubik, A., Parkin, D.M., Khlat, M., Erban, J., Polak, J. & Adamec, M. (1990) Lack of benefit from semi-annual screening for cancer of the lung. *Int. J. Cancer* (in press)

Kuroichi, T., Hirose, K., Nakagawa, N. & Tominaga, S. (1983) Comparison of the changes in the mortality from stomach cancer and the control areas (in Japanese). *Jpn. Soc. J. Gastroenterol. Mass Survey, 58*, 45-52

Läärä, E., Day, N.E. & Hakama, M. (1987) Trends in mortality from cervical cancer in the Nordic countries: association with organized screening programmes. *Lancet, i*, 1247-1249

La Vecchia, C., Franceschi, S., Decarli, A., Fasoli, M., Gentile, A. & Tognoni, G. (1984) Pap smear and the risk of cervical neoplasia: quantitative estimates from a case–control study. *Lancet, ii*, 779-782

MacGregor, J.E., Moss, S.M., Parkin, D.M. & Day, N.E. (1985) A case–control study of cervical cancer screening in north-east Scotland. *Br. Med. J., 290*, 1543-1546

Mackie, R.M., Freudenberger, T. & Aitchison, T.C. (1989) Personal risk-factor chart for cutaneous malignant melanoma. *Lancet, ii*, 487-490

Mehta, F.S., Gupta, M.B., Pindborg, J.J., Bhonsle, R.B., Jalhawalla, P.N. & Sinor, P.N. (1982) An intervention study of oral cancer and precancer in rural Indian populations: a preliminary report. *Bull. World Health Organ., 60*, 441-446

Melamed, M., Flehinger, B., Zaman, M., Heelan, R., Perchick, W. & Martini, N. (1984) Screening for early lung cancer: results of the Memorial Sloan-Kettering study in New York. *Chest, 86*, 44-53

Miller, A.B., ed. (1978) *Screening for Cancer*, Geneva, Interntional Union Against Cancer

Miller, A.B., Lindsay, J. & Hill, G.B. (1976) Mortality from cancer of the uterus in Canada and relationship to screening for cancer of the cervix. *Int. J. Cancer, 17*, 602-612

Miller, A.B., Chamberlain, J. & Tschechkovski, M. (1985) Self-examination in the early detection of breast cancer. A review of the evidence, with recommendations for further research. *J. Chronic Dis., 38*, 527-540

National Institutes of Health (1984) Consensus conference: precursors to malignant melanoma. *J. Am. Med. Assoc., 251*, 1864-1866

Oshima, A. (1988) Screening for stomach cancer: the Japanese program. In: Chamberlain, J. & Miller, A.B., eds, *Screening for Gastrointestinal Cancer*, Bern, Hans Huber, pp. 65-70

Oshima, A., Hirata, N., Ubukata, T., Umeda, K. & Fujimoto, I. (1986) Evaluation of a mass screening program for stomach cancer with a case control study design. *Int. J. Cancer, 38*, 829-833

Palli, D., Rosselli del Turco, M., Buiatti, E., Carli, S., Ciatto, S., Toscano, L. & Maltoni, G. (1986) A case control study of the efficacy of a non-randomised breast cancer screening program in Florence (Italy). *Int. J. Cancer, 38*, 501-504

Parkin, D.M., Nguyen-Dinh, X. & Day, N.E. (1985) The impact of screening on the incidence of cervix cancer in England and Wales. *Br. J. Obstet. Gynaecol., 92*, 150-157

Pedersen, E., Hoeg, K. & Kolsted, P. (1971) Mass screening for cancer of the uterine cervix in Østfold County, Norway: an experiment. Second Report of the Norwegian Cancer Society. *Acta Obstet. Gynaecol. Scand., 50*, 69-71

Prorok, P.C. & Miller, A.B., eds (1984) *Screening for Cancer. I. General Principles on Evaluation of Screening for Cancer and Screening for Lung, Bladder and Oral Cancer* (UICC Technical Report Series Vol. 76), Geneva, International Union Against Cancer

Prorok, P.C., Chamberlain, J., Day, N.E., Hakama, M. & Miller, A.B. (1984) UICC Workshop on the evaluation of screening programmes for cancer. *Int. J. Cancer, 34*, 1-4

Raymond, L., Obradovic, M. & Riotton, G. (1984) Une étude cas-témoins pour l'évaluation du dépistage cytologique du cancer du col utérin. *Rev. Epidemiol. Santé Publ., 32*, 10-15

Reynolds, P. & Austin, D.F. (1984) Epidemiologic-based screening strategies for malignant melanoma of the skin. *Prog. Clin. Biol. Res., 156*, 245-254

Rhodes, A.R., Weinstock, M.A., Fitzpatrick, T.B., Mihm, M.C. & Sober, A.J. (1987) Risk factors for cutaneous melanoma: a practical method of recognizing predisposed individuals. *J. Am. Med. Assoc., 253*, 3146-3154

Shapiro, S., Venet, W., Strax, P., Venet, L. & Roeser, R. (1982) Ten- to fourteen-year effect of screening on breast cancer mortality. *J. Natl Cancer Inst.*, *69*, 349-355

Shapiro, S., Venet, W., Strax, P. & Venet, L. (1988) Current results of the breast cancer screening randomized trial: the health insurance plan (HIP) of greater New York study. In: Day, N.E. & Miller, A.B., eds, *Screening for Breast Cancer*, Toronto, Hans Huber, pp. 3-15

Sobol, H., Narod, S.A., Nakamura, Y., Boneu, A., Calmettes, C., Chadenas, D., Charpentier, G., Chatal, J.F., Delepine, N., Delisle, M.J., Dupond, J.L., Gardet, P., Godefroy, H., Guillausseau, P.-J., Guillausseau-Scholer, C., Houdent, C., Lalau, J.D., Mace, G., Parmentier, C., Soubrier, F., Tourniaire, J. & Lenoir, G.M. (1989) Screening for multiple endocrine neoplasia type 2a with DNA-polymorphism analyses. *New Engl. J. Med.*, *321*, 996-1001

Sun, T., Yu, H., Hsia, C., Wang, N. & Huang, X. (1988) Evaluation of sero-survey trials for the early detection of hepatocellular carcinoma in area of high prevalence. In: Chamberlain, J. & Miller, A.B., eds, *Screening for Gastrointestinal Cancer*, Bern, Hans Huber, pp. 81-86

Tabar, L., Gad, A., Holmberg, L.H., Ljungquist, U., Fagerberg, C.J.G., Baldetorp, L., Gröntoft, O., Lundström, B., Manson, J.C., Eklund, G., Day, N.E. & Pettersson, F. (1985) Reduction in mortality from breast cancer after mass screening with mammography. *Lancet*, *i*, 829-832

Tabar, L., Fagerberg, G., Duffy, S.W. & Day, N.E. (1989) The Swedish two county trial of mammographic screening for breast cancer: recent results and calculation of benefit. *J. Epidemiol. Community Health*, *43*, 107-114

de-Thé, G. & Zheng, Y. (1986) Population screening for EBV markers toward improvement of nasopharyngeal carcinoma control. In: Epstein, M.A. & Achong, B.G., ed., *The Epstein-Barr Virus: Recent Advances*, London, William Heinemann

Tockman, M.S., Levin, M.L., Frost, J.K., Ball, W.C., Jr, Stitik, F.P. & Marsh, B.R. (1985) Screening and detection of lung cancer. In: Aisner, J., ed. *Lung Cancer* (Contemporary Issues in Clinical Oncology Vol. 3), New York, Churchill Livingstone, pp. 25-36

UK Trial of Early Detection of Breast Cancer Group (1988) First results on mortality reduction in the UK trial of early detection of breast cancer. *Lancet*, *ii*, 411-416

Verbeek, A.L., Hendriks, J.H., Holland, R., Mravunac, M., Sturmans, F. & Day, N.E. (1984) Reduction of breast cancer mortality through mass screening with modern mammography. First results of the Nijmegen project, 1975-1981. *Lancet*, *i*, 1222-1224

Verbeek, A.L.M., Hendriks, J.H.C.L., Holland, R., Mravunac, M. & Sturmans, F. (1985) Mammographic screening and breast cancer mortality: age-specific effects in Nijmegen project, 1975-1982 (Letter). *Lancet*, *i*, 865-866

Warnakulasuriya, K.A.A.S., Ekanayake, A.N., Sivayoham, S., Stjernswärd, J., Pindborg, J.J., Sobin, L.H. & Perea, K.S. (1984) Utilization of primary health care workers for early detection of cancer and precancer cases in Sri Lanka. *Bull. World Health Organ.*, *62*, 243-250

Waterhouse, R.L. & Resnick, M.I. (1989) The use of transrectal prostatic ultrasonography in the evaluation of patients with prostatic carcinoma. *J. Urol.*, *141*, 233-239

Winawer, S.J., Andrews, M., Flehinger, B., Sherlock, P., Schottenfeld, D. & Miller, D.G. (1980) Progress report on controlled trial of fecal occult blood testing for the detection of colorectal neoplasia. *Cancer*, *45*, 2959-2964

Zeng, Y., Zhang, L.G., Li, H.Y., Jan, M.G., Zhang, Q., Wu, Y.C., Wang, Y.S. & Su, G.R. (1982) Serological mass survey for early detection of nasopharyngeal carcinoma in Wuzhou city, China. *Int. J. Cancer*, *29*, 139-141

PART IV

THE CONTROL OF CANCER THROUGH PREVENTION AND EARLY DETECTION

The aim of this part is to make quantitative estimates of the potential effect of preventive measures. Two general types of preventive measure are considered – primary prevention and early detection in asymptomatic individuals (often called secondary prevention or screening). Primary prevention reduces the risk for cancer by reducing exposure to carcinogenic agents (which are reviewed in Part II) or by increasing resistance to them. Early detection aims at the elimination of disease at an early stage or preventing progression to more serious forms, as described in Part III. In both cases, quantification of effect is attempted only for those strategies for which there is clear evidence of effectiveness in practice and a sound basis for estimation.

The first chapter describes the type of epidemiological data required for, and how they are used in, estimating the effects of primary prevention and early detection.

Chapter 19. Quantification of effect

Quantification of strategies for primary prevention

Primary prevention of cancer can take a number of forms, including, for example, (i) complete removal of an agent from a workplace, as has happened in many countries with respect to some carcinogenic aromatic amines; (ii) partial removal of an agent from the environment, either by reducing exposure concentrations (e.g., the tar delivery of cigarettes) or by reducing the prevalence of exposure (e.g., reducing the proportion of smokers); and (iii) increasing resistance to carcinogenic agents (e.g., vaccination against hepatitis B virus). The effect of intervention is estimated ideally from observations on populations in which the intervention has occurred and its effect estimated directly (as in a controlled trial) or inferred by observation of subsequent trends in cancer (as a 'natural experiment' arising from changes in social, economic or cultural factors). However, there have been few randomized studies of primary prevention strategies, and natural experiments have occurred for only a very small number of exposures. It is therefore necessary to rely almost entirely on data from etiological studies of the exposure to which intervention is to be applied to estimate what the outcome of intervention might be.

For each primary prevention strategy, various aspects of the association between the exposure and the cancer must be known in order to estimate the effect. These features include the strength of the association at relevant exposure levels, the time expected to elapse between reduction in exposure and reduction in risk, and possible interactions with age and other factors.

Measures of associations between disease and exposure

The increase in risk associated with a given exposure is measured in terms of the observed increase in the incidence rate of the cancer in question. This increase can be expressed either in absolute terms – the extra number of cases per head of population per year, or in proportional terms – the proportional increase over the observed background incidence rate. For empirical reasons, the latter is often the more convenient measure. The reason is that background cancer incidence rates vary very widely by age and, to a lesser extent, among populations, and that for many exposures the excess risk is approximately proportional to the background risk. The proportional increase can then be simply expressed in quantitative terms, often by a single number. The absolute excess risk, on the other hand, often varies widely with age, and between populations, and is not portrayed adequately by a single figure.

The measure of proportional increase in risk that is usually used is the *relative risk*, defined simply as the ratio of the incidence rate in the exposed population to the incidence rate in the unexposed population. Relative risks are sometimes defined in terms of mortality rather than incidence rates, but the difference should be small.

Relative risk can be interpreted as the proportional decrease in risk for an exposed individual that would occur if the effect of a factor were removed, so that the quantitative value indicates the scope that exists for effective intervention. Illustrative examples of the degree of risk for specific cancers associated with a number of exposures is given in Table 34. The purpose of this table is to suggest in quantitative terms what might be considered weak, moderate and strong levels of effect for a risk factor for cancer.

Table 34. Risks for cancers at selected sites in association with certain exposures

Cancer site	Factor	High risk	Low risk	Reported relative risk
Stomach	Blood group	A	O	1.15
Nasopharynx	HLA system	BW46 antigen	Absence of BW46 antigen	1.8
Breast	Age at first birth	>30 years	<20 years	2.5
Breast	Ionizing radiation	>100 rads	No exposure	3.0
Pancreas	Cigarette smoking	>25 cigs/day	Nonsmokers	3.0
Bladder	Cigarette smoking	>25 cigs/day	Nonsmokers	5.0
Lung	Asbestos	Occupational exposure	No occupational exposure	5.0
Cervix	Cytological screening	Never screened	Negative result within three years	10
Oesophagus	Alcohol consumption	>100 g ethanol/day	<25 g ethanol/day – nonsmokers – smokers of 15-29 cigs/day	17.5 01.5[a]
Lung	Cigarette smoking	>25 cigs/day	Nonsmokers	30
Liver	Hepatitis B virus	Carriers	Noncarriers	>100[b]
Bladder	Benzidine and/or β-naphthylamine	Occupational exposure	No occupational exposure	500
Leukaemia	Melphalan	Ovarian cancer patients receiving > 600 mg	No chemotherapy	23
Mesothelioma	Asbestos	Occupational exposure	No occupational exposure	>200

[a] As compared to nonsmokers who drink <25 g alcohol/day
[b] As reported from a prospective study in Taiwan (Beasley *et al.*, 1981); case-control studies have produced lower estimates.

The relative risks in Table 34 indicate the reduction in risk from which exposed individuals might benefit. Thus, for a relative risk of r, elimination of the exposure would reduce an exposed individual's risk by a factor of $(r-1)/r$. That is to say, with a relative risk of 3, one can hope for a two-thirds reduction in absolute risk, while for a relative risk of 10 one can hope for a 90% reduction. For exposed individuals, this is the figure of interest, since it indicates the benefit that they can hope for from cessation of exposure (assuming their risk falls to that of an unexposed person after some reasonable interval from cessation of exposure).

These figures do not, however, provide measures of the amount of disease that might be removed from the population as a whole by the intervention. To calculate the population effect, that is the overall reduction in population rates of the disease, one needs also to know the proportion of the population that is exposed. For instance, for rare exposures, such as in a number of occupational situations, only a very small proportion of the population is exposed, so that, even though the relative risk is high, the population risk is low. If a proportion p of the population is exposed to a factor that increases risk by r-fold over the background incidence, 1, then the reduction in risk that would occur if the risk were removed is given by

$$p(r-1)/((1-p)+pr).$$

This quantity is known as the *population attributable risk* and expresses the proportion of cases in the population that can be attributed to the exposure. It represents the potential benefit that society as a whole might derive from intervention measures. Thus, the risk for cancer of the pancreas among heavy smokers could be calculated as follows: p, the proportion of the population exposed, is 0.2 or 20%, and r, the risk for pancreatic cancer, is 3.0. Then,

$$0.2(3-1)/((1-0.2)+(0.2\times3)) = 0.4/0.8+0.6 = 0.4/1.4 = 0.29 \text{ or about } 30\%.$$

In the next chapter, devoted to individual sites, the population attributable risk is used as a quantitative summary of the potential for primary prevention.

The attributable risk, as described above, is overly simple as a measure of potential prevention – for three reasons. Firstly, it supposes a dichotomy between exposed and unexposed, whereas for many agents there is a range from light to moderate to heavy exposure. Indeed, for some potential risk factors, such as consumption of dietary fat, an unexposed population does not exist. Intervention will not eliminate the exposure but will rather lead to an overall reduction in exposure levels (Wahrendorf, 1987). To predict the effect of such an intervention, not just one value of the relative risk is needed but the range of values associated with different levels of exposure; in other words, the dose–response relationship. Secondly, neither the relative nor the attributable risks of an exposure indicate how long after its removal or reduction an effect can be expected. While some measures reduce risk almost immediately, others may take decades to yield results. Reasonable estimates of when the benefits of intervention will appear are essential for a correct forecast of the effect. Finally, it ignores the possibility that the effect of exposure (or its removal) varies with age or some other factor, which may be differently distributed in the population experiencing the intervention than in the population from which the estimates of relative risk were derived.

Dose–response relationships

The difficulty of obtaining accurate data on levels of exposure to carcinogens in human populations has severely limited the number of agents for which the shape of the exposure–response curve is well documented. Figure 23 illustrates the increasing risk for lung cancer with increasing number of cigarettes smoked per day (Doll & Peto, 1978). The increase is nearly linear, with a slight tendency to upward curvature. Figures 24 and 25 show the increasing risk for cancer of the oesophagus with increasing alcohol and tobacco consumption, respectively. The former curves sharply upward, the latter is nearly flat after an initial increase (Breslow & Day, 1980). The approach to prevention is clearly different in these three cases. With a dose–response curve as in Figure 24, heavily exposed people form a group at particularly elevated risk; reducing the exposure of this group should clearly be the initial aim of intervention measures. If the situation is more like that described in Figure 25, however, simply reducing the exposure of the heavily exposed will have little effect. The only effective action is removal of the exposure, for those moderately as well as those heavily exposed. In the roughly linear situation of Figure 23, which is perhaps the most frequently encountered, all those exposed will benefit from a reduction in exposure, the benefit increasing proportionately to the degree of reduction. Although reduction of the proportion of the population most heavily exposed is important, one should not overlook the fact that a substantial reduction in risk may be obtained by reducing the proportion of people exposed at moderate levels, particularly when the latter group is substantial. The question also arises as to whether the initial target should be reduction or elimination of the exposure, since both may yield substantial decreases in risk, and the requisite measures may differ. An example is whether cigarettes with a high 'tar' content should be more actively discouraged than those with low 'tar' content, or whether the focus of action should be the complete cessation of smoking. The matter is complicated further, of course, when there are differently shaped exposure-response functions for different diseases caused by the same agent (as in Figures 23 and 25).

Figure 23. Dose–response relationship between lung cancer and daily cigarette consumption, standardized for age[a]

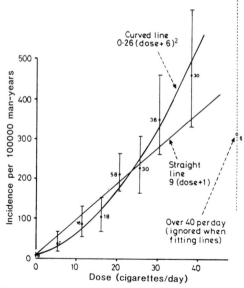

[a] From Doll & Peto (1978)

Figure 24. Relative risk for oesophageal cancer as a function of alcohol consumption[a]

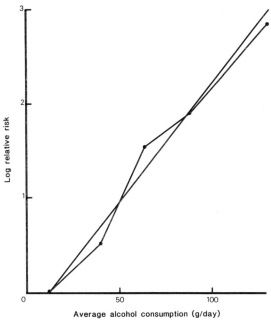

Average alcohol consumption (g/day)

[a] From Breslow & Day (1980)

Figure 25. Relative risk for oesophageal cancer as a function of tobacco consumption[a]

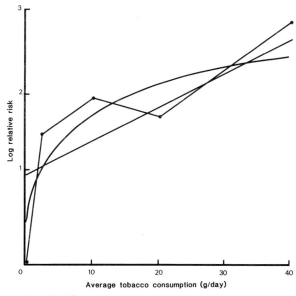

Average tobacco consumption (g/day)

[a] From Breslow & Day (1980)

Delay between reduction in exposure and decrease in risk

The consequences of introducing control measures to reduce exposure differ according to the nature of the exposure. Some studies have suggested that the high risk for endometrial cancer associated with oestrogen therapy disappears rapidly in absolute terms after exposure ceases. Cessation of smoking, however, does not result in a fall in the absolute incidence of lung cancer, but the incidence ceases to rise further with age, as it would do if smoking continued. The relative risk therefore falls rapidly after smoking stops, approaching a value of unity after some 20 years. At the other extreme, the incidence of mesothelioma continues to increase throughout life in people exposed to asbestos, although the incidence attained at any age depends on the 'dose' accumulated during the period of exposure. Thus, here too, cessation of exposure will be beneficial, although possibly not within the first 15 years.

There are two reasons why it would be important to know how quickly the effect of stopping exposure to a particular agent is likely to be manifested. The first is to allow one to predict the effect of intervention: unless one can predict what effect is likely to occur and when, it is difficult to set up a mechanism for judging whether the intervention is effective. Secondly, the type of intervention will to some extent be determined by the rapidity of its effect.

Quantification of the effects of strategies for early detection

Quantitative prediction of effect is easier for early detection than for primary prevention strategies. A secondary preventive measure can be demonstrated to be effective only through active implementation, whereas primary prevention by removal of a risk factor can be predicted once the factor has been shown to be causally related to disease – well before the result of its removal can be seen. Thus, the reduction in mortality or morbidity that will follow the introduction of a screening programme can be predicted only on the basis of data from a population in which the measure has actually been introduced (ideally by way of a randomized controlled trial). Limitations of studies of effectiveness are discussed in Part III (pp. 268–270). While the need for such data is restrictive, they will provide a much more solid basis for prediction than is afforded by the results of etiological studies.

Another way in which early detection measures lend themselves more readily to quantification is that their full effect is seen rather rapidly – usually within a few years of implementation. In contrast, primary prevention, even when fully implemented in a population, may take decades to have a visible effect if substantial exposure has occurred in the past and exerted its effects at an early stage in the process of carcinogenesis. It is the extent of exposure to agents that act at later stages of the process of carcinogenesis that determines the current incidence of specific cancers, and, for rapid results, it is exposure to the latter type of agent that should be controlled (Day & Brown, 1980). Finally, early detection through screening is, to a far greater extent than primary preventive measures, external to the cultural environment of the population to which it is applied. It is therefore less likely to set off a chain of interlinked countereffects, the impact of all of which must be taken into account in predicting the impact on cancer risk.

For example, reduction of betel-quid chewing through an active primary prevention programme in India could conceivably be accompanied by a compensatory increase in tobacco smoking unless adequate public health measures are taken in parallel. A screening programme, in contrast, would be unlikely to have effects of this kind.

The effect of population screening is usually quantified by measuring the 'relative protection', which is analogous to the relative risk in studies of cancer etiology. As described in Part III, it is simply the ratio of disease incidence or mortality among screened individuals, compared to that among those who are not screened. Thus, for a test which confers a relative protection of 0.60, the risk for disease is reduced by 40%.

In practice, a single number does not adequately summarize the effect of secondary prevention. It would do so only if the test were applied to an entire population. In fact, this is never the case. Screening is often targetted at high-risk groups, at least as defined by age. Even if a systematic programme is established, people slip through the net and miss being screened. Furthermore, the relative protection afforded by screening may actually differ with age and other factors, as has been clearly demonstrated for mammographic examination of the breast.

References

Beasley, R.P., Hwang, L.Y., Lin, C.C. & Chien, C.S. (1981) Hepatocellular carcinoma and hepatitis B virus. A prospective study of 22,707 men in Taiwan. *Lancet*, *ii*, 1129-1133

Breslow, N.E. & Day, N.E. (1980) *Statistical Methods in Cancer Research*, Vol. I, *The Analysis of Case-control Data* (IARC Scientific Publications No. 32), Lyon, IARC

Day, N.E. & Brown, C.C. (1980) Multistage models and primary prevention of cancer. *J. Natl Cancer Inst.*, *64*, 977-989

Doll, R. & Peto, R. (1978) Cigarette smoking and bronchial carcinoma: dose and time relationships among regular smokers and lifelong non-smokers. *J. Epidemiol. Community Health*, *32*, 303-313

Wahrendorf, J. (1987) An estimate of the proportion of colo-rectal and stomach cancers which might be prevented by certain changes in dietary habits. *Int. J. Cancer*, *40*, 625-628

Chapter 20. Site-by-site quantification of the effects of preventive measures

Each of the sections below is arranged as follows. Firstly, the potential for prevention is indicated on the basis of descriptive data on the cancer at the site in question, citing data on incidence in countries at high and low risk, as given by Muir *et al.* (1987) and summarized in Tables 6 and 7 (pp. 32–35) and the Appendix, and, when available, data from studies of migrants and of time trends. Secondly, we briefly review the important risk factors for cancers at selected sites and indicate those that are viewed as causal. For these factors, the population attributable risk, and, hence, the reduction in risk that would arise from reduction or elimination of the exposure, are estimated on the basis of the results of the available epidemiological studies, which are summarized in greater detail in Part II. For a limited number of interventions, further details regarding the delay of effects and other specific aspects are given. Secondary preventive measures that appear to be beneficial are reviewed, and the effect of their introduction is quantified when possible.

For practical reasons, quantification of population attributable risk is not attempted for primary preventive measures which involve only a tiny fraction of the people in any country, even if the agent involved conveys a very large increase in risk (see Table 34, p. 290). Examples are the leukaemogenic drugs, such as those used in cancer therapy (see p. 148), and occupational carcinogens, such as vinyl chloride, benzene and wood dust (see pp. 128, 130, 143), which induce liver angiosarcoma, leukaemia and nasal sinus cancer, respectively.

Cancer of the oral cavity

Oral cancer is defined here as cancers arising in the mouth, oropharynx and hypopharynx. The highest incidences of oral cancer in men occur in France (Bas-Rhin, 46.5) and India (Bombay, 32.7). The lowest male rates are seen among Israeli Jews (2.1) and in Japan (Miyagi Prefecture, 2.2). Males tend to have far higher rates than females; a number of registries have reported female rates below 1.0 (e.g., Japan, Miyagi, 0.7). Comparison of the rates in Bas-Rhin and among Israeli Jews indicates a potential preventability among men in Bas-Rhin of 95%. A more conservative comparison is that between Bas-Rhin and Navarra, Spain, where the population is ethnically closer to that of France but where the oral cancer rate in men is much lower (8.1), giving a potential for prevention of 83%. The potential for prevention among Indians in Bombay can be evaluated by comparing their rate (32.7) with that of 2.2 experienced by Indian males in Fiji; although the figures for Fiji are based on relatively few cases, they suggest that over 90% of the oral cancer in Bombay is preventable.

A large body of evidence, reviewed in Parts I (pp. 52–53) and II (pp. 170, 177, 181), shows that oral cancer is causally related to both the consumption of alcohol and the smoking and chewing of tobacco products and mixtures. However, the prevalence of these risk factors, and consequently their relative importance in the etiology of oral cancer, varies greatly by geographical region. In many western countries, especially those of southern Europe (including France), the level of consumption of alcoholic beverages is high (Estève *et al.*, 1984), while the use of chewed tobacco products (once common among men) is now relatively rare. Unfortunately, this situation appears to be changing, with increasing use of smokeless tobacco by teenagers and young adults in North America and elsewhere.

The chewing of tobacco quid, often mixed with betel nut, lime or other substances, is widespread in many parts of central and south-east Asia, where alcohol consumption is moderate or low. Because of these widely different profiles, we consider separately the two regions where most of the etiological studies have been performed, namely, central and south-east Asia and North America and Europe.

A number of large case–control studies of oral cancer have been carried out in the Indian subcontinent (see p. 177). Although it is difficult to obtain precise estimates of the risks for oral cancer associated with specific substances, it is clear that almost all of the risk is due to the smoking of tobacco and the chewing of quids of various kinds. Of 2433 cases of oral cancer reported in the four large studies (Sanghvi *et al.*, 1955; Shanta & Krishnamurthi, 1963; Wahi *et al.*, 1965; Jussawalla & Deshpande, 1971), only 168 reported that they neither smoked nor chewed, in contrast to 2767 out of 4257 controls. The crude relative risk represented by these figures is 25, corresponding to an attributable risk of over 90% under the assumption that half the population is habit-free. Even the most conservative estimate of relative risk, of around 5, from the studies of Jussawalla and Deshpande (1971) and Sanghvi *et al.* (1955), gives an attributable risk for these habits of 67%. This is consistent with the estimate of 70% arrived at by Jayant *et al.* (1977). With rather more conservative estimates of the prevalence of smoking and tobacco chewing in India, Notani *et al.* (1989) estimated the attributable risks associated with these habits as 61% for oral cancer (81% for males, 36% for females) and 79% for cancers of the pharynx and larynx (90% for males, 30% for females).

The most obvious and efficacious measure of control for oral cancer in central and south-east Asia would be the elimination of chewing and smoking habits. Although these customs are deeply rooted in the societies of the region, some attempts are being made towards this goal, and small intervention studies carried out in India show that leukoplakia, a possible precursor of oral cancer, does regress rapidly after cessation of betel chewing (Mehta *et al.*, 1982). Education programmes which reduced the prevalence of chewing and smoking tobacco also seem to have had an effect in reducing rates of leukoplakia (Gupta *et al.*, 1990).

A number of case–control studies of oral cancer have been carried out in different parts of North America and Europe (although none in the countries where rates are highest, namely France, Italy and Switzerland). These studies provide estimates of relative risk for various combinations of alcohol and tobacco consumption, and a number of authors have used them as the basis for

calculations of attributable risk. Both Wynder *et al.* (1957) and Rothman and
Keller (1972) concluded that about three-quarters of the cases of oral cancer in
the populations they studied could have been prevented had exposure to alcohol
and tobacco not occurred. The fraction of nondrinkers and nonsmokers reported
in the control series of these studies was generally less than 20%. Assuming a
relative risk of 3 for the consumption of alcohol and/or tobacco as compared to
consumption of neither gives an attributable risk of about 60% for the two habits,
but this choice of relative risk is almost certainly very conservative. Assuming that
the effects of drinking and smoking are multiplicative (see p. 175), relative risks
of 2.5 for drinking and 4 for smoking and prevalences of 15% nonsmoking
drinkers, 15% nondrinking smokers and 50% drinking smokers give a population
attributable risk of about 83% for both habits.

Cancer of the nasopharynx

An indication of the potential for primary prevention within Chinese ethnic
groups in south-east Asia and China, among whom the incidence of
nasopharyngeal cancer (NPC) is the highest, can be obtained by utilizing the
published incidence rates. The potential in Hong Kong Chinese in comparison to
Chinese in Los Angeles is thus 78% for males of all ages and 82% for those aged
35–64. For females, the estimates are more tenuous, being based on smaller
numbers of cases in Los Angeles; however, potential reductions in Hong Kong are
72% and 73%, respectively. In other populations, the incidence is very low, with
rates generally below 1 per 100 000.

NPC has been linked to a number of factors, including consumption of salted
fish during the weaning period (see p. 213), exposure to smoke and fumes and the
Epstein–Barr virus (see p. 189). Extremely high relative risks associated with
consumption of salted fish have been reported in Hong Kong, where it has been
suggested that a very large proportion (about 90%) of young cases of NPC could
be prevented by elimination of this practice (Yu *et al.*, 1986). In southern China,
however, the proportion of cases that can be attributed to consumption of salted
fish in childhood is much lower (between 10 and 40%); however, the estimates of
relative risk upon which the calculations of proportions were based depend on the
recall of long past events and may therefore be underestimates (Yu *et al.*, 1988,
1989). Rates among Chinese immigrants to the USA are about half of those of
Chinese in south-east Asia (see p. 53). Studies of occupational exposure to smoke
and fumes suggest that some reduction in risk for NPC would be achieved through
improvement of working conditions (Lin *et al.*, 1973; Henderson *et al.*, 1976;
Armstrong *et al.*, 1983), but quantification is not feasible. The Epstein–Barr virus
may play a role in the etiology of NPC, but there is so far insufficient evidence to
recommend preventive strategies based on vaccination or antibody testing.

Cancer of the oesophagus

The greater than 100-fold difference between northern China, Soviet Central
Asia and Iran at one end and the low rates in other areas (shown in the Appendix)
at the other indicate a large potential for preventing oesophageal cancer.
Although in the very high incidence areas of China and Iran, oesophageal cancer

appears to have been common for several centuries, rapid changes have been observed in other populations: an increase has been seen in France, England and Wales and Australia and among blacks in South Africa and the USA. In Scandinavia and Switzerland, by contrast, the rates have been decreasing.

In many parts of the world, alcohol consumption and smoking appear to be the major risk factors for oesophageal cancer (see p. 182). However, in several Asian regions the risk is extremely high although the level of consumption of these factors is moderate, and in those areas malnutrition would appear to be more important. In a case–control study in the USA by Wynder and Bross (1961), the two factors appeared to combine multiplicatively to increase risk, and the total proportion of the risk attributable to the two factors together was 75%. Two larger case–control studies conducted in northern France (Tuyns *et al.*, 1977, 1988; see p. 182 and Table 20) confirmed these findings; there was an exponential increase in risk associated with increasing alcohol intake (in contrast to the sublinear increase in risk with increasing tobacco smoking), indicating a dominant effect of alcohol at high exposure levels. Attributable risks of a similar order can be estimated from the case–control studies of Martinez (1969), carried out in Puerto Rico, and of Pottern *et al.* (1981), among the black male population of Washington DC, whose rate of oesophageal cancer is the highest reported in the USA. In the latter study, alcohol again appeared to play a more important role than tobacco. In contrast, among urban Africans in South Africa, several case–control studies have related oesophageal cancer far more strongly to use of tobacco than to alcohol consumption (Oettle, 1964; Bradshaw & Schonland, 1974; Rose & McGlashan, 1975). In Bombay, India, where oesophageal cancer is almost as common in women as in men, drinking of the local alcoholic brews and smoking of *bidi* cigarettes are both associated with particularly high risks in men, but chewing of tobacco quids, smoking and drinking explain only a small fraction of the incidence in women (Jussawalla, 1971). Notani *et al.* (1989) estimated that 34% of oesophageal cancer in India is related to tobacco use, although the percentages for males (50%) and females (13%) are very different.

A common theme running through the results of many analytical studies of the epidemiology of oesophageal cancer is the association of the disease with poverty and a restricted diet. Studies in France and the USA have implicated low consumption of meat, dairy products, fruit and vegetables (Wynder & Bross, 1961; Ziegler *et al.*, 1981; Tuyns *et al.*, 1987), and, as described in Part II, (pp. 210, 217), in areas of extremely high oesophageal cancer risk, such as northern Iran and parts of China, low intake of vegetables, fruit and foods of animal origin have been reported. It seems likely that a substantial fraction of oesophageal cancer in several parts of Asia could be prevented by improving nutrition, with provision of fresh fruit and vegetables as an important component of the diet.

Several other risk factors have been investigated in epidemiological studies, including opium use (in eastern and central Asia), *N*-nitroso compounds and thermal injury from the drinking of hot beverages such as tea (Iran/IARC Cancer Study Group, 1977) and maté (Vassallo *et al.*, 1985; Victora *et al.*, 1987; see p. 215), but for the moment their role is not sufficiently clear to provide a basis for prevention.

Cancer of the stomach

The potential for preventing stomach cancer can be estimated on the basis of the 20-fold difference in rates between Japan and Kuwait. There has been a dramatic decrease in the rates of gastric cancer in most populations over the last four to five decades (see Part I, p. 56), indicating a reduction in exposure to as yet unidentified agents or the introduction of a protective agent. Studies of migrant populations have shown that the risk for stomach cancer changes, albeit rather slowly, in populations who move from high-risk to low-risk countries (see p. 56).

Case–control and cohort studies in a wide variety of populations have shown increased risk associated with more frequent use of starchy foods (such as corn, wheat, rice, potatoes and beans), smoked, salted and fried foods, and a decreased risk associated with the more frequent intake of green leafy vegetables, citrus fruits and dairy products (see Table 25, p. 212). These findings are compatible with an association between the decline in gastric cancer seen in the last 40 years and the decreasing dependence of populations on stored, heavily preserved and starchy foods and their greater access to green vegetables and citrus fruits, often all the year round.

Several hypotheses have been proposed to interpret the associations between dietary factors and stomach cancer risk. Those studied most extensively are high intake of salt, and the role of nitrate and nitrite in the endogenous formation of *N*-nitroso compounds (Correa & Haenszel, 1982). Laboratory research and studies in humans have indicated the possible preventive effect of vitamin C and other antioxidants, which inhibit the endogenous formation of *N*-nitroso compounds; however, definitive proof is still lacking (Bartsch *et al.*, 1988). In recent case–control studies in Canada, Greece, Poland, Italy and China, fruits and vegetables were identified as major protective factors (see Table 25). Although it would be difficult to provide a reliable estimate of the proportion of risk for stomach cancer that could be prevented by a diet rich in fresh fruits and vegetables, daily consumption of several servings of these foods has been associated with a 50% lower risk for stomach cancer as compared to rare consumption.

The concentrations of preformed *N*-nitroso compounds in foods and beverages have also been of some concern. The levels in beer have been reduced in some countries by introducing changes in malting processes. Levels of added and residual nitrites have been reduced in foods such as bacon, and nitrosation inhibitors such as vitamin C have been added. For instance, the contamination of bacon in the USA with *N*-nitrosopyrrolidine was reduced from 20–1000 ng/kg in 1971–72 to average levels of 5–15 ng/kg in 1977 (Havery *et al.*, 1978).

Cancers of the colon and rectum

The incidence of and mortality from cancer of the colon and rectum are highest in developed countries in North America, northern and western Europe and New Zealand. The lowest rates are found in Africa and Asia (see p. 57). Even without the data for Africa, there is still a large difference in risk between populations at high and low risk. In general, studies of migrants suggest that the risk changes relatively rapidly towards that of the host country and that environmental factors play a major role in the pathogenesis of colorectal cancer. Most such studies have been based on populations moving from low-risk to high-risk areas, such as Chinese and Japanese to Hawaii and other parts of the USA. The incidence of colorectal cancer generally approximates that in the new country in the second generation after emigration (Kolonel *et al.*, 1980; Shimizu *et al.*, 1987).

A large number of epidemiological studies indicate that diet is by far the most important exogenous factor so far identified in the etiology of cancer of the colon and rectum. The information is provided by about 20 case–control studies and three prospective cohort studies (see Table 23, p. 204), although there are important differences in the methods used to investigate dietary habits and to estimate nutrient intake (see pp. 201–202). They provide, nevertheless, considerable agreement concerning the evidence that two groups of foods or nutrients are associated in opposite ways with risk for cancer of the colon and rectum. Protective factors are represented by vegetables and – although the evidence is less consistent – fibre; the factors that may increase the risk are represented by total and saturated fats, animal and total proteins and total energy.

The association between cancer of the colon and rectum and fat intake was evaluated in 11 case–control studies. Eight studies found an increased risk for intake of total or saturated fat: the relative risk for subjects with a fat intake above the median was of the order of 1.5–2.0 in most studies conducted in developed countries, where fat intake is relatively high. This estimate indicates that some 15–25% of colorectal cancers could be attributed to high fat intake. The results also suggest, however, that high intake of vegetables or of fibre may reduce the risk for cancers of the colon and rectum to about one-half or one-third. This would suggest that about 25–35% of colorectal cancers might be prevented by high intake of vegetables and fibre. It has also been suggested (Newmark *et al.*, 1984) that the damaging effect of secondary bile acids on the colonic epithelium could be prevented by adequate concentrations of calcium in the colon.

Taking into consideration only these two groups of factors, and keeping in mind that the observed relative and attributable risks may be underestimated substantially due to random errors in dietary assessment, it might be postulated that up to one-half of colorectal cancers that occur in developed countries could be prevented by a low-fat, high-vegetable diet. The scientific evidence supporting this conclusion is not yet definitive, however. Dietary habits that conform to the recommendations for prevention of cardiovascular disease (National Research Council, 1989) are generally consistent with those indicated by case–control studies for colorectal cancer.

For populations of developing countries who do not at present have a high incidence of or mortality from colorectal cancer, it would be desirable to assess carefully any change in nutritional habits that may be occurring and, if necessary and possible, take corrective actions now. Although it should be recognized that the first priority may often be to correct undernutrition, this aim should still be compatible with prevention of a potential increase in the frequency of colorectal cancer.

Other factors that have been found occasionally to be associated with risk for cancer of the colorectum are certain occupational exposures, aspects of reproductive history, reduced physical activity and a history of cholecystectomy. The impact of these exposures on the total number of cases arising in high-incidence populations is likely to be small, either because of the rarity of the exposure, because the relative risk associated with the factor is small or because of both.

Cancer of the liver

Incidence data show that the highest rates among males have been recorded in southern Africa and south-east Asia and the lowest rates in populations originating in western Europe (Nova Scotia, Canada, 0.7; New South Wales, Australia, 1.2; south-western UK, 1.2) and among Indian populations (e.g., Madras, India, 2.1). This indicates a potential preventability of over 98%, although ethnic differences play an important role in the variation. The Israeli cancer registry shows that the incidence rates for hepatocellular carcinoma (HCC), the most frequently occurring malignancy of the liver, in Jewish migrants tend to reflect the incidence in their place of birth. This strongly suggests that exposure during early life is one of the main determinants of the risk for HCC later in life. Hepatitis B viral infection, ingestion of aflatoxin and alcohol consumption are all believed to play causal roles.

A considerable number of epidemiological studies have established a strong, specific association between infection with hepatitis B virus (HBV) and HCC (see p. 184). The attributable risk in high-risk countries of Asia, estimated from case–control studies, is 60–80% (Muñoz & Bosch, 1987). So far, no study of comparable quality is available for Africa, the other high-risk area for HCC. In low-risk countries, such as those of western Europe, the attributable risk is possibly below 5%.

Several safe and effective vaccines against HBV have been developed which are currently being used in large-scale trials and in vaccination campaigns (Szmuness et al., 1980; Maupas et al., 1981; Beasley et al., 1983; The Gambia Hepatitis Study Group, 1987). For countries with high or intermediate incidence rates of HCC, vaccination after birth has been recommended (World Health Organization, 1984).

In Asian and African countries with high rates of both HCC and the carrier state of hepatitis B surface antigen (HBsAg), most infection takes place early in life (Coursaget et al., 1987). This indicates that vaccination must occur even earlier, followed by a booster at 12 months. Table 35 summarizes the estimated reduction in the incidence of HCC expected after mass vaccination programmes aimed at all infants from high-risk populations but in which various degrees of coverage are achieved. The assumptions underlying these estimates are: (1) The attributable risk for HBV in high-risk countries is at least 80%. (2) About 10% of newborns who develop the HBsAg carrier state are infected perinatally, and only 50% of them will be protected by vaccination. (3) Antibody response to HBV vaccine is 20%, 80% and 95% after one, two and three doses of vaccine, respectively. Under these assumptions, the routine introduction of HBV vaccine in parts of Africa and Asia is likely to achieve a reduction of about 60–65% of HCC cases. If HBV is in fact responsible for 90% of HCC cases, the expected reduction in HCC will increase to over 70%. Even if the protection given by the HBV vaccine against hepatitis B decreases over time, it is expected that the protection against HCC will remain.

Table 35. Predicted effect of four different hepatitis B virus vaccination coverages on reducing the incidence of hepatocellular carcinoma (HCC)

Vaccination programme	Coverage of newborns (%)				Reduction in incidence (%)
	Full (3 doses)	Partial (2 doses)	Partial (1 dose)	Unvac- cinated	
I	80	10	5	5	65
II	75	5	5	15	58
III	50	10	10	30	44
IV	25	15	15	45	29

Once the appropriate vaccine is widely available and administered, the effect of mass vaccination on incidence or mortality will be detectable only after a minimal period of 20 years in areas with extremely high rates, such as Mozambique, and after 30–40 years in most high-risk countries. In low-risk countries, some cases might be prevented by HBV vaccination of selected high-risk groups. These include the newborn of HBsAg-positive mothers, hospital personnel, dialysis patients, haemophilic patients, drug addicts, male homosexuals, and persons with accidental percutaneous exposure or sexual contacts with carriers of HBsAg or actively infected people. Assuming that virtually all newborns of HBsAg-positive mothers are properly vaccinated, the impact on HCC incidence will be only as large as the estimates of the attributable risk, that is to say about 5–15% of HCC cases.

Aflatoxins, which are produced by fungal contaminants of certain foodstuffs, are potent liver carcinogens in animals and have recently been evaluated as human liver carcinogens (p. 126) on the basis of the results of correlation studies in several countries. In only one study (Peers *et al.*, 1987), carried out in Swaziland, was an attempt made to estimate the effect of aflatoxins and HBV simultaneously. It appeared that, although exposure to HBV was extremely high, the variation in HCC risk across the country was better explained by the estimated levels of exposure to aflatoxin. These results suggest that both factors play important roles.

The importance of reducing contamination of food by mycotoxins such as aflatoxin is obvious, since, apart from their potential as carcinogens, they are also acute toxic hazards. Such contamination is primarily a problem in developing countries, where agriculture is based mainly on small subsistence farms. The measures that reduce contamination of foodstuffs by aflatoxins – improved methods of harvesting and storage – will also reduce food losses due to insect and rodent damage and should therefore have general appeal for administrators. It is difficult to estimate the effect that such interventions would have on the incidence of liver cancer; however, the results of correlation studies performed in countries with high prevalences of hepatitis B infection (Bosch & Muñoz, 1989), indicate that a halving of the median daily aflatoxin intake might be equivalent to a 40% lower incidence of liver cancer.

Consumption of alcoholic beverages has been associated with liver cancer (see p. 182): in western countries where case–control studies have been carried out, the relative risk has been estimated at about 4 for consumption of more than 80 g of alcohol daily (Yu *et al.*, 1983), giving an attributable risk of about 13% for heavy consumption. In other studies, somewhat higher relative risks have been found, so that this proportion estimated to be preventable is probably the minimum.

Cancer of the pancreas

An estimate of the potential for preventing pancreatic cancer in people of European stock based on the highest rate in males of 10.4 in Neuchâtel, Switzerland, and the lowest rate of 3.1 in Tarragona, Spain, indicates a potential for prevention of 70%. In females, the highest rate is in Denmark (7.0) and the lowest (1.9) in Doubs, France, indicating a potential for prevention in Danish females of 73%. Comparisons between rates in blacks in the USA and in Dakar, Senegal, suggest an even greater potential for prevention in blacks in the USA.

Currently, the only factor to emerge consistently as a risk factor for pancreatic cancer is tobacco smoking (see p. 171; Table 17). In the major cohort studies of smoking, mortality from pancreatic cancer was almost always elevated in smokers compared to nonsmokers. The results of these studies are summarized in *IARC Monographs* Volume 38 (IARC, 1986a). In the study of Doll and Peto (1976), assuming that 50% of males are cigarette smokers, an attributable risk of 13% can be calculated. However, in the study of US veterans (Rogot & Murray, 1980), 459 deaths were observed from pancreatic cancer as compared to 256 expected in nonsmokers, giving a ratio of observed to expected of 1.8 and an attributable risk of 44%. Largely on the basis of this study, but using the estimated rate of death in nonsmokers from the study of the American Cancer Society (Garfinkel, 1980), Doll and Peto (1981) estimated an attributable risk of 40% in men and of 25% in women. Case–control studies in the USA give rise to estimates of attributable risk varying from 23% to 55% for men and 14% to 25% for women (Wynder *et al.*, 1973; MacMahon *et al.*, 1981; Wynder *et al.*, 1983; Mack *et al.*, 1986; Raymond *et al.*, 1987; Cuzick & Babicker, 1989). It seems likely, therefore, that in the studied populations, mostly in the USA, up to 40% of pancreatic cancer in males and 20% in females can be attributed to cigarette smoking.

Cancer of the larynx

The potential for prevention in males in Navarra, Spain, where the rate is 17.2, in comparison with the lowest rate reported for European populations of 2.8 in Sweden, would be of the order of 84%. Nearly all reported rates in females are low, and therefore similar comparisons have not been attempted.

Laryngeal cancer shares with oesophageal and oral cancer the major risk factors – alcohol and tobacco consumption (see pp. 170, 175, 181). The major cohort studies on tobacco have almost invariably found a substantially increased risk for laryngeal cancer in smokers compared to nonsmokers. In none of these studies, however, was alcohol consumption assessed, and they can be used only indirectly to estimate population attributable risks. In a case–control study, Wynder *et al.* (1976) estimated a relative risk for laryngeal cancers in persons who had ever smoked of 13.2. With a proportion exposed of 0.8, the attributable risk was over 90% in males; the corresponding findings for females were 9.0, 0.4 and 76% respectively. The authors noted that the combined effect of alcohol and tobacco seemed to be multiplicative, as confirmed in a reanalysis of the data by Flanders and Rothman (1982). Subsequent case–control studies (Hinds *et al.*, 1979; Burch *et al.*, 1981; Graham *et al.*, 1981; Elwood *et al.*, 1984) produced similar conclusions. The relative risk was generally far higher for smoking than for alcohol consumption, and the attributable risk for the two habits either singly or combined was in the range of 80–90%.

Jayant *et al.* (1977) estimated the proportion of cases of laryngeal cancer in Bombay, India, that could be attributed to chewing tobacco quid and/or smoking. The population attributable risk for these two exposures combined was 78%; 28% of the cases occurred in chewers who were nonsmokers, 38% in smokers who did not chew and 34% in cases who admitted to both habits. The smokers mostly smoked *bidis* and the chewers used *pan*, a preparation incorporating betel nut, tobacco and lime. Only 11% of the cases were nonchewers and nonsmokers compared to 46% of the population controls.

Cancer of the lung

The highest rates for cancer of the bronchus and trachea in people of European stock are 100.4 in males in western Scotland and 33.3 among white females in the San Francisco Bay Area; the lowest rates are found in Iceland in males (24.7) and in Doubs, France, in females (2.8), indicating a potential for prevention of 75% in males in western Scotland, and 92% in females in San Francisco. The highest rate in a black population was that in New Orleans and the lowest that in Senegal; the percentage difference indicates an even greater potential for prevention in New Orleans blacks than in whites.

Tobacco smoking

The major cohort studies of mortality in relation to smoking have provided consistent evidence of a substantially increased risk for lung cancer among male (e.g., Hammond, 1966; Kahn, 1966; Doll & Peto, 1976; Rogot & Murray, 1980) and female smokers (Doll *et al.*, 1980). These studies are summarized in IARC (1986a) and discussed on pp. 169–176 of this book. Although the study populations were not random samples of the general population, and the data cannot therefore be used to estimate directly the attributable proportion of lung cancer due to tobacco use, the relative risks observed within these groups can be regarded as indicative of the risk that is present for the general population from similar levels of tobacco use. Thus, using prevalence data on the extent of smoking in the general population, an estimate of the population attributable risk in the general population can be derived. As all of the studies tend to agree on a relative risk of about 10 for use compared to non-use of tobacco, and as in many populations with relatively stable smoking rates the prevalence in males has been of the order of 50% or greater, the population attributable risk from tobacco use is at least 80%. Recent temporal trends in smoking prevalence and lung cancer rates are discussed in Part I, pp. 61–64.

Data on lung cancer risk in women are less extensive than for men. In most countries, smoking is a more recently established habit among women, so that estimates of relative risk for current smokers tend to be lower than those for men. However, result from cohort studies in populations in which smoking by women is well established (Doll *et al.*, 1980; Garfinkel & Stellman, 1988) suggest that the risks are the same as those for men. Thus, assuming a relative risk of 10 (as above) and a prevalence of cigarette smoking in the female population of 0.35, the attributable risk is approximately 76%. Estimates for the USA in 1985, when 27.8% of women were current smokers and 16.9% former smokers, suggest that the attributable risk is 58% for current smoking and 24% for former smoking – that is, 82% of lung cancer deaths in women are caused by tobacco.

A more direct estimate of attributable risk can be obtained if the mortality rate in nonsmokers is known from the results of a cohort study. This allows calculation of the number of deaths that would have been expected in a population if no one had smoked. The most reliable data are those of the American Cancer Society for the nonsmoking population of the USA. Table 36 gives estimates for five countries, where American Cancer Society rates have been used to calculate expected deaths in nonsmokers. Attributable risks are 83–94% in males and 57–83% in females.

Table 36. Lung cancer deaths attributable to smoking in five countries, 1985

Country	Sex	No. of deaths	Expected deaths[a] (non-smokers)	Mortality rate age ≥ 35		Attributable to smoking	
				Observed	In non-smokers	Deaths	%
Canada	M	8278	639	156.5	11.7	7639	92
	F	3164	593	54.7	10.2	2571	81
England &	M	25 994	1591	219.7	13.4	24 403	94
Wales	F	9798	1692	72.1	12.4	8106	83
Japan	M	20 837	3201	71.9	10.8	17 636	85
	F	7753	2948	24.1	9.1	4805	62
Sweden	M	1879	313	85.4	14.0	1566	83
	F	706	304	29.4	12.6	402	57
USA	M	83 854	6274	172.1	12.5	77 580	93
	F	38 702	6389	68.1	11.3	32 313	83

[a] Using mortality in nonsmokers estimated from American Cancer Society rates (IARC, 1986a; Table 70, p. 232)

In many developed countries, there have been major changes in the types of cigarettes used in the last two decades (see p. 174), including the adoption of filters and the use of tobacco containing less 'tar'. It is of considerable importance to know whether such changes result in a reduction in the relative risk for lung cancer due to smoking. A large case–control study in a number of European countries addressed this issue (Lubin *et al.*, 1984). The relative risk for any tobacco use by males was 7.6, and for females 3.5; however, life-time smokers of filter cigarettes appeared to have approximately half the relative risk of those in other categories. The study indicates a lung cancer risk approximately 50% lower for low-tar cigarette smokers. Use of filter, low-tar cigarettes was associated with a slightly smaller reduction of risk. The study also indicated a less harmful effect for lifetime smokers of low-tar cigarettes; however, there was no evidence of reduced risk for those who changed from high- to low-tar cigarettes. Thus, while there is clear evidence that stopping smoking reduces the risk for lung cancer, it is not yet evident that switching to low-tar cigarettes after a substantial number of years of smoking those with a high-tar level results in any reduction in the risk for lung cancer. Although filter and/or low-tar cigarettes may confer a lower risk for lung cancer, however, they do not appear to result in a lower risk for other diseases, such as chronic respiratory disease and cardiovascular disease (Stellman, 1986).

The study of Lubin *et al.* (1984) seems to suggest similar orders of risk for light and dark tobacco. This was confirmed in a population-based case–control study in Italy (Pastorino *et al.*, 1984). In Cuba, where dark tobacco is used extensively (Joly *et al.*, 1983), the relative risk for smokers compared to nonsmokers was 14.1 in males and 7.3 in females. Smoking of pipes and cigars is not risk free (p. 173), and people who switch from cigarettes to pipes or cigars and continue to inhale, continue to increase their risks for all of the cancers that are associated with tobacco smoking.

Benefits of stopping smoking

Broadly speaking, three types of study can be drawn upon to evaluate the results of stopping or reducing smoking on the risk for cancer. These are population (ecological) studies, observational studies of individuals (cohort and case–control studies) and intervention studies. Population studies are done to compare changes in smoking prevalence with lung cancer incidence in either entire populations or subsets of them such as birth cohorts. Their results tend to confirm that, for western populations at least, time trends in lung cancer incidence, including recent declines observed in Finland, the UK and the USA, can be quite well expiained by changes in smoking habits, particularly if the tar content of the cigarettes smoked is taken into account (see p. 62).

The second type of evidence derives from epidemiological studies of individuals, including substantial numbers of ex-smokers, whose risk for cancer was examined in relation to the length of time since quitting and the duration and intensity of smoking beforehand. These studies were reviewed in IARC (1986a) and by Shopland (1989). The major prospective (cohort) studies, which started in the 1950s and 1960s, provide information on the mortality risk in relation to years since stopping smoking (Table 37). The relationship is strong, but, at least in the first three studies listed, the risk did not decline to that of lifetime nonsmokers. It is noticeable that the risk of persons who have stopped recently (one to four years) appears to be higher than that of continuing smokers – this is almost certainly due to the fact that some smokers stop because they are diagnosed as having lung cancer, or have early symptoms of it, e.g., cough or haemoptysis, and they die from the disease soon afterwards. In a more recent prospective study of 1.2 million individuals in the USA (the American Cancer Society 50-state study), Garfinkel and Stellman (1988) analysed the results of quitting smoking among women with no history of cancer or cardiovascular disease, and among all women. Among the 'healthy' quitters, the risk for lung cancer was reduced within two years of stopping, although the early rise was seen when all women were included.

Table 37. Lung cancer mortality ratios in ex-smokers of cigarettes, by number of years since stopping smoking[a]

Study population	Time since stopping smoking (years)	Mortality ratio	Reference
British doctors	1-4	16.0	Doll & Peto (1976);
	5-9	5.9	Doll *et al.* (1980)
	10-14	5.3	
	≥ 15	2.0	
	Current smoker	14.0	
US veterans[b]	1-4	18.8	Rogot & Murray (1980)
	5-9	7.7	
	10-14	4.7	
	15-19	4.8	
	≥ 20	2.1	
	Current smoker	11.3	
Japanese men	1-4	4.7	Hirayama (1975)
	5-9	2.5	
	≥ 10	1.4	
	Current smoker	3.8	
Men aged 50-69 years in 25 US states	< 1 (1-19 cigs/day)	7.2	Hammond *et al.* (1977)
	(≥ 20 cigs/day)	29.1	
	1-4 (1-19 cigs/day)	4.6	
	(≥ 20 cigs/day)	12.0	
	5-9 (1-19 cigs/day)	1.0	
	(≥ 20 cigs/day)	7.2	
	> 10 (1-19 cigs/day)	0.4	
	(≥ 20 cigs/day)	1.1	
	Current smoker (1-19 cigs/day)	6.5	
	(≥ 20 cigs/day)	13.7	

[a] From US Department of Health and Human Services (1982)
[b] Includes data only for smokers who stopped smoking other than on their doctor's orders

In a large case–control study in five European countries, Lubin *et al.* (1984) were also able to investigate the risk for lung cancer in relation to length of time since stopping smoking, but in addition to see how this varied with the total duration of smoking or amount smoked before quitting (Table 38). The relative benefits of cessation were much greater in individuals who had smoked for relatively short periods – for instance, smokers of less than 20 years' duration had risks about the same as those of nonsmokers ten years after quitting, whereas for those who had smoked for over 50 years the relative benefits of stopping were much smaller. In the American Cancer Society 50-state study (Garfinkel & Stellman, 1988), the risk among women who were light smokers (1–20 cigarettes per day) returned almost to the level of the nonsmokers after 16 years – as in the earlier 25-state study in men. These findings are in keeping with those of the autopsy studies of Auerbach (1962, 1979), who found that atypical changes observed in the bronchial epithelium of smokers had largely disappeared in ex-smokers.

Table 38. Relative risk for developing lung cancer by time since stopping smoking and total duration of smoking habit[a]

Time since stopping smoking (years)	Duration of smoking habit (years)			
	1-19	20-39	40-49	>50
Men				
0	1.0[b]	2.2	2.8	3.0
1-4	1.1	2.1	3.3	3.8
5-9	0.4	1.5	2.2	2.8
>10	0.3	1.0	1.6	2.7
Women				
0	1.0[c]	2.1	2.7	5.2
1-4	1.0	2.3	2.1	7.1
5-9	0.4	2.0	1.1	1.7
>10	0.4	0.3	2.3	

[a] From Lubin *et al.* (1984)
[b] Baseline category: risk for men who had never smoked relative to that for current smokers who had smoked for one to 19 years was 0.6.
[c] Baseline category: risk for women who had never smoked relative to that for current smokers who had smoked for one to 19 years was 0.3.

The aim of intervention studies is to reduce smoking in populations of individuals, in contrast to the observational studies discussed above, where those who had stopped were self-selected. No intervention study has been designed to find out whether the risk for cancer is decreased by inducing people to stop or to reduce smoking. Those that have been performed were concerned primarily with prevention of cardiovascular disease, in which several preventive measures (e.g., weight reduction, diet) were applied in addition to smoking cessation. These studies have been reviewed recently (Hakama *et al.*, 1989). In two small studies – one in Oslo (Hjerman *et al.*, 1981) and one London (Rose *et al.*, 1982) – reduction in smoking was achieved by individual counselling. A much larger trial in the USA (the Multiple Risk Factor Intervention Trial, MRFIT) also included reduction in blood pressure by drugs and dietary changes (Friedewald *et al.*, 1989). In none of these trials was a reduction in mortality from lung cancer observed after five to ten years of follow-up. A similarly negative result emerged from an intervention trial in which workers in 80 factories in four European countries were randomized as controls or to receive special interventions to reduce smoking, body weight, blood pressure and serum cholesterol (WHO Collaborative Group, 1989). Although these results are disappointing, they can be explained in terms of the small numbers of subjects (particularly in the Oslo and London studies), the relatively short periods of follow-up, and the smaller than anticipated differences in smoking between intervention and control groups – many subjects in the latter opting to give up smoking.

The largest intervention so far attempted is the community trial in northern Karelia, Finland, involving 180 000 individuals, the aim of which was to change dietary and smoking habits by public health education and by reorganizing community and health services (Hakulinen *et al.*, 1989). Although this was not a randomized trial, the expected numbers of cases of different cancers were estimated from incidence data for the rest of Finland. It was concluded that, over a 14-year period, a 10% reduction in lung cancer had been achieved.

Other causes

Many specific occupations and occupational exposures have been associated with elevated risks for lung cancer, and in a number of cases the link has been clearly established to be causal. A detailed review of this evidence is given on pp. 141–146. Clearly identified occupational lung carcinogens are asbestos, coal-tars and soots, chromium, arsenic and nickel compounds, mustard gas, bischloromethyl ether and radon. Increased risks for lung cancer have also been found to be causally associated with occupational exposure in aluminium production, in the manufacture of auramine, in coal gasification and coke production, in iron and steel founding, in the manufacture of isopropyl alcohol by the strong-acid process, in boot and shoe manufacture and repair, in the manufacture of magenta, in the rubber industry, in underground haematite mining with exposure to radon and in furniture and cabinet-making. Substantial questions remain, however, with regard to the carcinogenicity of various dusts, fumes and other exposures which occur in many working environments.

Estimations of attributable risks in people in certain occupations can be made either by considering specific exposures, if the proportion of the population exposed is known, or by evaluating the relative risks of various occupations, adjusted for smoking, in case–control studies of lung cancer. The latter approach has been used on several occasions. Risks attributable to exposure in the work place were found by Pike *et al.* (1978) in Los Angeles county, USA (36%), by Pastorino *et al.* (1984) in Milan, Italy (33%), and by Kvåle *et al.* (1986) in Norway (13–27%). Simonato *et al.* (1988) reviewed the case–control studies of lung cancer in relation to occupation and found a wide range of estimates of attributable risk (1–40%). The estimates depended on both the geographical location of the study and the method used to define occupational exposure.

Several occupational carcinogens appear to interact multiplicatively with tobacco, particularly radiation and asbestos (see pp. 157, 175). For an individual exposed to these agents, a major component of risk would be reduced by cessation of cigarette smoking. Thus, although the attributable risk from occupation in some areas may be of the order of 10-30%, this is due largely to an interaction with smoking (Pastorino *et al.*, 1984), and the additional contribution of occupation over and above that of tobacco is probably less than 9%.

Malignant melanoma of the skin

The incidence of melanoma is high among Caucasian populations living at tropical and temperate latitudes. Australia (Queensland: males, 30.9; females, 28.5) records the highest rates among the registries covered by Muir *et al.* (1987). Non-Caucasian populations generally have rates below 1.0, indicating a potential for prevention (ignoring racial differences) of over 95% in Australia, depending on the registry chosen. However, because of the clear importance of constitutional and other genetic factors in the etiology of the disease (see below), a more appropriate comparison would be that with the UK, from where most of the Australian population originates. The rates are 2.2 in men and 3.8 in women in England and Wales, indicating potentials for prevention in Queensland of 93% and 87%, respectively.

Studies in migrants indicate that people who move to sunny environments acquire an increased risk for melanoma, which is related to the duration of residence in the new country, or perhaps to age at migration (see Part I, p. 67).

Although there is substantial evidence that exposure to the sun increases the risk for melanoma (see p. 163), the relationship is clearly not a simple one. For example, melanoma is as likely to occur on intermittently exposed areas such as the back, chest and legs as on the face and hands. Secondly, indoor occupations carry a risk equal to and sometimes higher than that of outdoor occupations; however, in one study, the effect disappeared after adjusting for socioeconomic status (Cooke *et al.*, 1984), and, in another study, the higher risk for melanoma in office workers was restricted to those melanomas occurring on areas of skin usually covered by clothing (Vagero *et al.*, 1986). The results, while not fully consistent, suggest that short-term exposure to intense sunlight increases the risk for melanoma, while long-term, constant exposure may have a smaller effect. A study by Elwood *et al.* (1985) permits estimation of attributable risks associated with different patterns of exposure to the sun; e.g., people with four or more 'sunny vacations' per decade had a relative risk of about 1.7 compared to individuals who had none. The fraction of the population exposed at this level was 0.1, giving an attributable risk of about 40%. From the population-based study of Green *et al.* (1985) conducted in Queensland, Australia, it is possible to calculate attributable risks for numbers of severe sunburns in a life time; the relative risk was 2.7, the proportion of the controls exposed, 0.30, and thus the attributable risk was more than 30%.

The attributable risks calculated from these studies do not approach the potential for prevention indicated by the differences in incidence in descriptive epidemiology, perhaps because the most appropriate exposure index for predicting melanoma risk has not been discovered.

The potential for reducing mortality from malignant melanoma by regular surveillance of high-risk populations is described on p. 274.

Other cancers of the skin

The incidence of skin cancers other than melanoma is difficult to calculate accurately (see p. 68). The potentially preventable fraction of cases cannot therefore be estimated reliably. Comparing the rates in Tasmania, Australia, with those in Hamburg, Federal Republic of Germany, suggests a potential preventability of 97% in males in Tasmania.

A relationship with exposure to the sun has been suggested by a number of observations. Firstly, there is a gradient of increasing incidence with decreasing latitude among Caucasian populations (Urbach, 1971; Daniels, 1975) – much stronger than that noted for melanoma. Secondly, the cancers arise predominantly on parts of the body that are exposed to the sun – notably the face and hands (Scotto & Fraumeni, 1982). Thirdly, outdoor workers, such as farmers and fishermen, have elevated rates of skin cancer in contrast to a lower than average rate of melanoma. Finally, there seems to be a strong relationship between risk and life-time exposure to the sun (Fears *et al.*, 1977). Nevertheless, there is no reliable case–control or cohort study that allows an estimation of the risk associated with different levels or types of exposure to the sun; it is therefore not possible to quantify the effect of interventions other than total elimination of exposure. The obvious preventive measure of sun avoidance is being strongly promoted in some countries such as Australia, where skin cancer rates are the highest in the world. The wearing of hats and sun-screen creams during recreational and occupational sun exposure is encouraged. In order to evaluate the efficacy of such programmes in preventing skin cancer, it is essential that routine registration be established, at least on a limited basis.

Occupational exposures to soots, tars and mineral oils have been recognized as being responsible for skin cancer ever since the classic finding of scrotal cancer in chimney sweeps by Percivall Pott (see p. 141). However, the general improvement in working conditions during this century has probably reduced the number of skin cancers from this cause to a low level.

Because of the low rate of fatality from skin cancer other than melanoma, there is perhaps a less dramatic need for early detection measures. High-risk groups (i.e., fair-skinned Caucasians living at low latitudes) should be made aware of the possibility of skin cancer, so that they can present any suspicious lesion to their general practitioner for examination at an early stage, thus limiting the surgery required. The effects of such education on subsequent morbidity and mortality from skin cancer remain to be evaluated.

Cancer of the breast

The highest rate of breast cancer that has been recorded in women of European origin is 87.0 in whites in the San Francisco Bay area, USA, and the lowest, 18.4 in Nowy Sacz, Poland, indicating a potential for prevention in San Francisco whites of 79%. However, comparable rates exist in populations of non-European origin who have migrated to countries of predominantly European populations. In San Francisco, the rate among Japanese is 48.9, as compared to that in Japan where the rate in the Miyagi rural region is 18.6, indicating a potential for prevention in San Francisco Japanese of 62%.

The most clearly established risk factors for breast cancer are reproductive, including age at first birth, parity, age at menarche and age at menopause (see pp. 240–243). Two studies provide data that permit calculation of attributable risks of 17% for breast cancer in relation to age over 25 years at the time of first full-term pregnancy (MacMahon *et al.*, 1970; Henderson *et al.*, 1974). However, even if childbearing patterns are associated with risk, they offer little scope for practicable preventive measures, both because the attributable risks are certainly not large and because it is unlikely that a woman would modify childbearing with the goal of preventing breast cancer. Nevertheless, population control policies in operation in certain countries may have the unfortunate side effect of increasing the risk for breast cancer. Similarly, in many developed countries where diminishing proportions of women have children at younger ages, the incidence of breast cancer may be expected to increase in the future. A decline in risk following induced cessation of ovarian function has been observed (see p. 240), which offers theoretical, but ethically problematic, possibilities for intervention.

The possible role of diet in the causation of breast cancer is reviewed in some detail in Chapter 12. There is a suggestion from several case–control studies that a diet rich in fat and protein of animal origin increases the risk for breast cancer. In all of these studies, information on diet was available only for periods a few years before diagnosis. Some studies have indicated a stronger association with fat and protein for postmenopausal women, while in others the risks were similar for pre- and postmenopausal women. The interpretation of these studies is still uncertain, also in view of the lack of association seen in some prospective studies. If the observed association with risk for breast cancer were real, the implications for public health would be to recommend moderate intake of fat, and particularly of saturated fat. These recommendations were adopted recently by an expert committee appointed by the US National Academy of Sciences (National Research Council, 1989).

A number of recent studies have suggested that alcohol consumption of more than 30 g per day is associated with a 1.5– to 2–fold increase in the risk for breast cancer (see p. 183) . The results of 16 epidemiological studies were reviewed by Longnecker *et al.* (1988): overall, the data are consistent in indicating an increase in risk for breast cancer associated with consumption of alcoholic beverages. Recent studies of populations characterized by a relatively high consumption of wine and other alcoholic beverages (Toniolo *et al.*, 1989) support the hypothesis that the risk is associated with total ethanol intake, independently of the type of beverage. While there are many good medical reasons for recommending only moderate alcohol consumption, even in countries where alcohol consumption is common among women the proportion of cases of breast cancer attributable to alcohol drinking is probably very modest – in the order of 5% or less.

A number of studies have indicated the potential importance of both height and weight in increasing the risk for breast cancer after the menopause (e.g., de

Waard & Baanders van Halewijn, 1974; de Waard *et al.*, 1977; Lew & Garfinkel, 1979). A study in California (Paffenbarger *et al.*, 1980) showed a significant effect of obesity in increasing the risk for breast cancer in postmenopausal but not in premenopausal women. An attributable risk of 18% for an obesity index (weight (kg)/height^2 (m)) of 21.5 or more can be estimated.

In the San Francisco Bay area of California, the proportion of breast cancer occurring in women over the age of 55 is 0.63 (Muir *et al.*, 1987). Therefore, the proportion of all breast cancers that might be prevented in that population by reducing obesity is approximately 11%. This is similar to the estimate of 13% made by Miller (1978). Lubin *et al.* (1985) evaluated the effect of obesity on risk for breast cancer in Israel and estimated an attributable risk of 30% for excess weight in their population.

A number of other agents are known or suspected to increase the risk for breast cancer. These include ionizing radiation (see p. 157), to which the breast may be exposed for diagnostic and therapeutic purposes, and using combined oral contraceptives at young ages or before the first pregnancy (see p. 153). Long-term use of menopausal oestrogens may increase the risk for breast cancer (p. 152), and in some areas, notably the west of the USA where their use was common, a limited proportion of breast cancers in postmenopausal women may be attributable to them. Although the overall contribution of these agents to the total number of cases of breast cancer is probably small, the medical benefits of their use should be weighed against their potential hazard in each case.

With regard to early prevention, a woman aged 50 or more who undergoes regular screening can reduce her risk of dying from breast cancer by at least 40% (see Part III, pp. 275–278). This effect is less than the effect of regular screening for cervical cancer, but in many countries the relative incidences of the two malignancies are such that breast cancer screening would have a larger absolute effect. The dose of radiation to the breast during modern mammography is less than 0.0002 Gy per visit, if properly controlled, and for women over age 50 the radiation received from screening once every two years represents a negligible carcinogenic hazard.

Nevertheless, the requirements of a full-scale mammographic screening programme are not inconsiderable, and so far in few countries have decisions been taken to mount centralized programmes. In the USA, it has been accepted as an objective that, by the year 2000, 80% of women aged 50–70 should be receiving annual physical examinations and annual mammography – substantial increases from the 1983 estimates of 45% and 15%, respectively (Greenwald & Sondik, 1986). Such policies could be expected to have major impacts on mortality from breast cancer after a delay of only about five years. A UICC workshop concluded, 'In countries where breast cancer is common and where the necessary resources are available, screening using mammography only or mammography plus physical examination is applicable as public health policy. The greatest initial benefit would be obtained by concentrating screening on women aged 50–69.'(Day *et al.*, 1986).

Cancer of the uterine cervix

Cervical cancer rates tend to be highest in Asia, South America and Africa. The highest rates are seen in Recife, Brazil (83.2 per 100 000), Cali, Colombia (48.2) and São Paulo, Brazil (35.1) and in New Zealand Maoris (28.9). The lowest rates occur in Israel (Jews, 4.0; non-Jews, 3.0), indicating a potential for prevention of over 95%, if possible ethnic differences in susceptibility are ignored.

The most clearly defined risk factors for cervical cancer in western populations are age at first intercourse, which is inversely related to cervical cancer risk, and, independently, the number of sexual partners throughout life (see pp. 243). The epidemiological data strongly implicate a venereally transmitted factor in the etiology of cervical cancer (see pp. 185–189) and suggest that primary prevention could be implemented by modifying the patterns of sexual behaviour that facilitate its diffusion. Such modification, in particular the use of condoms, would be consistent with recommendations for the prevention of AIDS, but its effect would be difficult to predict on the basis of current data, especially in many developing countries where information on sexual behaviour is limited.

In addition, it seems probable that high parity confers an additional risk, independent of these sexual variables (p. 243). Limitations of family size by effective family planning programmes might therefore be expected to decrease the incidence of cervical carcinoma. In a recent study in Latin America (Brinton *et al.*, 1989), the risk for four to five live births was 1.4, that for six to 11 was 1.7 and that for 12 or more, 2.5, compared with three or fewer children. Since more than 60% of control women had had more than three live-born children, about 30% of cervical cancer in this population can be attributed to their high fertility.

The etiological role of some types of human papilloma and other viruses is currently being investigated. If this is confirmed, then a vaccine against such viruses might substantially change the perspective for primary prevention.

An association between cigarette smoking and cervical carcinoma, in-situ carcinoma and dysplasia has been reported repeatedly (see p. 173). In most studies, the level of risk of smokers compared to nonsmokers is about 2, although in some studies it is substantially higher. Should that estimate be in the right range, the risk attributable to smoking in populations in which a substantial proportion of the female population are current smokers would be quite substantial (i.e., 20–25% in several European countries, the USA, Canada and Australia), but it would be far smaller in countries where the prevalence of smoking among women has been low (i.e., China, south-east Asia and northern parts of Africa).

The strong evidence in favour of the effectiveness of cervical cytology screening in reducing the incidence of and mortality from cervical cancer is outlined in Part III (pp. 278–281). The relative protection given by different degrees of screening, as estimated in a recent collaborative study (IARC, 1986b; IARC Working Group, 1986) is given in Table 39.

In using these results to estimate the life-time protection a woman would acquire if she attended regularly for screening, we assume that the precancerous lesions detected by cervical cytology can be treated effectively to prevent progression to an invasive tumour. Follow-up studies of women registered with treated in-situ carcinoma of the cervix suggest that these people are still at higher risk than the general population for developing an invasive cervical cancer.

Table 39. Relative protection against cervical cancer obtained from different degrees of screening[a]

Time since last negative smear (months)	No. of cases	Relative protection
0-11	25	15.3
12-23	23	11.9
24-35	25	8.0
36-47	30	5.3
48-59	30	2.8
60-71	16	3.6
72-119	6	1.6
$\geq$ 120	7	0.8[b]

[a] From IARC (1986b) and IARC Working Group (1986)
[b] Based on data from only two centres

The degree of protection that a woman would receive from different screening regimens is given in Table 40, assuming western European incidence rates. Screening every three years between the ages of 25 and 64 (13 tests) gives about 90% protection; screening every five years between the ages of 35 and 64 (six tests) gives 70% protection. The predicted percentage reductions are similar for a country such as Colombia, where incidence rates are two to three times higher. The only difference is seen when screening is begun at the age of 35, since in high-risk countries the incidence of invasive cancer increases rapidly before this age. Even screening every ten years between ages 35 and 64 should give more than 50% protection, a figure important to bear in mind for countries with limited resources.

It is clear that screening before the age of 25 brings little extra benefit, because screening is aimed at preventing invasive disease, and the disease is very rare in women under the age of 25. Recommendations that screening should start at age 18 for sexually active girls appear to be based on the premise that women under age 25 with detectable precancerous lesions may form an ultra-high-risk group. Thus, if the opportunity presents itself (by their attendance for oral contraceptives or for antenatal or postnatal care) to include them in screening programmes, they can be placed on special surveillance if lesions have already developed (Task Force, 1982).

The effect of the introduction of mass screening can be predicted by the use of simulation models, which incorporate (among other factors) the frequency of screening, the target age group and the degree of compliance (see Parkin, 1985, for example). Although it may be possible to reduce the incidence of invasive cervical cancer by more than 90%, more realistic goals are closer to the 60% obtained by a national mass screening programme in Finland, in which women aged 35–60 are tested every five years.

Table 40. Effects on cervical cancer incidence of different screening policies, starting at age 20[a]

Screening schedule	Cumulative rate 20-64, per 10^5	Reduction in rate (%)	No. of tests	No. of cases prevented per 10^5 tests
None	1575			
Every 10 years, 25-64	581.5	63.1	4	248
Every 10 years, 35-64	709.6	54.9	3	288
Every 5 years, 20-64	257.6	83.6	9	146
Every 5 years, 25-64	286.7	81.8	8	161
Every 5 years, 35-64	478.8	69.6	6	132
Every year, 20-34, then every 5 years, 35-64	232.3	85.5	21	64
Every 3 years, 20-64	137.8	91.2	15	96
Every 3 years, 25-64	161.0	89.8	13	109
Every 3 years, 35-64	352.8	77.6	10	122
Every year, 20-34, then every 3 years, 35-64	131.2	91.7	25	59
Every year, 20-64	105.0	93.3	35	33

[a] From IARC Working Group (1986); assuming western European incidence rates: at ages 20-24, $5/10^5$; at 25-29, $15/10^5$; at 30-34, $25/10^5$; and at 35-64, $45/10^5$

Cancer of the endometrium

Endometrial cancer is most common among white women in the USA (annual incidence, 30–40 per 100 000 per year) and in some European countries (15–30 cases per 100 000 per year). It is rare (2 per 100 000 per year) in most countries of Asia and Africa; the rates in eastern Europe and Latin America are slightly higher (3–6 per 100 000). The potential for prevention in the USA is thus near 90% in comparison with eastern Europe and over 95% in comparison with the lowest rates in the world.

case–control studies of endometrial cancer have implicated both endogenous and exogenous hormonal factors (see pp. 151–153, 244–245). Women with endometrial carcinoma are more often obese than their controls; other characteristics found frequently in these patients are late menopause and low parity. The risk of developing endometrial carcinoma is also strongly enhanced among women exposed to oestrogen therapy for menopausal and postmenopausal symptoms. Relative risks of 4–8 have been observed in a number of studies in the USA. With a relative risk of 6, and a prevalence of use of exogenous oestrogens of 15% among postmenopausal women, one can calculate an attributable risk of 40%.

The effect on the frequency of endometrial cancer of reducing the use of replacement oestrogens has appeared relatively rapidly, in contrast to many other carcinogens. The incidence of endometrial carcinoma in the USA rose dramatically following the increase in use of oestrogens for menopausal symptoms (Weiss *et al.*, 1976; Greenwald *et al.*, 1977), and Jick *et al.* (1979, 1980) described a sharp downward trend in the incidence of endometrial cancer from July 1975 to July 1977 in the Seattle, WA, USA, area. Thus, Jick *et al.* (1979) studied a group of 11 000 women aged 50–64 with intact uteri, following widespread reports of the potential risks of replacement oestrogens and a reduction in their use, and observed 51 cases of endometrial cancer in 1975 and 16 in 1976. On the basis of the estimated rate of disease in nonusers, it can be calculated that the risk attributable to use of oestrogens was 78% in 1975 and 54% in 1976. Similar observations have come from studies of time trends and other descriptive studies. A similar effect was seen in California (Austin & Roe, 1982). Contrasting results, however, come from the study of Shapiro *et al.* (1985): in one of the largest case–control studies of endometrial cancer, the effect of postmenopausal oestrogen therapy persisted for up to 15 years following cessation.

Sequential oral contraceptives have also been found to increase the risk for endometrial cancer (see p. 153). Observations of substantial relative risks (Weiss & Sayvetz, 1980; Henderson *et al.*, 1983) contributed to the elimination of these formulations from contraceptive use in the USA. In contrast, use of combination oral contraceptives is associated with a consistent, highly significant reduction in the risk for developing endometrial carcinoma, of the order of 40% (Weiss & Sayvetz, 1980; Kelsey *et al.*, 1982; Centers for Disease Control, 1983; Henderson *et al.*, 1983).

A number of studies have shown increases of two to five fold in risk for endometrial cancer in obese women. In North American populations, the attributable risk was in the range 15–30%, depending on the definition of obesity (Mack *et al.*, 1976; Elwood *et al.*, 1977; Kelsey *et al.*, 1982; Henderson *et al.*, 1983). Other studies showed smaller increases in risk associated with use of replacement oestrogens in obese than in nonobese women (Ziel & Finkle, 1975; Mack *et al.*, 1976; Hoogerland *et al.*, 1978; Hulka *et al.*, 1980; Kelsey *et al.*, 1982). The study of Henderson *et al.* (1983), on women aged 45 or less, suggests that the proportion of endometrial cancer that might be prevented in younger women by weight reduction is greater than that in older women.

High correlations between endometrial cancer and high fat intake have been found in international studies (see p. 209), and there is some evidence from case–control studies that fat consumption is related to increased risk. Dietary factors, over and above those resulting in obesity, may be responsible for a proportion of the disease, so it is possible that some reduction in the frequency of endometrial cancer could result from following the general dietary changes recommended for the primary prevention of colorectal cancers; i.e., limiting fat consumption and avoiding excess energy intake.

Cancer of the ovary

The highest reported rate for cancer of the ovary in women of European stock is 15.3 in Norway, and the lowest is 5.4 in Zaragoza, Spain. This suggests a potential for prevention in Norwegian women of 65%; in most other relatively high-risk European populations, the potential appears to be nearer 50%.

Ovarian cancer appears to share certain risk factors with cancers of the breast and endometrium (see p. 244). Nulliparous women are at higher risk than parous women, and factors associated with suppression of ovulation appear to be protective. An association with dietary fat intake was noted in population correlation studies (Armstrong & Doll, 1975) and in two epidemiological studies (see p. 209).

As reviewed on p. 153, use of combined oral contraceptives may substantially reduce the risk for ovarian cancer. The possible reduction may be up to 40% for women over the age of 40 (Rosenberg *et al.*, 1982).

Cancer of the prostate

An indication of the potential for preventing prostatic cancer can be obtained by comparing incidence rates in men of European stock: the highest rate was 70.2 in Utah, USA, and the lowest 9.8 in Cluj County, Romania, indicating a potential for prevention of 86% in men in Utah. However, the very high rates in most registries in the USA may reflect diagnoses of latent prostatic cancer. If the rate in men in Utah is reduced by one-third to account for this effect, the resultant 46.8 (closer to rates in registries with high rates in Canada and Europe as well as New York State) still indicates, in comparison with Romania, a potential for prevention of nearly 80%.

The risk factors proposed for prostatic cancer are hormones, sexual activity and diet (see pp. 209, 246). No clear picture has yet emerged, and it is not therefore possible to make any recommendation concerning preventive measures.

Cancer of the urinary bladder

Among Caucasians, the highest reported rate of bladder cancer in males is in Basel, Switzerland (27.8) and the lowest in Vas, Hungary (7.7), indicating a potential for prevention in Basel of 72%. In females, the highest reported rate is in Connecticut, USA (7.4), and the lowest also in Vas (1.2), indicating a potential for prevention in Connecticut white women of 84%.

A substantial body of evidence implicates tobacco smoking (p. 170) and occupational exposure to aromatic amines (p. 129) as causes of bladder cancer; and in countries of North Africa and the Middle East, schistosomiasis infection plays an important role (p. 194).

The major cohort studies on smoking and cancer agree in showing an approximately two-fold elevation in mortality from bladder cancer in smokers compared to nonsmokers. In the the study of British doctors (Doll & Peto, 1976), the risk in current male smokers relative to nonsmokers after 20 years of follow-up was 1.8, which, if applied to a prevalence of smokers in the general population of 50%, would indicate an attributable risk of around 30%. In the 16-year follow-up of US veterans (Rogot & Murray, 1980), the ratio of observed deaths to those expected in nonsmokers was 2.2 and the difference between observed and expected, 1.75, giving an attributable risk in that population of about 50%. Doll and Peto (1981) calculated that possibly 3811 excess deaths from bladder cancer due to tobacco use occurred in the USA in 1978, giving an attributable risk of 56%. Results from case–control studies are generally consistent with these findings.

Morrison *et al.* (1984) conducted simultaneous population-based case–control studies in Boston, USA, Manchester, UK, and Nagoya, Japan, using similar methods and determined population attributable risks for tobacco use in males and females of 44% and 56% in Boston, 46% and 14% in Manchester, and 34% and 24% in Nagoya, respectively. In the population-based case–control study of Mommsen *et al.* (1983), the attributable risk for smoking among women was 32%. The relative risk for bladder cancer due to smoking black tobacco may be substantially higher (up to five or six fold) than that for blond tobacco (Vineis *et al.*, 1984). Thus, in countries where black tobacco has predominated, such as France, Italy and Spain, the attributable risk could be substantially higher than that in the USA and other countries where most of the tobacco smoked is blond. Vineis *et al.* attributed 70% of male cases and 22% of female cases in Turin to tobacco smoking.

A number of cohort and case–control studies have indicated elevated risks for bladder cancer following certain occupational exposures (see pp. 129, 141–146). One of the first estimates of population attributable risk was derived by Cole (1973) from his population-based study in the Boston, MA, USA, area: an estimate of 18% for certain high-risk occupations was derived for males and 6% for females. Vineis and Simonato (1986) reviewed all case–control studies of bladder cancer in relation to occupation and estimated that the risk attributable to work-place exposures ranged from 0 to 19%. It can be assumed that this range reflects the different distribution of industries and occupations in the populations studied, as well as the methods of defining exposure.

One of the main problems in conducting case–control studies of schistosomiasis as a risk factor is the difficulty in measuring past infection in healthy controls (Cheever, 1978). However, if it is assumed that the transitional-cell form of bladder cancer is not related to infection by *Schistosoma haematobium*, it is possible to view those cases as controls and to calculate the relative risk of infection accordingly. Table 41 summarizes three studies from different parts of Africa, on the basis of which this calculation is made. There is remarkable agreement in the relative risks estimated, despite the widely differing prevalence of infection across the studies. If schistosomiasis is in fact somehow involved in the etiology of transitional-cell cancer, or if there has been misclassification of cell type or infection status, these relative risks will be underestimates. The same data can be used to estimate attributable risk, if the percentage of cases of transitional-cell carcinoma with ova detected is used to estimate the proportion of the population exposed. These estimates are also somewhat consistently around 50%, except for the low estimate from Iraq due to the low estimated prevalence of exposure.

Control of schistosomiasis-related bladder cancer can presumably be achieved most effectively by controlling schistosomiasis infection, which is clearly a desirable goal in itself. Schistosomiasis is now endemic in 74 countries of the world; it is estimated that more than 200 million people living in rural agricultural areas are infected and that 500-600 million people are exposed to infection because of poverty, ignorance, substandard housing and the availability of few, if any, sanitary facilities (Doumenge *et al.*, 1987). Control has been attempted in a number of ways. Molluscicides have been used against the snail hosts, but the agents are expensive and require prolonged, extensive use to be effective; furthermore, control of transmission fell from favour in the 1970s. Various drugs are used to kill the parasites in infected individuals. Safe, effective chemotherapeutic agents, such as metrifonate, oxamniquine and praziquantel, are available (World Health Organization, 1983) and are the basis of the modern method for controlling morbidity in infected populations. Other essential methods of control involve installation of water supplies to minimize contact with infected water, provision of adequate sanitary facilities and education programmes aimed at altering the exposure of people in endemic areas.

Table 41. Bladder cancer cell type and presence of *Schistosoma haematobium* ova in three case-control studies in Africa

Country	No. of patients examined	Squamous-cell tumours (%)	Transitional-cell tumours (%)	Relative risk for association between cell type and presence of ova	Reference
Egypt	1095	73	14	2.8	El-Bolkainy *et al.* (1981)
Malawi	375	80	6	3.6	Lucas (1982)
Iraq	1704	53	37	3.0	Al-Fouadi & Parkin (1984)

Many successes have been reported in various national control programmes (World Health Organization, 1985). In one area of Egypt, with a population of over one million, the combination of widespread molluscicide application and chemotherapy reduced the prevalence of *S. haematobium* infection from 46% to 6% over a nine-year period. A similar programme in Iran resulted in a reduction in infection from 8% to 0.7% over nine years (Iarotski & Davis, 1981). The full effectiveness of such programmes in preventing cancer of the bladder, however, can be estimated only if long-term cancer registration is established in endemic areas where major control campaigns are being implemented.

Cancer of the kidney

The highest rate of cancer of the kidney in men of European origin is 12.2 in Iceland, and the lowest is 1.7 in Cluj County, Romania, suggesting a potential for prevention in Iceland of 86%. In females, the highest rate was 7.6 in Iceland and the lowest 1.3 in Cluj County, suggesting a potential for prevention in Icelandic females of 83%.

For this site, the major risk factor identified is cigarette smoking. Although (as indicated on p. 150), abusers of phenacetin-containing analgesics have an increased risk for cancer of the renal pelvis, the attributable risk is likely to be very low. Increased mortality from kidney cancer has been identified in all of the major cohort studies of tobacco smoking, with relative risks for smokers compared to nonsmokers of 2.7 in the study of British doctors (Doll & Peto, 1976) and 1.4 in the study of US veterans (Rogot & Murray, 1980). Assuming a population prevalence of cigarette smoking of 50%, an attributable risk of the order of 17% to 45% can be estimated for cigarette smoking.

In a hospital-based study of renal adenocarcinoma, Wynder *et al.* (1974) found a dose–response relationship with tobacco smoking in both men and women; the highest risks were 2.2 in people of each sex who smoked more than 20 cigarettes/day. From these data, attributable risks of 35% in men and 15% in women can be calculated. McLaughlin *et al.* (1983, 1984) reported the findings of a large population-based case–control study of cancer of the renal pelvis and kidney adenocarcinoma. Clear dose–response relationships were found for people of each sex with cigarette smoking. Attributable risks for renal pelvic cancer were 82% in men and 61% in women, and those for renal adenocarcinoma were 30% among men and 24% among women. For all renal cancers, the attributable risks for cigarette smoking were about 40% in men and 30% in women.

Leukaemia and lymphoma

The variation in incidence of these malignancies is generally rather less than for most solid tumours. For leukaemia, the incidence in populations of European origin varies from 11.6 in males in Ontario, Canada, to 3.0 in Szabolcs, Hungary, suggesting that up to 75% of male cases are potentially preventable. Differential exposures to the known endogenous causes of leukaemia – ionizing radiation (see Chapter 8), mutagenic drugs (Chapter 7) and chemicals (Chapter 5) and the human T-cell lymphotropic type 1 retrovirus (pp. 191–192), may account for some of the geographic variation; however, population exposure levels to these agents are usually too low to account for more than a small percentage of cases.

The considerable variation in incidence rates of Hodgkin's disease between countries, and the changes within countries for migrant populations and over time (p. 81), suggest important environmental factors in etiology. No practical preventive measure is, however, known. The same is broadly true for the non-Hodgkin's lymphomas, although a small proportion may be attributable to occupational and industrial exposures to herbicides (IARC, 1987) or infection with the human immunodeficiency viruses (p. 192). Burkitt's lymphoma (BL) is common in many parts of sub-Saharan Africa, with incidence rates of up to 80 per million children, compared with 1–3 per million in European populations (Parkin *et al.*, 1988). Since BL in Africa is associated with endemic malaria, and there is some evidence that successful chemotherapy of malaria is associated with a reduced incidence of disease (Geser *et al.*, 1989), it is possible that up to 96% of BL in African children would disappear if successful eradication of malaria were possible.

References

Al-Fouadi, A. & Parkin, D.M. (1984) Cancer in Iraq; seven years' data from the Baghdad Tumour Registry. *Int. J. Cancer*, *34*, 207-213

Armstrong, B.K. (1988) The epidemiology and prevention of cancer in Australia. *Aust. N.Z. J. Surg.*, *58*, 179-187

Armstrong, B. & Doll, R. (1975) Environmental factors and cancer incidence and mortality in different countries, with special reference to dietary practices. *Int. J. Cancer*, *15*, 617-631

Armstrong, R.W., Armstrong, M.J., Yu, M.C. & Henderson, B.E. (1983) Salted fish and inhalants as risk factors for nasopharyngeal carcinoma in Malaysian Chinese. *Cancer Res.*, *43*, 2967-2970

Auerbach, O., Stout, A.P., Hammond, E.C. & Garfinkel, L. (1962) Bronchial epithelium in former smokers. *New Engl. J. Med.*, *267*, 119-125

Auerbach, O., Hammond, E.C. & Garfinkel, L. (1979) Changes in bronchial epithelium in relation to cigarette smoking 1955-1960 vs 1970-1977. *New Engl. J. Med.*, *300*, 381-386

Austin, D.F. & Roe, K.M. (1982) The decreasing incidence of endometrial cancer. Public health implications. *Am. J. Public Health*, *72*, 65-68

Bartsch, H., Ohshima, H. & Pignatelli, B. (1988) Inhibitors of endogenous nitrosation. Mechanisms and implications in human cancer prevention. *Mutat. Res.*, *202*, 307-324

Beasley, R.P., Hwang, L.Y., Lee, C.G.Y., Lan, C.C., Roan, C.H., Huang, F.Y. & Chen, C.L. (1983) Prevention of perinatally transmitted hepatitis B virus infection with hepatitis B immune globulin and hepatitis B vaccine. *Lancet*, *ii*, 1099-1102

Bosch, F.X. & Muñoz, N. (1989) Epidemiology of hepatocellular carcinoma. In: Bannasch, P., Keppler, D. & Weber, G., eds, *Liver Cell Carcinoma* (Falk Symposium 51), Dordrecht, Kluwer Academic Publishers, pp. 3-14

Bradshaw, E. & Schonland, M. (1974) Smoking, drinking and oesophageal cancer in African males of Johannesburg, South Africa. *Br. J. Cancer*, *30*, 157-163

Brinton, L.A., Reeves, W.C., Brenes, M.M., Herrero, R., de Britton, R.C., Gaitan, E., Tenorio, F., Garcia, M. & Rawls, W.E. (1989) Parity as a risk factor for cervical cancer. *Am. J. Epidemiol.*, *130*, 486-496

Burch, J.D., Howe, G.R., Miller, A.B. & Semenciw, R. (1981) Tobacco, alcohol, asbestos and nickel in the etiology of cancer of the larynx: a case-control study. *J. Natl Cancer Inst.*, *67*, 1219-1224

Centers for Disease Control (1983) Cancer. A steroid hormone study. Oral contraceptive use and the risk of endometrial cancer. *J. Am. Med. Assoc.*, *249*, 1600-1604

Cheever, A.M. (1978) Schistosomiasis and neoplasia. *J. Natl Cancer Inst.*, *61*, 13-18

Cole, P. (1973) A population based study of bladder cancer. In: Doll, R. & Vodopija, I., eds, *Host Environment Interactions in the Etiology of Cancer in Man* (IARC Scientific Publications No. 7), Lyon, IARC, pp. 83-87

Cooke, K.R., Skegg, C. & Fraser, J. (1984) Socioeconomic status, indoor and outdoor work, and malignant melanoma. *Int. J. Cancer*, *34*, 57-62

Correa, P. & Haenszel, W. (1982) Epidemiology of gastric cancer. In: Correa, P. & Haenszel, W., eds, *Epidemiology of Cancer of the Digestive Tract* (Developments in Oncology 6), The Hague, Martinus Nijhoff, pp. 59-84

Coursaget, P., Yvonnet, B., Chotard, J., Vincelot, P., Sarr, M., Diouf, C., Chiron, J.P. & Diop-Mor, I. (1987) Age- and sex-related study of hepatitis B virus chronic carrier state in infants from an endemic area (Senegal). *J. Med. Virol.*, *22*, 1-5

Cuzick, J. & Babiker, A.G. (1989) Pancreatic cancer, alcohol, diabetes mellitus and gallbladder disease. *Int. J. Cancer*, *43*, 415-421

Daniels, F., Jr (1975) Sunlight. In: Schottenfeld, D., ed., *Cancer Epidemiology and Prevention: Current Concepts*, Springfield, IL, C.C. Thomas, pp. 126-152

Day, N.E., Baines, C.J., Chamberlain, J., Hakama, M., Miller, A.B. & Prorok, P. (1986) UICC project on screening for cancer: report of the workshop on screening for breast cancer. *Int. J. Cancer*, *38*, 303-308

Doll, R. & Peto, R. (1976) Mortality in relation to smoking: 20 years' observations on male British doctors. *Br. Med. J.*, *ii*, 1525-1536

Doll, R. & Peto, R. (1981) The causes of cancer: quantitative estimates of avoidable risks of cancer in the United States today. *J. Natl Cancer Inst.*, *66*, 1191-1308

Doll, R., Gray, R., Hafner, B. & Peto, R. (1980) Mortality in relation to smoking: 22 years' observations on female British doctors. *Br. Med. J.*, *280*, 967-971

Doumenge, J.P., Mott, M.E., Cheung, C., Villenave, D., Chapuis, O., Perrin, M.F. & Réaud-Thomas, G. (1987) *Atlas of the Global Distribution of Schistosomiasis*, Geneva, World Health Organization

El-Bolkainy, M.N., Mkhtar, N.M., Ghoneim, M.A. & Hussein, M.H. (1981) The impact of schistosomiasis on the pathology of bladder carcinoma. *Cancer*, *48*, 2643-2648

Elwood, J.M., Cole, P., Rothman, K.J. & Kaplan, S.D. (1977) Epidemiology of endometrial cancer. *J. Natl Cancer Inst.*, *59*, 1055-1060

Elwood, J.M., Pearson, J.C.G., Skippen, D.H. & Jackson, S.M. (1984) Alcohol, smoking, social and occupational factors in the aetiology of cancer of the oral cavity, pharynx and larynx. *Int. J. Cancer*, *34*, 603-612

Elwood, J.M., Gallagher, R.P., Hill, G.B. & Pearson, J.C.G. (1985) Cutaneous melanoma in relation to intermittent and constant sun exposure - the western Canada melanoma study. *Int. J. Cancer*, *35*, 427-433

Estève, J., Tuyns, A.J., Raymond, L. & Vineis, P. (1984) Tobacco and the risk of cancer. Importance of kinds of tobacco. In: O'Neill, I.K., von Borstel, R.C., Miller, C.T., Long, J. & Bartsch, H., eds, *N-Nitroso Compounds: Occurrence, Biological Effects and Relevance to Human Cancer* (IARC Scientific Publications No. 57), Lyon, IARC, pp. 867-876

Fears, T.R., Scotto, J. & Schneiderman, M.A. (1977) Mathematical models of age and ultraviolet effects on the incidence of skin cancer among whites in the United States. *Am. J. Epidemiol.*, *105*, 420-427

Flanders, W.D. & Rothman, K.J. (1982) Interaction of alcohol and tobacco in laryngeal cancer. *Am. J. Epidemiol.*, *115*, 371-379

Friedewald, W.T., Kuller, L.H. & Ockene, J.K. (1989) Primary prevention of cancer, relevant Multiple Risk Factor Intervention Trial results. In: Hakama, M., Beral, V., Cullen, J. & Parkin, D.M., eds, *Evaluating Effectiveness of Primary Prevention of Cancer* (IARC Scientific Publications No. 103), Lyon, IARC (in press)

Garfinkel, L. (1980) Cancer mortality in nonsmokers; prospective study by the American Cancer Society. *J. Natl Cancer Inst.*, *65*, 1169-1173

Garfinkel, L. & Stellman, S.D. (1988) Smoking and lung cancer in women: findings in a prospective study. *Cancer Res.*, *48*, 6951-6955

Geser, A., Brubaker, G. & Draper, C.C. (1989) Effect of malaria suppression program on the incidence of African Burkitt's lymphoma. *Am. J. Epidemiol.*, *129*, 740-752

Graham, S., Mettlin, C., Marshall, J., Priore, R., Rzepka, T. & Shedd, D. (1981) Dietary factors in the epidemiology of cancer of the larynx. *Am. J. Epidemiol.*, *113*, 675-680

Green, A., Siskind, V., Bain, C. & Alexander, J. (1985) Sunburn and malignant melanoma. *Br. J. Cancer*, *51*, 393-397

Greenwald, P. & Sondik, E., eds (1986) *Cancer Control Objectives for the Nation: 1985-2000* (Natl Cancer Inst. Monogr. No. 2), Washington DC, US Department of Health and Human Services

Greenwald, P., Caputo, T.A. & Wolfgang, P.E. (1977) Endometrial cancer after menopausal use of oestrogens. *Obstet. Gynecol.*, *50*, 239-243

Gupta, P.C., Mehta, F.S., Pindborg, J.J., Daftary, D.K., Aghi, M.B., Bhonsle, R.B. & Murti, P.R. (1990) A primary prevention study of oral cancer among Indian villagers. Eight-year follow-up results. In: Hakama, M., Beral, V., Cullen, J. & Parkin, D.M., eds, *Evaluating Effectiveness of Primary Prevention of Cancer* (IARC Scientific Publications No. 103), Lyon, IARC (in press)

Hakama, M., Beral, V., Cullen, J. & Parkin, D.M., eds (1989) *Evaluating Effectiveness of Primary Prevention of Cancer* (IARC Scientific Publications No. 103), Lyon, IARC (in press)

Hakulinen, T., Pukkala, E., Kenward, M., Teppo, L., Puska, P., Tuomilehto, J. & Kuulasmaa, K. (1989) Changes in cancer incidence in north Karelia, an area with a comprehensive preventive cardiovascular programme. In: Hakama, M., Beral, V., Cullen, J. & Parkin, D.M., eds, *Evaluating Effectiveness of Primary Prevention of Cancer* (IARC Scientific Publications No. 103), Lyon, IARC (in press)

Hammond, E.C. (1966) Smoking in relation to the death rates of one million men and women. *Natl Cancer Inst. Monogr.*, *19*, 127-204

Hammond, E.C., Garfinkel, L., Seidman, H. & Law, E.A. (1977) Some recent findings concerning cigarette smoking. In: Hiatt, H.H., Watson, J.D., Winsten, J.A., eds, *Origins of Human Cancer*, Book A, *Incidence of Cancer in Humans*, Cold Spring Harbor, NY, CSH Press, pp. 101-112

Havery, D.C., Fazio, T. & Howard, J.W. (1978) Trends in levels of *N*-nitrosopyrrolidine in fried bacon. *J. Assoc. Off. Anal. Chem.*, *61*, 1379-1382

Henderson, B.E., Powell, D., Rosario, I., Keys, C., Hanisch, R., Young, M., Casagrande, J., Gerkins, V. & Pike, M.C. (1974) An epidemiologic study of breast cancer. *J. Natl Cancer Inst.*, *53*, 609-614

Henderson, B.E., Louie, E., Soo Hoo Jing, J., Buell, P. & Gardner, M.B. (1976) Risk factors associated with nasopharyngeal carcinoma. *New Engl. J. Med.*, *295*, 1101-1106

Henderson, B.E., Casagrande, J.T., Pike, M.C., Mack, T., Rosario, I. & Duke, A. (1983) The epidemiology of endometrial cancer in young women. *Br. J. Cancer*, *47*, 749-756

Hinds, M.W., Thomas, D.B. & O'Reilly, H.P. (1979) Asbestos, dental X-rays, tobacco, and alcohol in the epidemiology of laryngeal cancer. *Cancer*, *44*, 1114-1120

Hirayama, T. (1975) Smoking and cancer: a prospective study on cancer epidemiology based on a census population in Japan. In: Steinfeld, J., Griffiths, W., Ball, K. *et al.*, eds, *Proceedings of the 3rd World Conference on Smoking and Health*, Vol. II, Washington DC, US Department of Health, Education, and Welfare, pp. 65-72

Hjerman, I., Holme, I., Velve Byre, K. & Leren, P. (1981) Effect of diet and smoking intervention on the incidence of coronary heart disease: report from the Oslo Study Group of a randomized trial in healthy men. *Lancet*, *ii*, 1303-1310

Hoogerland, D.L., Buchler, D.A., Crowley, J.J. & Carr, W.F. (1978) Estrogen use - risk of endometrial cancer. *Gynecol. Oncol.*, *6*, 451-458

Hulka, B.S., Fowler, W.C., Kaufman, D.G., Grimson, R.C., Greenberg, B.G., Hogue, C.J., Berger, G.S. & Pulliam, C.C. (1980) Estrogens and endometrial cancer: cases and two control groups from North Carolina. *Am. J. Obstet. Gynecol.*, *137*, 92-101

IARC (1986a) *IARC Monographs on the Evaluation of the Carcinogenic Risk of Chemicals to Humans*, Vol. 38, *Tobacco Smoking*, Lyon

IARC (1986b) Screening for squamous cervical cancer: duration of low risk after negative results of cervical cytology and its implication for screening policies. *Br. Med. J.*, *293*, 659-664

IARC (1987) *IARC Monographs on the Evaluation of Carcinogenic Risks to Humans*, Suppl. 7, *Overall Evaluations of Carcinogenicity: An Updating of* IARC Monographs *Volumes 1 to 42*, Lyon

IARC Working Group (1986) Summary chapter. In: Hakama, M., Miller, A.B. & Day, N.E., eds, *Screening for Cancer of the Uterine Cervix* (IARC Scientific Publications No. 76), Lyon, IARC, pp. 133-144

Iarotski, L. & Davis, A. (1981) The schistosomiasis problem in the world: results of a WHO questionnaire survey. *Bull. World Health Organ.*, *59*, 115-127

Iran/IARC Cancer Study Group (1977) Esophageal cancer studies in the Caspian littoral of Iran: results of population studies - a prodrome. *J. Natl Cancer Inst.*, *59*, 1127-1138

Jayant, K., Balakrishnan, V., Sanghvi, L.D. & Jussawalla, D.J. (1977) Quantification of the role of smoking and chewing tobacco in oral, pharyngeal, and esophageal cancers. *Br. J. Cancer*, *35*, 232-235

Jick, H., Watkins, R.N., Hunter, J.R., Dinan, B.J., Madsen, S., Rothman, K.J. & Walker, A.M. (1979) Replacement estrogens and endometrial cancer. *New Engl. J. Med.*, *300*, 218-222

Jick, H., Walker, A.M., Rothman, K.J. (1980) The epidemic of endometrial cancer: a commentary. *Am. J. Public Health*, *70*, 264-267

Joly, O.G., Lubin, J.H. & Caraballoso, M. (1983) Dark tobacco and lung cancer in Cuba. *J. Natl Cancer Inst.*, *70*, 1033-1039

Jussawalla, D.J. (1971) Epidemiological assessment of aetiology of oesophageal cancer in Greater Bombay. In: Jussawalla, J.D. & Doll, R., eds, *International Seminar on the Epidemiology of Oesophageal Cancer, Bangalore, 4 November 1971*, Bombay, Indian Cancer Society, pp. 20-30

Jussawalla, D.J. & Deshpande, V.A. (1971) Evaluation of cancer risk in tobacco chewers and smokers: an epidemiologic assessment. *Cancer, 28*, 244-252

Kahn, H.A. (1966) The Dorn study of smoking and mortality among US veterans. Report on eight and one-half years of observation. *Natl Cancer Inst. Monogr., 19*, 1-125

Kelsey, J.L., LiVolsi, V.A., Holford, T.R., Fischer, D.B., Mostow, E.D., Schwartz, P.E., O'Connor, T. & White, C. (1982) A case–control study of cancer of the endometrium. *Am. J. Epidemiol., 116*, 333-342

Kolonel, L.N., Hinds, M.W. & Hankin, J.H. (1980) Cancer patterns among migrant and native-born Japanese in Hawaii in relation to smoking, drinking and dietary habits. In: Gelboin, H.V., MacMahon, B., Matsushima, T., Sugimura, T., Takayama, S. & Takebe, H., eds, *Genetic and Environmental Factors in Experimental and Human Cancer*, Tokyo, Japan Scientific Societies Press, pp. 327-340

Kvåle, G., Bjelke, E. & Heuch, I. (1986) Occupational exposure and lung cancer risk. *Int. J. Cancer, 37*, 185-193

Lew, E.A. & Garfinkel, L. (1979) Variations in mortality by weight among 750,000 men and women. *J. Chronic Dis., 32*, 563-576

Lin, T.M., Chen, K.P., Lin, C.C., Hsu, M.M., Tu, S.M., Chiang, T.C., Jung, P.F. & Hirayama, T. (1973) Retrospective study on nasopharyngeal carcinoma. *J. Natl Cancer Inst., 51*, 1403-1408

Longnecker, M.P., Berlin, J.A., Orza, M.J. & Chalmers, T.C. (1988) A meta-analysis of alcohol consumption in relation to risk of breast cancer. *J. Am. Med. Assoc., 260*, 252-256

Lubin, J.H., Blot, W.J., Berrino, F., Lamant, F., Gilles, C.R., Kunze, M., Schmahl, D. & Visco, G. (1984) Modifying risk of developing lung cancer by changing habits of cigarette smoking. *Br. Med. J., 288*, 1953-1956

Lubin, F., Ruder, A.M., Wax, Y. & Modan, B. (1985) Overweight and changes in weight throughout adult life in breast cancer etiology. A case–control study. *Am. J. Epidemiol., 122*, 579-588

Lucas, S.B. (1982) Bladder tumours in Malawi. *Br. J. Urol., 54*, 275-279

Mack, T.M., Pike, M.C., Henderson, B.E., Pfeffer, R.I., Gerkins, V.R., Arthur, M. & Brown, S.E. (1976) Estrogens and endometrial cancer in a retirement community. *New Engl. J. Med., 294*, 1262-1267

Mack, T.M., Yu, M.C., Hanisch, R. & Henderson, B.E. (1986) Pancreas cancer and smoking, beverage consumption, and past medical history. *J. Natl Cancer Inst., 76*, 49-60

MacMahon, B., Cole, P., Lin, T.M., Lowe, C.R., Mirra, A.P., Ravnihar, B., Salber, E.J., Valaoras, V.G. & Yuasa, S. (1970) Age at first birth and breast cancer risk. *Bull. World Health Organ., 43*, 209-221

MacMahon, B., Yen, S., Trichopoulos, D., Warren, K. & Nardi, G. (1981) Coffee and cancer of the pancreas. *New Engl. J. Med., 304*, 630-633

Martinez, I. (1969) Factors associated with cancer of the oesophagus, mouth and pharynx in Puerto Rico. *J. Natl Cancer Inst., 42*, 1069-1094

Maupas, P., Chiron, J.-P., Barin, F., Coursaget, P., Goudeau, A., Perrin, J., Denis, F. & Diop Mor, I. (1981) Efficacy of hepatitis B vaccine in prevention of early HBsAg carrier state in children - controlled trial in an endemic area (Senegal). *Lancet, i*, 289-292

McLaughlin, J.K., Blot, W.J., Mandel, J.S., Schuman, L.M., Mehl, E.S. & Fraumeni, J.F., Jr (1983) Etiology of cancer of the renal pelvis. *J. Natl Cancer Inst., 71*, 287-291

McLaughlin, J.K., Mandel, J.S., Blot, W.J., Schuman, L.M., Mehl, E.S. & Fraumeni, J.F., Jr (1984) A population-based case–control study of renal cell carcinoma. *J. Natl Cancer Inst., 72*, 275-284

Mehta, F.S., Gupta, M.B., Pindborg, J.J., Bhonsle, R.B., Jalhawalla, P.N. & Sinor, P.N. (1982) An intervention study of oral cancer and precancer in rural Indian populations: a preliminary report. *Bull. World Health Organ., 60*, 441-446

Miller, A.B. (1978) An overview of hormone-associated cancers. *Cancer Res., 38*, 3985-3990

Mommsen, S., Aagaard, J. & Sell, A. (1983) A case–control study of female bladder cancer. *Eur. J. Cancer Clin. Oncol., 19*, 725-729

Morrison, A.S., Buring, J.E., Verhoek, W.G., Aoki, K., Leck, I., Ohno, Y. & Obata, K. (1984) An international study of smoking and bladder cancer. *J. Urol., 131*, 650-654

Muir, C., Waterhouse, J., Mack, T., Powell, J. & Whelan, S., eds (1987) *Cancer Incidence in Five Continents, Vol. V* (IARC Scientific Publications No. 88), Lyon, IARC

Muñoz, N. & Bosch, F.X. (1987) Epidemiology of hepatocellular carcinoma. In: Okuda, K. & Ishak, K.G., eds, *Neoplasms of the Liver*, Tokyo, Springer, pp. 3-19

National Research Council (1989) *Diet and Health. Implications for Reducing Chronic Disease Risk*, Washington DC, National Academy Press

Newark, H.L., Wargovich, M.J. & Bruce, W.R. (1984) Colon cancer and dietary fat, phosphate and calcium: a hypothesis. *J. Natl Cancer Inst.*, 72, 1323-1325

Notani, P., Jayant, K. & Sanghvi, L.D. (1989) Assessment of morbidity and mortality due to tobacco usage in India. In: Sanghvi, L.D. & Notani, P., eds, *Tobacco and Health. The Indian Scene*, Bombay, Tata Memorial Centre

Oettle, A.G. (1964) Cancer in Africa. Especially in regions south of the Sahara. *J. Natl Cancer Inst.*, 33, 383-439

Paffenbarger, R.S., Kampert, J.B. & Chang, H.-G. (1980) Characteristics that predict risk of breast cancer before and after the menopause. *Am. J. Epidemiol.*, 112, 258-268

Parkin, D.M. (1985) A computer simulation model for the practical planning of cervical cancer screening programmes. *Br. J. Cancer*, 51, 551-568

Parkin, D.M., Stiller, C.A., Draper, G.J., Bieber, C.A., Terracini, B. & Young, J.L., eds (1988) *International Incidence of Childhood Cancer* (IARC Scientific Publications No. 89), Lyon, IARC

Pastorino, U., Berrino, F., Gervasio, A., Pesenti, V., Riboli, E. & Crosignani, P. (1984) Proportion of lung cancers due to occupational exposure. *Int. J. Cancer*, 33, 231-237

Peers, F., Bosch, F.X., Kaldor, J., Linsell, A. & Pluijmen, M. (1987) Aflatoxin exposure, hepatitis B virus infection and liver cancer in Swaziland. *Int. J. Cancer*, 39, 545-553

Pike, M.C., Jing, J.S., Rosario, I.P., Henderson, B.E. & Menck, H.R. (1978) Occupation: 'explanation' of an apparent air pollution related localized excess of lung cancer in Los Angeles County. In: Breslow, N. & Whittemore, A., eds, *Energy and Health*, Philadelphia, SIAM, pp. 3-16

Pottern, L.M., Morris, L.E., Blot, W.J., Ziegler, R.G. & Fraumeni, J.F., Jr (1981) Esophageal cancer among black men in Washington, DC. Alcohol, tobacco and other risk factors. *J. Natl Cancer Inst.*, 67, 777-783

Raymond, L., Infante, F., Tuyns, A.J., Voirol, M. & Lowenfels, A.B. (1987) Alimentation et cancer du pancréas. *Gastroenterol. Clin. Biol.*, 11, 488-492

Rogot, E., Murray, J.L. (1980) Smoking and causes of death among US veterans: 16 years of observation. *Public Health Rep.*, 95, 213-222

Rose, E.F. & McGlashan, N.D. (1975) The spatial distribution of oesophageal carcinoma in the Transkei, South Africa. *Br. J. Cancer*, 31, 197-206

Rose, G., Hamilton, P., Colwell, L. & Shapely, M. (1982) A randomized controlled trial of anti-smoking advice: 10 year results. *J. Epidemiol. Community Health*, 36, 102-108

Rosenberg, L., Shapiro, S., Slone, D., Kaufman, D.W., Helmrich, S.P., Miettinen, O.S., Stolley, P.D., Rosenshein, N.B., Schottenfeld, D. & Engle, R.L., Jr (1982) Epithelial ovarian cancer and combination oral contraceptives. *J. Am. Med. Assoc.*, 247, 3210-3212

Rothman, K. & Keller, A. (1972) The effect of joint exposure to alcohol and tobacco on risk of cancer of the mouth and pharynx. *J. Chronic Dis.*, 25, 711-716

Sanghvi, L.D., Rao, K.C.M. & Khanolkar, V.R. (1955) Smoking and chewing of tobacco in relation to cancer of the upper alimentary tract. *Br. Med. J.*, i, 1111-1114

Scotto, J. & Fraumeni, J.F., Jr (1982) Skin (other than melanoma). In: Schottenfeld, D. & Fraumeni, J.F., Jr, eds, *Cancer Epidemiology and Prevention*, Philadelphia, Saunders, pp. 996-1011

Shanta, V. & Krishnamurthi, S. (1963) Further study in aetiology of carcinomas of the upper alimentary tract. *Br. J. Cancer*, 17, 8-23

Shapiro, S., Kelly, J.P., Rosenberg, L., Kaufman, D.W., Helmrich, S.P., Rosenshein, N.B., Lewis, J.L., Jr, Knapp, R.C., Stolley, P.D. & Schottenfeld, D. (1985) Risk of localized and widespread endometrial cancer in relation to recent and discontinued use of conjugated estrogens. *New Engl. J. Med.*, 31, 969-972

Shimizu, H., Mack, T., Ross, R.K. & Henderson, B.E. (1987) Cancer of the gastrointestinal tract among Japanese and white immigrants in Los Angeles county. *J. Natl Cancer Inst.*, 78, 223-228

Shopland, D.R. (1989) Changes in lung cancer risk following smoking cessation. In: Hakama, M., Beral, V., Cullen, J. & Parkin, D.M., eds, *Evaluating Effectiveness of Primary Prevention of Cancer* (IARC Scientific Publications No. 103), Lyon, IARC (in press)

Simonato, L., Vineis, P. & Fletcher, A.C. (1988) Estimates of the proportion of lung cancer attributable to occupational exposure. *Carcinogenesis*, *9*, 1159-1165

Stellman, S.D. (1986) Influence of cigarette yield on coronary heart disease and chronic obstructive pulmonary disease. In: Zaridze, D. & Peto, R., eds, *Tobacco: A Major International Health Hazard* (IARC Scientific Publications No. 74), Lyon, IARC, pp. 237-249

Szmuness, W., Stevens, C.E., Harley, E.J., Zang, E.A., Oleszko, W.R., William, D.C., Sadovsky, R., Morrison, J.M. & Kellner, A. (1980) Hepatitis B vaccine: demonstration of efficacy in a controlled trial in a high-risk population in the United States. *New Engl. J. Med.*, *30*, 833-841

Task Force (1982) Cervical cancer screening programs: summary of the 1982 Canadian Task Force report. *Can. Med. Assoc. J.*, *127*, 531-589

The Gambia Hepatitis Study Group (1987) The Gambia hepatitis intervention study. *Cancer Res.*, *47*, 5782-5787

Toniolo, P., Riboli, E., Protta, F., Charrel, M. & Cappa, A.P.M. (1989) Alcohol and wine consumption and risk of breast cancer in northern Italy. *Cancer Res.*, *49*, 5203-5206

Tuyns, A.J., Péquignot, G. & Jensen, O.M. (1977) Le cancer de l'oesophage en Ille-et-Vilaine en fonction des niveaux de consommation d'alcool et de tabac. Des risques qui se multiplient. *Bull. Cancer*, *64*, 45-60

Tuyns, A.J., Riboli, E., Doornbos, G. & Péquignot, G. (1987) Diet and esophageal cancer in Calvados (France). *Nutr. Cancer*, *9*, 81-92

Tuyns, A.J., Estève, J., Raymond, L., Berrino, F., Benhamou, E., Blanchet, F., Boffetta, P., Crosignani, P., del Moral, A., Lehmann, W., Merletti, F., Péquignot, G., Riboli, E., Sancho-Garnier, H., Terracini, B., Zubiri, A. & Zubiri, Z. (1988) Cancer of the larynx/hypopharynx, tobacco and alcohol. *Int. J. Cancer*, *41*, 483-491

Urbach, F. (1971) Geographic distribution of skin cancer. *J. Surg. Oncol.*, *3*, 219-234

US Department of Health and Human Services (1982) *The Health Consequences of Smoking: Cancer. A Report of the Surgeon General*, Washington DC, US Public Health Service

US Department of Health and Human Services (1989) *Reducing the Health Consequences of Smoking: 25 Years of Progress. A Report of the Surgeon General* (DHSS Publication No (CDC) 89-8411), Washington DC, US Public Health Service

Vagero, D., Ringback, G. & Kiviranta, H. (1986) Melanoma and other tumors of the skin among office, other indoor and outdoor workers in Sweden, 1961-1979. *Br. J. Cancer*, *53*, 507-512

Vassallo, A., Correa, P., De Stefani, E., Cendan, M., Zavala, D., Chen, V., Carzoglio, J. & Deneo-Pellegrini, H. (1985) Esophageal cancer in Uruguay: a case-control study. *J. Natl Cancer Inst.*, *75*, 1005-1009

Victora, C.G., Muñoz, N., Day, N.E., Barcelos, L.B., Peccin, D.A. & Braga, N.M. (1987) Hot beverages and oesophageal cancer in southern Brazil: a case-control study. *Int. J. Cancer*, *39*, 710-716

Vineis, P. & Simonato, L. (1986) Estimates of the proportion of bladder cancers attributable to occupation. *Scand. J. Work Environ. Health*, *12*, 55-60

Vineis, P., Estève, J. & Terracini, B. (1984) Bladder cancer and smoking in males: types of cigarettes, age at start, effect of stopping and interaction with occupation. *Int. J. Cancer*, *34*, 165-170

de Waard, F. & Baanders van Halewijn, E.A. (1974) A prospective study in general practice on breast cancer risk in postmenopausal women. *Int. J. Cancer*, *14*, 153-160

de Waard, F., Cornelis, J.P., Aoki, K. & Yoshida, M. (1977) Breast cancer incidence according to weight and height in two cities of the Netherlands and in Aichi prefecture Japan. *Cancer*, *40*, 1269-1275

Wahi, P.N., Kehar, U. & Lahiri, B. (1965) Factors influencing oral and oropharyngeal cancers in India. *Br. J. Cancer*, *19*, 642-660

Weiss, N.S. & Sayvetz, T.A. (1980) Incidence of endometrial cancer in relation to the use of oral contraceptives. *New Engl. J. Med.*, *302*, 551-554

Weiss, N.S., Szekely, D.R. & Austin, D.F. (1976) Increasing incidence of endometrial cancer in the United States. *New Engl. J. Med.*, *294*, 1259-1262

WHO Collaborative Group (1989) WHO European collaborative trial in the multifactorial prevention of coronary heart disease. In: Hakama, M., Beral, V., Cullen, J. & Parkin, D.M., eds, *Evaluating Effectiveness of Primary Prevention of Cancer* (IARC Scientific Publications No. 103), Lyon, IARC (in press)

World Health Organization (1983) *The Role of Chemotherapy in Schistosomiasis Control* (WHI SCHISTO/83.70), Geneva

World Health Organization (1984) WHO viral hepatitis programme. *Bull. World Health Organ.*, *62*, 849-852

World Health Organization (1985) *The Control of Schistosomiasis* (World Health Organ. Tech. Rep. Ser. 728), Geneva

Wu, A.H., Henderson, B.E., Pike, M.C. & Yu, M.C. (1985) Smoking and other risk factors for lung cancer in women. *J. Natl Cancer Inst.*, *74*, 747-751

Wynder, E.L. & Bross, I.J. (1961) A study of etiological factors in cancer of the esophagus. *Cancer*, *14*, 389-413

Wynder, E.L., Bross, I.J. & Feldman, R.M. (1957) A study of the etiological factors in cancer of the mouth. *Cancer*, *10*, 1300-1322

Wynder, E.L., Mabuchi, K., Maruchi, N. & Fortner, J.G. (1973) Epidemiology of cancer in the pancreas. *J. Natl Cancer Inst.*, *50*, 645-667

Wynder, E.L., Mabuchi, K. & Whitmore, W.F., Jr (1974) Epidemiology of adenocarcinoma of the kidney. *J. Natl Cancer Inst.*, *53*, 1619-1634

Wynder, E.L., Covey, L.S., Mabuchi, K. & Mushinski, M. (1976) Environmental factors in cancer of the larynx. A second look. *Cancer*, *38*, 1591-1601

Wynder, E.L., Hall, N.E.L. & Polansky, M. (1983) Epidemiology of coffee and pancreatic cancer. *Cancer Res.*, *43*, 3900-3906

Yu, M.C., Mack, T., Hanisch, R., Peters, R.L., Henderson, B.E. & Pike, M.C. (1983) Hepatitis, alcohol consumption, cigarette smoking, and hepatocellular carcinoma in Los Angeles. *Cancer Res.*, *43*, 6077-6079

Yu, M.C., Ho, J.H.C., Lai, S.H. & Henderson, B.E. (1986) Cantonese-style salted fish as a cause of nasopharyngeal carcinoma: report of a case–control study in Hong Kong. *Cancer Res.*, *46*, 956-961

Yu, M.C., Mo, C.-C., Chong, W.-X., Yeh, F.-S. & Henderson, B.E. (1988) Preserved foods and nasopharyngeal carcinoma: a case–control study in Guangxi, China. *Cancer Res.*, *48*, 1954-1959

Yu, M.C., Huang, T.-B. & Henderson, B.E. (1989) Diet and nasopharyngeal carcinoma: a case–control study in Guangzhou, China. *Int. J. Cancer*, *43*, 1077-1082

Ziegler, R.G., Morris, L.E., Blot, W.J., Pottern, L.M., Hoover, R. & Fraumeni, J.F., Jr (1981) Esophageal cancer among black men in Washington, DC. II. Role of nutrition. *J. Natl Cancer Inst.*, *67*, 1199-1206

Ziel, H.K. & Finkle, W.D. (1975) Increased risk of endometrial carcinoma among users of conjugated estrogens. *New Engl. J. Med.*, *293*, 1167-1170

CONCLUSION

In the last chapter, we summarized the available evidence on the preventability of human cancer, either through primary prevention (reducing exposure to environmental risk factors or increasing resistance to them) or by programmes of early detection and treatment. Some indication of the potential size of the reduction in incidence or mortality was given, when this was possible. For primary prevention, precise estimates require information on the magnitude of the excess risk for, and the prevalence of exposure to, the environmental agents concerned. Similarly, for screening, if there is information on the reduction in incidence or mortality in relation to different screening intensities, an estimate of the probable benefit of a programme can be made. For some countries where there has been a large volume of epidemiological research, and where population surveys have been conducted so that the prevalence of exposure to possible carcinogens is known, reasonable quantitative estimates of the preventability of cancer are possible. For example, such estimates were used in preparing targets for cancer control in the USA (Doll & Peto, 1981; Greenwald & Sondik, 1986) and in Australia (Armstrong, 1988). This type of exercise is less easy elsewhere where populations are less well characterized, and for many countries, particularly in the developing world, it is virtually impossible.

Table 42 attempts to summarize in very general terms the preventability of the major cancers of the world, on the basis of the data presented in this book. While no 'bottom line' estimate of preventability of either morbidity or death can be made, it is clear that high proportions of cancer are both potentially and actually preventable given present knowledge. That said, there remains a series of challenges for cancer research and public health: to gain an understanding of the causes of those common cancers, such as cancer of the ovary and of the prostate, that are as yet poorly understood; to increase the certainty with which we can advocate preventive measures for any other cancers; and to apply prevention in practice for those cancers over which some certainty of understanding prevails, so that the benefits of over 100 years of research on cancer etiology can be fully realized.

Table 42. Theoretical preventability and estimated reduction in risk for cancers at selected sites

Site	Estimated no. of cases worldwide (1980)	Differences in risk between highest and lowest recorded incidences in Table 7 (%; M/F)	Preventive measure	Regions or countries to which data apply	Potential reduction in incidence or mortality
Oral cavity & pharynx	378 500	95/88	Elimination of tobacco smoking and chewing	Asia	60 – 80%
			Elimination of tobacco smoking and reduction in alcohol consumption	Europe, Americas	60 – 80%
			Avoidance of salted fish [for nasopharynx]	Southern Chinese populations	10 – 90%
Oesophagus	310 400	96/94	Elimination of tobacco smoking and reduction in alcohol consumption	USA, Caribbean, southern Europe, India	75%
			General improvement in nutrition (micro-nutrients?)	Central Asia, China	35%
					Uncertain
Stomach	669 400	86/85	High consumption of fresh vegetables and fruit	Worldwide	up to 50%[a]
			Screening by photofluorography	Japan	up to 50%[a,b]
Colon/Rectum	572 100	80/80	Low fat and animal protein consumption; high vegetable consumption	'Western' countries	up to 35%[a]
			Screening by proctosigmoidoscopy or for occult blood in faeces	'Western' countries	Uncertain[b]
Liver	251 200	93/90	Vaccination against hepatitis B virus	Sub-Saharan Africa, south-east Asia	70%
			Reduction of aflatoxin contamination	Sub-Saharan Africa, south-east Asia	40%[a]
			Reduction of alcohol consumption	'Western' countries	15%[a]
Pancreas	137 400	70/73	Elimination of tobacco smoking	Worldwide	30%
Larynx	120 000	84/87	Elimination of tobacco smoking and reduction in alcohol consumption	Worldwide	85%
Lung	660 500	75/92	Elimination of tobacco smoking	Worldwide	80 – 90% males / 60 – 80% females[c]
			Elimination of certain occupational exposures	Industrialized countries	10%
			Reduction of air pollution	Industrialized countries and large urban areas	Uncertain

Cancer site	Incidence		Intervention	Region	Estimated reduction
Melanoma	(70 000)[d]	96/95	Reduction in recreational sun exposure and use of sun-screens	Europe, North America, Australia/New Zealand	>40%
			Surveillance of high-risk groups	Europe, North America, Australia/New Zealand	Uncertain[b]
Non-melanoma skin cancer	?	97/99	Reduction in sun exposure	Europe, North America, Australia/New Zealand	Uncertain, but high
Breast	572 100	79	Low fat and animal protein consumption	'Western' countries	Uncertain
			Weight reduction for the obese	Worldwide	10%[e]
			Screening by mammography every two years at 50 or more years of age	'Western' countries	35 – 40%[b,c]
Cervix	465 600	78	Elimination of tobacco smoking	'Western' countries	Uncertain
			Reduction in high parity	Developing countries	30%[b]
			Use of barrier contraceptives	Worldwide	Uncertain
			Reduction in infection rate of sexually transmitted diseases	Worldwide	50%
			Cytological screening:		
			3 yearly at ages 35–64	'Western' countries	80%
			10 yearly at ages 35–64	Developing countries	55%
Endometrium	148 800	83	Weight reduction for the obese	Worldwide	25%
			Elimination of use of post-menopausal oestrogens	USA, Europe	40%[f]
Ovary	137 600	65	Uncertain	–	–[g]
Prostate	235 800	86	Uncertain	–	–[g]
Bladder	219 400	72/84	Elimination of tobacco smoking	Worldwide	30 – 70%
			Elimination of certain occupational exposures	Industrialized countries	10 – 20%
			Elimination of schistosomal infection	Africa, eastern Mediterranean	50%
Kidney	(100 000)[d]	86/83	Elimination of tobacco smoking	'Western' countries	30 – 40%
Lymphoma	237 900	79/87	Control of malaria	Sub-Saharan Africa	25%[a]
Leukaemia	188 200	74/66	Avoidance of unnecessary exposure to radiation and benzene	Worldwide	Uncertain

[a] Estimate very approximate
[b] Refers to reduction in mortality *only* (no change in incidence)
[c] Uncertain (but less) for women in China
[d] Estimated using incidence rates in the Appendix
[e] Women over 50 years of age
[f] Reduction in relation to a situation of the 1960s and 1970s
[g] Evidence of a reduced risk following use of combination oral contraceptives

Appendix. Age-standardized incidence rates per 100 000 for selected registries by site (with ICD-9 code) and sex[a]

Registry	Lip (140)		Tongue (141)		Salivary gland (142)		Mouth (143–5)		Naso-pharynx (147)	
	M	F	M	F	M	F	M	F	M	F
Senegal, Dakar[b]	0,2	0,4	0.9	0,3	0.5	–	1.0	1.3	0,1	–
Brazil, São Paulo	5.4	1.3	7.4	0.9	1.7	1.1	8.0	2.2	1.4	0.4
Colombia, Cali	1.0	0,3	1.8	0.5	1.2	1.0	1.9	1.6	0,4	0,4
USA, Puerto Rico	0.8	0.2	5.7	1.2	0.6	0.5	6.4	1.8	0.6	0.2
USA, SEER registries: whites[c]	3.3	0.3	2.8	1.3	1.0	0.7	4.0	2.1	0.6	0.2
USA, SEER registries: blacks[c]	0,1	0,1	2.7	1.3	0.7	0.7	7.2	2.4	0.9	0.4
China, Shanghai	0.2	0.1	0.5	0.5	0.5	0.5	1.2	0.8	4.4	2.0
India, Bombay	0.3	0.2	9.4	3.4	0.5	0.4	6.5	5.0	0.8	0.3
Israel: Jews	3.6	0.8	0.7	0.4	0.6	0.6	0.9	0.6	1.2	0.4
Israel: non-Jews	2.7	0,2	0,5	0,3	0,2	0,2	1.9	0,4	1,0	0,2
Japan, Miyagi	0,1	0,0	1.1	0.4	0.5	0.3	0.5	0.2	0.5	0.2
Philippines, Rizal	0,1	0,2	1.4	1.6	0.5	0.4	3.1	4.5	4.7	2.6
Czechoslovakia, Slovakia	6.6	0.8	2.8	0.2	0.6	0.4	3.4	0.4	0.5	0.2
Sweden	2.5	0.3	0.9	0.5	0.7	0.7	1.5	0.6	0.5	0.2
France, Bas-Rhin	0.7	–	7.4	0.8	0.8	0.6	13.5	0.8	1.1	0,1
Spain, Navarra	7.7	0.7	2.9	0,2	0,5	0,4	2.8	0,4	1.1	0,2
UK, England & Wales	0.7	0.1	1.0	0.5	0.5	0.4	1.2	0.5	0.4	0.2
Australia, New South Wales	4.2	0.8	2.0	0.9	0.9	0.4	2.5	1.1	0.8	0.3
New Zealand: Maoris	–	–	0,3	0,5	1,6	0,7	0,9	1,3	1,9	0,6
USA, Hawaii: Hawaiians	0,0	0,0	1,8	1,1	0,7	1,1	2,0	1,9	0,6	1,1

Registry	Oropharynx, hypopharynx & pharynx unspeci-fied (146,148,149)		Oesophagus (150)		Stomach (151)	
	M	F	M	F	M	F
Senegal, Dakar[b]	0,5	–[d]	0,2	0,2	3.7	2.0
Brazil, São Paulo[b]	8.1	1.1	16.2	4.0	53.6	25.1
Colombia, Cali	2.1	1.0	3.1	1.9	49.6	26.3
USA, Puerto Rico	9.0	1.1	11.9	3.7	17.6	8.6
USA, SEER registries: whites[c]	3.9	1.5	4.2	1.4	10.0	4.3
USA, SEER registries: blacks[c]	8.7	2.6	18.1	5.3	19.2	7.2
China, Shanghai	0.6	0.3	20.8	8.9	58.3	24.6
India, Bombay	16.8	4.3	14.7	10.3	8.9	6.0
Israel:Jews	0.5	0.2	1.9	1.4	16.2	9.3
Israel: non-Jews	0,4	0,6	1,0	0,9	7.9	4.9
Japan, Miyagi	0.6	0.1	13.3	3.1	79.6	36.0
Philippines, Rizal	2.3	1.9	1.9	1.6	9.4	6.7
Czechoslovakia, Slovakia	3.7	0.3	4.1	0.3	31.7	14.5
Sweden	1.3	0.4	3.0	0.8	15.0	7.5
France, Bas-Rhin	25.6	0.9	16.7	1.0	15.5	7.4
Spain, Navarra	2.4	0,3	6.9	0.7	31.6	13.5
UK, England & Wales	1.4	0.7	5.9	3.1	18.5	7.8
Australia, New South Wales	3.0	0.7	3.7	1.9	12.9	5.9
New Zealand: Maoris	1.8	0,7	7.4	1,4	29.8	19.7
USA, Hawaii: Hawaiians	2,4	1,2	11.0	1,7	31.2	14.9

Registry	Colon (153)		Rectum (154)		Liver (155)		Pancreas (157)	
	M	F	M	F	M	F	M	F
Senegal, Dakar[b]	0,6	0.7	1.5	1.0	25.6	9.0	1.0	1,0
Brazil, São Paulo	13.0	12.0	9.0	9.1	3.8	2.6	7.3	4.6
Colombia, Cali	5.2	6.3	3.4	3.7	2.8	1.4	5.2	3.6
USA, Puerto Rico	10.3	9.7	7.4	5.4	3.1	1.6	4.9	3.4
USA, SEER Registries: whites[c]	33.2	26.9	17.0	11.0	2.3	1.0[e]	9.4	6.4
USA, SEER registries: blacks[c]	34.0	31.0	13.6	8.8	4.8	1.7[f]	14.6	9.5
China, Shanghai	8.5	7.6	9.4	7.1	34.4	11.6	5.5	3.8
India, Bombay	3.4	2.9	4.5	2.5	4.9	2.5	2.1	1.3
Israel: Jews	16.2	15.0	16.6	13.4	3.4	1.8	8.9	5.9
Israel: non-Jews	4.7	4.5	3.0	2.4	2.9	1.7	3.1	2.1
Japan, Miyagi	9.8	9.4	9.9	7.4	11.2	4.0	9.0	5.1
Philippines, Rizal	4.8	4.1	5.0	3.4	17.5	7.1	3.3	2.3
Czechoslovakia, Slovakia	11.8	9.3	15.2	8.8	5.1	2.8	8.3	4.5
Sweden	16.8	15.8	11.6	7.8	4.7	2.7	8.7	6.3
France, Bas-Rhin	23.1	14.6	18.0	8.5	6.9	1.2	5.5	2.2
Spain, Navarra	11.2	8.1	11.2	7.5	7.9	4.7	5.2	2.9
UK, England & Wales	16.6	14.7	13.7	7.9	1.6	0.8	7.9	4.9
Australia, New South Wales	23.7	20.1 .	15.4	9.3	1.2	0.4	7.5	4.4
New Zealand: Maoris	10.5	11.5	11.6	4.8	11.2	4.2	12.1	5.0
USA, Hawaii: Hawaiians	19.9	12.0	16.1	6.9	7.3	2,7	9.0	7.8

Registry	Larynx (161)		Lung (162)		Pleura (163)	
	M	F	M	F	M	F
Senegal, Dakar[b]	1.3	0,1	1.1	0,1	–	–
Brazil, São Paulo	17.8	1.3	36.5	7.9	–	–
Colombia, Cali	5.5	1.2	25.4	9.7	0,8	0,3
USA, Puerto Rico	7.0	0.7	18.1	6.5	0,1	0,1
USA, SEER Registries: whites[c]	7.8	1.5	72.6	27.2[g]	1.1	0.2
USA, SEER Registries: blacks[c]	11.5	2.0	109.0	28.4	0.5	0.1
China, Shanghai	3.1	0.7	54.7	18.5	0.1	0.1
India, Bombay	10.0	2.0	15.7	3.5	0.2	0.2
Israel: Jews	5.5	0.6	27.9	9.0	0.2	0.1
Israel: non-Jews	4.9	0,5	23.4	3.6	0,3	–
Japan, Miyagi	2.2	0.2	29.6	8.7	0,1	0,1
Philippines, Rizal	3.5	0.6	36.9	8.7	0,1	0,0
Czechoslovakia, Slovakia	10.5	0.4	70.0	6.8	0.3	0.2
Sweden	2.8	0.3	25.3	7.6	2.3	0.7
France, Bas-Rhin	12.4	0.5	60.2	3.9	0.4	0,1
Spain, Navarra	17.2	0,2	34.9	4.0	0.8	0,4
UK, England & Wales	4.0	0.7	72.0	19.0	0.8	0.2
Australia, New South Wales	5.6	0.6	53.4	11.3	1.2	0.1
New Zealand: Maoris	4.2	0,4	101.3	68.1	0,4	0,4
USA, Hawaii: Hawaiians	6.0	1,5	82.8	39.7	0,4	0,0

Registry	Bone (170)		Connective tissue (171)		Melanoma (172)	
	M	F	M	F	M	F
Senegal, Dakar[b]	0,2	0,3	2.7	1.5	1.2	1.3
Brazil, São Paulo	2.6	1.8	3.6	3.0	3.5	4.0
Colombia, Cali	1.3	0.7	3.1	2.8	3.3	3.0
USA, Puerto Rico	0.7	0.4	1.5	1.2	1.4	1.0
USA, SEER Registries:						
whites[c]	0.9	0.7	2.2	1.6[h]	9.7	8.6
USA, SEER Registries:						
blacks[c]	0.6	0.6	2.4	1.9[h]	0.8	0.5
China, Shanghai	2.1	1.5	1.5	1.4	0.3	0.2
India, Bombay	0.9	0.7	1.5	1.0	0.2	0.2
Israel: Jews	1.6	1.1	2.2	1.9	5.8	7.4
Israel: non-Jews	0.6	1.1	1.6	1.5	0,3	0,4
Japan, Miyagi	0.9	0.7	1.1	0.9	0.6	0.3
Philippines, Rizal	1.0	0.5	1.5	0.9	0.5	0,2
Czechoslovakia, Slovakia	1.1	0.8	1.8	1.4	3.0	3.4
Sweden	1.0	1.5	2.0	1.8	7.2	8.2
France, Bas-Rhin	1.6	1.2	1.3	1.7	3.1	4.6
Spain, Navarra	1.1	1.0	2.8	2.0	2.2	2.4
UK, England & Wales	0.9	0.7	1.4	1.1	2.2	3.8
Australia, New South Wales	0.9	0.7	2.2	1.4	17.1	16.1
New Zealand: Maoris	1.4	1,4	1.6	1,7	3.7	1,3
USA, Hawaii: Hawaiians	0,5	1,5	4.3	1,6	1,2	1,2

Registry	Other skin (173)		Breast (174)		Cervix (180)	Placenta (181)
	M	F	M	F	F	F
Senegal, Dakar[b]	10.3	7.9	0,7	11.8	17.2	0.9
Brazil, São Paulo	62.4	55.9	0.8	65.5	35.1	0.4
Colombia, Cali	56.2	58.9	0.0	34.8	48.2	0,0
USA, Puerto Rico	2.3	1.5[c,i]	0.3	35.1	15.6	0,0
USA, SEER Registries: whites[c]	10.7	9.1[l]	0.7	82.7	8.9	
USA, SEER Registries: blacks[c]	1.9	1.4[i]	1.0	70.0	19.3	
China, Shanghai	1.8	1.2	0.3	19.1	8.5	0.5
India, Bombay	1.5	1.4	0.4	24.1	20.6	0.3
Israel: Jews			0.8	61.3	4.0	0.3
Israel: non-Jews			0.3	14.0	3.0	0,1
Japan, Miyagi	1.6	1.3	0.1	22.0	10.0	0.4
Philippines, Rizal	3.3	2.6	0.4	29.8	16.6	0.7
Czechoslovakia, Slovakia	31.9	24.6	0.4	31.2	15.0	0.1
Sweden	8.0	3.5[j]	0.4	60.7	9.9	0.1
France, Bas-Rhin	11.4	6.2[j]	0.6	62.4	15.7	0,1
Spain, Navarra	30.7	14.9	0.5	38.7	5.7	0,1
UK, England & Wales	30.1	19.3	0.5	54.0	11.7	0.1
Australia, New South Wales			0.7	53.1	10.9	0.2
New Zealand: Maoris			0.4	59.5	28.9	0,1
USA, Hawaii: Hawaiians			0,6	93.9	12.3	0,0

Registry	Corpus (182)	Ovary (183)	Prostate (185)	Testis (186)
	F	F	M	M
Senegal, Dakar[b]	1.5	4.3	4.3	0,2
Brazil, São Paulo	13.7	10.1	33.0	2.0
Colombia, Cali	6.0	7.8	30.6	1.5
USA, Puerto Rico	8.0	5.9	30.7	1.0
USA, SEER Registries: whites[c]	23.4	12.9[k]	61.3	4.5
USA, SEER Registries: blacks[c]	12.0	9.1[k]	100.2	1.0
China, Shanghai	3.0	5.0	1.8	0.7
India, Bombay	2.0	7.2	8.2	1.0
Israel: Jews	9.8	11.9	18.8	2.2
Israel: non-Jews	3.1	3.8	6.5	0,7
Japan, Miyagi	2.8	4.2	6.3	1.0
Philippines, Rizal	3.5	7.0	11.1	0.6
Czechoslovakia, Slovakia	13.7	9.2	15.8	2.7
Sweden	13.2	15.2	45.9	3.3
France, Bas-Rhin	12.7	11.2	27.4	4.3
Spain, Navarra	12.5	6.4	20.5	1.2
UK, England & Wales	8.2	11.1	20.9	3.3
Australia, New South Wales	8.3	8.9	33.8	3.5
New Zealand: Maoris	15.4	10.9	35.4	7.9
USA, Hawaii: Hawaiians	25.2	14.1	40.9	3.3

Registry	Penis (187.1-4)	Bladder (188)		Kidney and renal pelvis (189.0-1)	
	M	M	F	M	F
Senegal, Dakar[b]	0,4	3.0	1.7	0,5	0.6
Brazil, São Paulo	2.5	15.7	3.7	3.4	2.0
Colombia, Cali	2.4	9.6	2.7	2.1	1.8
USA, Puerto Rico	3.6	9.6	3.1	2.7	1.4
USA, SEER Registries: whites[c]	0.6	25.4	6.7	9.1	4.1
USA, SEER Registries: blacks[c]	1.1	12.7	4.6	8.7	4.2
China, Shanghai	0.6[l]	7.1	1.7	1.8	1.0[m]
India, Bombay	2.1	4.3	1.0	1.4	0.5
Israel: Jews	0,0	20.3	4.3	6.0	3.8
Israel: non-Jews	0,1	12.5	1.5	1.7	0,8
Japan, Miyagi	0.5	6.4	1.9	3.0	1.4
Philippines, Rizal	0.9	2.8	0.9	1.4	1.0
Czechoslovakia, Slovakia	0.8	11.9	2.0	6.1	3.1
Sweden	0.9[l]	15.5	4.2	11.3	6.4[m]
France, Bas-Rhin	0.6	22.0	3.7	9.8	4.5
Spain, Navarra	0.8[l]	21.5	2.7	5.6	1.9[m]
UK, England & Wales	0.8	16.9	4.5	4.7	2.3
Australia, New South Wales	0.6[l]	17.1	5.0	7.2	4.4[m]
New Zealand: Maoris	0,7	4.6	3,2	6.0	2.3
USA, Hawaii: Hawaiians	0,4	10.0	4.5	7.4	2,0

Registry	Eye (190)		Brain, nervous system (191–2)		Thyroid (193)	
	M	F	M	F	M	F
Senegal, Dakar[b]	1.5	0.9	2.0	1.3	0,6	1.1
Brazil, São Paulo	1.2	1.2	6.9	5.5	2.0	5.3
Colombia, Cali	0,5	0.5	4.6	2.6	1.4	5.3
USA, Puerto Rico	0.7	0.4	3.4	2.1	1.1	3.2
USA, SEER Registries: whites[c]	0.9	0.7	7.0	4.9	2.2	5.6
USA, SEER Registries: blacks[c]	0.4	0,2	4.2	2.8	1.3	3.4
China, Shanghai	0.1	0.3	3.6	2.9	1.2	3.3
India, Bombay	0.3	0.1	2.1	1.5	0.6	1.7
Israel: Jews	0.6	0.5	9.0	8.5	2.5	6.0
Israel: non-Jews	0,8	0,8	5.5	3.3	1.3	2.5
Japan, Miyagi	0,2	0.4	2.0	1.7	1.1	3.9
Philippines, Rizal	0.3	0.3	1.4	1.1	2.0	4.7
Czechoslovakia, Slovakia	0.9	0.6	4.9	3.4	0.9	2.3
Sweden	0.9	0.6	9.4	9.3	1.6	4.3
France, Bas-Rhin	0,4	0,4	5.9	4.0	1.0	2.8
Spain, Navarra	1.0	0,3	7.9	5.7	0,3	2.7
UK, England & Wales	0.5	0.5	5.2	3.6	0.6	1.5
Australia, New South Wales	0.9	0.5	6.4	4.7	1.2	3.5
New Zealand: Maoris	0,6	0,3	9.1	4.8	2.3	3.1
USA, Hawaii: Hawaiians	0,0	0,4	3.0	4.1	5.9	10.5

Registry	Hodgkin's disease (201)		Non–Hodgkin lymphoma (200,202)		Multiple myeloma (203)		Leukaemia (204–8)	
	M	F	M	F	M	F	M	F
Senegal, Dakar[b]	1.4	0.7	3.5	1.2	*0,2*	*0,2*	0.7	*0,2*
Brazil, São Paulo	3.2	2.2	7.1	5.8	1.9	1.6	6.2	4.1
Colombia, Cali	2.9	1.1	5.4	4.5	2.1	1.5	6.1	5.4
USA, Puerto Rico	2.5	1.6	5.3	4.1	2.9	2.4	6.0	4.5
USA, SEER Registries: whites[c]	3.4	2.4	11.4	8.4	3.7	2.6	11.8	6.9
USA, SEER Registries: blacks[c]	2.6	1.3	8.1	5.2	9.0	6.2	9.9	6.5
China, Shanghai	0.5	0.3	3.5	2.1	0.7	0.4	5.4	4.7
India, Bombay	1.1	0.5	3.6	2.0	1.2	1.0	3.9	2.6
Israel: Jews	2.5	2.0	9.9	7.1	3.1	2.1	8.5	6.1
Israel: non–Jews	1.9	0.6	6.6	4.2	1.6	1.4	5.1	1.8
Japan, Miyagi	0.5	0.3	4.1	2.1	1.4	1.1	5.4	4.4
Philippines, Rizal	1.1	0.5	4.5	2.7	0.4	0.4	4.1	4.0
Czechoslovakia, Slovakia	2.6	1.7	5.5	2.6	2.0	1.5	8.4	5.5
Sweden	2.3	1.5	7.4	4.9	3.5	2.3	8.4	5.8
France, Bas–Rhin	2.1	2.2	7.5	5.5	2.4	1.5	8.7	5.4
Spain, Navarra	2.4	1.2	5.5	3.4	1.8	1.3	8.5	5.1
UK, England & Wales	2.7	1.7	5.8	3.9	2.5	1.8	6.8	4.4
Australia, New South Wales	2.3	1.5	9.3	6.7	3.4	1.9	9.7	5.9
New Zealand: Maoris	2.5	*1,1*	7.9	5.2	5.6	4.3	10.9	7.1
USA, Hawaii: Hawaiians	*1,6*	*0,6*	10.1	6.5	5.3	5.4	8.7	5.0

[a] Data from Muir *et al.* (1987), except where otherwise noted. For rates based on fewer than ten cases among all age groups, the decimal is given by a comma, not a point, and the figure is printed in italics; 0.0/0,0 = a rate greater than 0 but less than 0.05; –, no case registered although data for the site were collected; blank, not available

[b] Data from Waterhouse *et al.* (1982)

[c] Data from the US Surveillance, Epidemiology and End Results (SEER) Program 1978–82

[d] Excludes 149

[e] Includes 159.0

[f] 155.0 only

[g] 162.2–162.9

[h] Includes 164.1

[i] Excludes basal– and squamous–cell carcinoma

[j] Excludes basal–cell carcinoma

[k] 183.3 only

[l] Includes 'Other male genital organs'

[m] Includes 'Other urinary organs'

Subject Index

PUBLICATIONS OF THE INTERNATIONAL
AGENCY FOR RESEARCH ON CANCER
Scientific Publications Series

(Available from Oxford University Press through local bookshops)

No. 1 **Liver Cancer**
1971; 176 pages (*out of print*)

No. 2 **Oncogenesis and Herpesviruses**
Edited by P.M. Biggs, G. de-Thé and L.N. Payne
1972; 515 pages (*out of print*)

No. 3 **N–Nitroso Compounds: Analysis and Formation**
Edited by P. Bogovski, R. Preussman and E.A. Walker
1972; 140 pages (*out of print*)

No. 4 **Transplacental Carcinogenesis**
Edited by L. Tomatis and U. Mohr
1973; 181 pages (*out of print*)

No. 5/6 **Pathology of Tumours in Laboratory Animals, Volume 1, Tumours of the Rat**
Edited by V.S. Turusov
1973/1976; 533 pages; £50.00

No. 7 **Host Environment Interactions in the Etiology of Cancer in Man**
Edited by R. Doll and I. Vodopija
1973; 464 pages; £32.50

No. 8 **Biological Effects of Asbestos**
Edited by P. Bogovski, J.C. Gilson, V. Timbrell and J.C. Wagner
1973; 346 pages (*out of print*)

No. 9 **N–Nitroso Compounds in the Environment**
Edited by P. Bogovski and E.A. Walker
1974; 243 pages; £21.00

No. 10 **Chemical Carcinogenesis Essays**
Edited by R. Montesano and L. Tomatis
1974; 230 pages (*out of print*)

No. 11 **Oncogenesis and Herpesviruses II**
Edited by G. de-Thé, M.A. Epstein and H. zur Hausen
1975; Part I: 511 pages
Part II: 403 pages; £65.00

No. 12 **Screening Tests in Chemical Carcinogenesis**
Edited by R. Montesano, H. Bartsch and L. Tomatis
1976; 666 pages; £45.00

No. 13 **Environmental Pollution and Carcinogenic Risks**
Edited by C. Rosenfeld and W. Davis
1975; 441 pages (*out of print*)

No. 14 **Environmental N–Nitroso Compounds. Analysis and Formation**
Edited by E.A. Walker, P. Bogovski and L. Griciute
1976; 512 pages; £37.50

No. 15 **Cancer Incidence in Five Continents, Volume III**
Edited by J.A.H. Waterhouse, C. Muir, P. Correa and J. Powell
1976; 584 pages; (*out of print*)

No. 16 **Air Pollution and Cancer in Man**
Edited by U. Mohr, D. Schmähl and L. Tomatis
1977; 328 pages (*out of print*)

No. 17 **Directory of On–going Research in Cancer Epidemiology 1977**
Edited by C.S. Muir and G. Wagner
1977; 599 pages (*out of print*)

No. 18 **Environmental Carcinogens. Selected Methods of Analysis. Volume 1: Analysis of Volatile Nitrosamines in Food**
Editor-in-Chief: H. Egan
1978; 212 pages (*out of print*)

No. 19 **Environmental Aspects of N–Nitroso Compounds**
Edited by E.A. Walker, M. Castegnaro, L. Griciute and R.E. Lyle
1978; 561 pages (*out of print*)

No. 20 **Nasopharyngeal Carcinoma: Etiology and Control**
Edited by G. de-Thé and Y. Ito
1978; 606 pages (*out of print*)

No. 21 **Cancer Registration and its Techniques**
Edited by R. MacLennan, C. Muir, R. Steinitz and A. Winkler
1978; 235 pages; £35.00

No. 22 **Environmental Carcinogens. Selected Methods of Analysis. Volume 2: Methods for the Measurement of Vinyl Chloride in Poly(vinyl chloride), Air, Water and Foodstuffs**
Editor-in-Chief: H. Egan
1978; 142 pages (*out of print*)

No. 23 **Pathology of Tumours in Laboratory Animals. Volume II: Tumours of the Mouse**
Editor-in-Chief: V.S. Turusov
1979; 669 pages (*out of print*)

Prices, valid for January 1990, are subject to change without notice

No. 24 Oncogenesis and Herpesviruses III
Edited by G. de-Thé, W. Henle and F. Rapp
1978; Part I: 580 pages, Part II: 512 pages (*out of print*)

No. 25 Carcinogenic Risk. Strategies for Intervention
Edited by W. Davis and C. Rosenfeld
1979; 280 pages (*out of print*)

No. 26 Directory of On-going Research in Cancer Epidemiology 1978
Edited by C.S. Muir and G. Wagner
1978; 550 pages (*out of print*)

No. 27 Molecular and Cellular Aspects of Carcinogen Screening Tests
Edited by R. Montesano, H. Bartsch and L. Tomatis
1980; 372 pages; £29.00

No. 28 Directory of On-going Research in Cancer Epidemiology 1979
Edited by C.S. Muir and G. Wagner
1979; 672 pages (*out of print*)

No. 29 Environmental Carcinogens. Selected Methods of Analysis. Volume 3: Analysis of Polycyclic Aromatic Hydrocarbons in Environmental Samples
Editor-in-Chief: H. Egan
1979; 240 pages (*out of print*)

No. 30 Biological Effects of Mineral Fibres
Editor-in-Chief: J.C. Wagner
1980; **Volume 1:** 494 pages; **Volume 2:** 513 pages; £65.00

No. 31 N-Nitroso Compounds: Analysis, Formation and Occurrence
Edited by E.A. Walker, L. Griciute, M. Castegnaro and M. Börzsönyi
1980; 835 pages (*out of print*)

No. 32 Statistical Methods in Cancer Research. Volume 1. The Analysis of Case-control Studies
By N.E. Breslow and N.E. Day
1980; 338 pages; £20.00

No. 33 Handling Chemical Carcinogens in the Laboratory
Edited by R. Montesano, et al.
1979; 32 pages (*out of print*)

No. 34 Pathology of Tumours in Laboratory Animals. Volume III. Tumours of the Hamster
Editor-in-Chief: V.S. Turusov
1982; 461 pages; £39.00

No. 35 Directory of On-going Research in Cancer Epidemiology 1980
Edited by C.S. Muir and G. Wagner
1980; 660 pages (*out of print*)

No. 36 Cancer Mortality by Occupation and Social Class 1851-1971
Edited by W.P.D. Logan
1982; 253 pages; £22.50

No. 37 Laboratory Decontamination and Destruction of Aflatoxins B_1, B_2, G_1, G_2 in Laboratory Wastes
Edited by M. Castegnaro, et al.
1980; 56 pages; £6.50

No. 38 Directory of On-going Research in Cancer Epidemiology 1981
Edited by C.S. Muir and G. Wagner
1981; 696 pages (*out of print*)

No. 39 Host Factors in Human Carcinogenesis
Edited by H. Bartsch and B. Armstrong
1982; 583 pages; £46.00

No. 40 Environmental Carcinogens. Selected Methods of Analysis. Volume 4: Some Aromatic Amines and Azo Dyes in the General and Industrial Environment
Edited by L. Fishbein, M. Castegnaro, I.K. O'Neill and H. Bartsch
1981; 347 pages; £29.00

No. 41 N-Nitroso Compounds: Occurrence and Biological Effects
Edited by H. Bartsch, I.K. O'Neill, M. Castegnaro and M. Okada
1982; 755 pages; £48.00

No. 42 Cancer Incidence in Five Continents, Volume IV
Edited by J. Waterhouse, C. Muir, K. Shanmugaratnam and J. Powell
1982; 811 pages (*out of print*)

No. 43 Laboratory Decontamination and Destruction of Carcinogens in Laboratory Wastes: Some N-Nitrosamines
Edited by M. Castegnaro, et al.
1982; 73 pages; £7.50

No. 44 Environmental Carcinogens. Selected Methods of Analysis. Volume 5: Some Mycotoxins
Edited by L. Stoloff, M. Castegnaro, P. Scott, I.K. O'Neill and H. Bartsch
1983; 455 pages; £29.00

No. 45 Environmental Carcinogens. Selected Methods of Analysis. Volume 6: N-Nitroso Compounds
Edited by R. Preussmann, I.K. O'Neill, G. Eisenbrand, B. Spiegelhalder and H. Bartsch
1983; 508 pages; £29.00

No. 46 Directory of On-going Research in Cancer Epidemiology 1982
Edited by C.S. Muir and G. Wagner
1982; 722 pages (*out of print*)

No. 47 **Cancer Incidence in Singapore 1968–1977**
Edited by K. Shanmugaratnam, H.P. Lee and N.E. Day
1983; 171 pages (*out of print*)

No. 48 **Cancer Incidence in the USSR (2nd Revised Edition)**
Edited by N.P. Napalkov, G.F. Tserkovny, V.M. Merabishvili, D.M. Parkin, M. Smans and C.S. Muir
1983; 75 pages; £12.00

No. 49 **Laboratory Decontamination and Destruction of Carcinogens in Laboratory Wastes: Some Polycyclic Aromatic Hydrocarbons**
Edited by M. Castegnaro, *et al.*
1983; 87 pages; £9.00

No. 50 **Directory of On-going Research in Cancer Epidemiology 1983**
Edited by C.S. Muir and G. Wagner
1983; 731 pages (*out of print*)

No. 51 **Modulators of Experimental Carcinogenesis**
Edited by V. Turusov and R. Montesano
1983; 307 pages; £22.50

No. 52 **Second Cancers in Relation to Radiation Treatment for Cervical Cancer: Results of a Cancer Registry Collaboration**
Edited by N.E. Day and J.C. Boice, Jr
1984; 207 pages; £20.00

No. 53 **Nickel in the Human Environment**
Editor-in-Chief: F.W. Sunderman, Jr
1984; 529 pages; £41.00

No. 54 **Laboratory Decontamination and Destruction of Carcinogens in Laboratory Wastes: Some Hydrazines**
Edited by M. Castegnaro, *et al.*
1983; 87 pages; £9.00

No. 55 **Laboratory Decontamination and Destruction of Carcinogens in Laboratory Wastes: Some N–Nitrosamines**
Edited by M. Castegnaro, *et al.*
1984; 66 pages; £7.50

No. 56 **Models, Mechanisms and Etiology of Tumour Promotion**
Edited by M. Börzsönyi, N.E. Day, K. Lapis and H. Yamasaki
1984; 532 pages; £42.00

No. 57 **N–Nitroso Compounds: Occurrence, Biological Effects and Relevance to Human Cancer**
Edited by I.K. O'Neill, R.C. von Borstel, C.T. Miller, J. Long and H. Bartsch
1984; 1013 pages; £80.00

No. 58 **Age–related Factors in Carcinogenesis**
Edited by A. Likhachev, V. Anisimov and R. Montesano
1985; 288 pages; £20.00

No. 59 **Monitoring Human Exposure to Carcinogenic and Mutagenic Agents**
Edited by A. Berlin, M. Draper, K. Hemminki and H. Vainio
1984; 457 pages; £27.50

No. 60 **Burkitt's Lymphoma: A Human Cancer Model**
Edited by G. Lenoir, G. O'Conor and C.L.M. Olweny
1985; 484 pages; £29.00

No. 61 **Laboratory Decontamination and Destruction of Carcinogens in Laboratory Wastes: Some Haloethers**
Edited by M. Castegnaro, *et al.*
1985; 55 pages; £7.50

No. 62 **Directory of On-going Research in Cancer Epidemiology 1984**
Edited by C.S. Muir and G. Wagner
1984; 717 pages (*out of print*)

No. 63 **Virus–associated Cancers in Africa**
Edited by A.O. Williams, G.T. O'Conor, G.B. de-Thé and C.A. Johnson
1984; 773 pages; £22.00

No. 64 **Laboratory Decontamination and Destruction of Carcinogens in Laboratory Wastes: Some Aromatic Amines and 4–Nitrobiphenyl**
Edited by M. Castegnaro, *et al.*
1985; 84 pages; £6.95

No. 65 **Interpretation of Negative Epidemiological Evidence for Carcinogenicity**
Edited by N.J. Wald and R. Doll
1985; 232 pages; £20.00

No. 66 **The Role of the Registry in Cancer Control**
Edited by D.M. Parkin, G. Wagner and C.S. Muir
1985; 152 pages; £10.00

No. 67 **Transformation Assay of Established Cell Lines: Mechanisms and Application**
Edited by T. Kakunaga and H. Yamasaki
1985; 225 pages; £20.00

No. 68 **Environmental Carcinogens. Selected Methods of Analysis. Volume 7. Some Volatile Halogenated Hydrocarbons**
Edited by L. Fishbein and I.K. O'Neill
1985; 479 pages; £42.00

No. 69 **Directory of On-going Research in Cancer Epidemiology 1985**
Edited by C.S. Muir and G. Wagner
1985; 745 pages; £22.00

No. 70 **The Role of Cyclic Nucleic Acid Adducts in Carcinogenesis and Mutagenesis**
Edited by B. Singer and H. Bartsch
1986; 467 pages; £40.00

No. 71 **Environmental Carcinogens. Selected Methods of Analysis. Volume 8: Some Metals: As, Be, Cd, Cr, Ni, Pb, Se Zn**
Edited by I.K. O'Neill and, P. Schuller and L. Fishbein
1986; 485 pages; £42.00

No. 72 **Atlas of Cancer in Scotland, 1975–1980. Incidence and Epidemiological Perspective**
Edited by I. Kemp, P. Boyle, M. Smans and C.S. Muir
1985; 285 pages; £35.00

No. 73 **Laboratory Decontamination and Destruction of Carcinogens in Laboratory Wastes: Some Antineoplastic Agents**
Edited by M. Castegnaro, *et al.*
1985; 163 pages; £10.00

No. 74 **Tobacco: A Major International Health Hazard**
Edited by D. Zaridze and R. Peto
1986; 324 pages; £20.00

No. 75 **Cancer Occurrence in Developing Countries**
Edited by D.M. Parkin
1986; 339 pages; £20.00

No. 76 **Screening for Cancer of the Uterine Cervix**
Edited by M. Hakama, A.B. Miller and N.E. Day
1986; 315 pages; £25.00

No. 77 **Hexachlorobenzene: Proceedings of an International Symposium**
Edited by C.R. Morris and J.R.P. Cabral
1986; 668 pages; £50.00

No. 78 **Carcinogenicity of Alkylating Cytostatic Drugs**
Edited by D. Schmähl and J.M. Kaldor
1986; 337 pages; £25.00

No. 79 **Statistical Methods in Cancer Research. Volume III: The Design and Analsis of Long–term Animal Experiments**
Edited by J.J. Gart, D. Krewski, P.N. Lee, R.E. Tarone and J. Wahrendorf
1986; 213 pages; £20.00

No. 80 **Directory of On–going Research in Cancer Epidemiology 1986**
Edited by C.S. Muir and G. Wagner
1986; 805 pages; £22.00

No. 81 **Environmental Carcinogens: Methods of Analysis and Exposure Measurement. Volume 9: Passive Smoking**
Edited by I.K. O'Neill, K.D. Brunnemann, B. Dodet and D. Hoffmann
1987; 383 pages; £35.00

No. 82 **Statistical Methods in Cancer Research. Volume II: The Design and Analysis of Cohort Studies**
By N.E. Breslow and N.E. Day
1987; 404 pages; £30.00

No. 83 **Long–term and Short–term Assays for Carcinogens: A Critical Appraisal**
Edited by R. Montesano, H. Bartsch, H. Vainio, J. Wilbourn and H. Yamasaki
1986; 575 pages; £48.00

No. 84 **The Relevance of N-Nitroso Compounds to Human Cancer: Exposure and Mechanisms**
Edited by H. Bartsch, I.K. O'Neill and R. Schulte–Hermann
1987; 671 pages; £50.00

No. 85 **Environmental Carcinogens: Methods of Analysis and Exposure Measurement. Volume 10: Benzene and Alklated Benzenes**
Edited by L. Fishbein and I.K. O'Neill
1988; 327 pages; £35.00

No. 86 **Directory of On–going Research in Cancer Epidemiology 1987**
Edited by D.M. Parkin and J. Wahrendorf
1987; 676 pages; £22.00

No. 87 **International Incidence of Childhood Cancer**
Edited by D.M. Parkin, C.A. Stiller, C.A. Bieber, G.J. Draper. B. Terracini and J.L. Young
1988; 401 pages; £35.00

No. 88 **Cancer Incidence in Five Continents Volume V**
Edited by C. Muir, J. Waterhouse, T. Mack, J. Powell and S. Whelan
1987; 1004 pages; £50.00

No. 89 **Method for Detecting DNA Damaging Agents in Humans: Applications in Cancer Epidemiology and Prevention**
Edited by H. Bartsch, K. Hemminki and I.K. O'Neill
1988; 518 pages; £45.00

No. 90 **Non–occupational Exposure to Mineral Fibres**
Edited by J. Bignon, J. Peto and R. Saracci
1989; 500 pages; £45.00

No. 91 **Trends in Cancer Incidence in Singapore 1968–1982**
Edited by H.P. Lee , N.E. Day and K. Shanmugaratnam
1988; 160 pages; £25.00

No. 92 **Cell Differentiation, Genes and Cancer**
Edited by T. Kakunaga, T. Sugimura, L. Tomatis and H. Yamasaki
1988; 204 pages; £25.00

No. 93 **Directory of On–going Research in Cancer Epidemiology 1988**
Edited by M. Coleman and J. Wahrendorf
1988; 662 pages (*out of print*)

No. 94 **Human Papillomavirus and Cervical Cancer**
Edited by N. Muñoz, F.X. Bosch and O.M.Jensen
1989; 154 pages; £19.00

No. 95 **Cancer Registration: Principles and Methods**
Edited by O.M. Jensen, D.M. Parkin, R. MacLennan, C.S. Muir and R. Skeet
Publ. due 1990; approx. 300 pages

No. 96 **Perinatal and Multigeneration Carcinogenesis**
Edited by N.P. Napalkov, J.M. Rice, L. Tomatis and H. Yamasaki
1989; 436 pages; £48.00

No. 97 **Occupational Exposure to Silica and Cancer Risk**
Edited by L. Simonato, A.C. Fletcher, R. Saracci and T. Thomas
Publ. due 1990; approx. 160 pages; £19.00

No. 98 **Cancer Incidence in Jewish Migrants to Israel, 1961–1981**
Edited by R. Steinitz, D.M. Parkin, J.L. Young, C.A. Bieber and L. Katz
1988; 320 pages; £30.00

No. 99 **Pathology of Tumours in Laboratory Animals, Second Edition, Volume 1, Tumours of the Rat**
Edited by V.S. Turusov and U. Mohr
Publ. due 1990; approx. 700 pages; £85.00

No. 100 **Cancer: Causes, Occurrence and Control**
Edited by L. Tomatis
1990; approx. 350 pages; £24.00

No. 101 **Directory of On–going Research in Cancer Epidemiology 1989–90**
Edited by M. Coleman and J. Wahrendorf
1989; 818 pages; £36.00

No. 102 **Patterns of Cancer in Five Continents**
Edited by S.L. Whelan and D.M. Parkin
Publ. due 1990; approx. 150 pages; £25.00

No. 103 **Evaluating Effectiveness of Primary Prevention of Cancer**
Edited by M. Hakama, V. Beral, J.W. Cullen and D.M. Parkin
Publ. due 1990; approx. 250 pages; £32.00

No. 104 **Complex Mixtures and Cancer Risk**
Edited by H. Vainio, M. Sorsa and A.J. McMichael
Publ. due 1990; approx. 450 pages; £38.00

No. 105 **Relevance to Human Cancer of N–Nitroso Compounds, Tobacco Smoke and Mycotoxins**
Edited by I.K. O'Neill, J. Chen, S.H. Lu and H. Bartsch
Publ. due 1990; approx. 600 pages

IARC MONOGRAPHS ON THE EVALUATION OF CARCINOGENIC RISKS TO HUMANS

(Available from booksellers through the network of WHO Sales Agents*)

Volume 1 Some Inorganic Substances, Chlorinated Hydrocarbons, Aromatic Amines, N–nitroso Compounds, and Natural Products
1972; 184 pages (*out of print*)

Volume 2 Some Inorganic and Organometallic Compounds
1973; 181 pages (*out of print*)

Volume 3 Certain Polycyclic Aromatic Hydrocarbons and Heterocyclic Compounds
1973; 271 pages (*out of print*)

Volume 4 Some Aromatic Amines, Hydrazine and Related Substances, N–nitroso Compounds and Miscellaneous Alkylating Agents
1974; 286 pages;
Sw. fr. 18.–/US $14.40

Volume 5 Some Organochlorine Pesticides
1974; 241 pages (*out of print*)

Volume 6 Sex Hormones
1974; 243 pages (*out of print*)

Volume 7 Some Anti–Thyroid and Related Substances, Nitrofurans and Industrial Chemicals
1974; 326 pages (*out of print*)

Volume 8 Some Aromatic Azo Compounds
1975; 375 pages;
Sw. fr. 36.–/US $28.80

Volume 9 Some Aziridines, N–, S– and O–Mustards and Selenium
1975; 268 pages;
Sw. fr. 27.–/US $21.60

Volume 10 Some Naturally Occurring Substances
1976; 353 pages (*out of print*)

Volume 11 Cadmium, Nickel, Some Epoxides, Miscellaneous Industrial Chemicals and General Considerations on Volatile Anaesthetics
1976; 306 pages (*out of print*)

Volume 12 Some Carbamates, Thiocarbamates and Carbazides
1976; 282 pages;
Sw. fr. 34.–/US $27.20

Volume 13 Some Miscellaneous Pharmaceutical Substances
1977; 255 pages;
Sw. fr. 30.–/US $24.00

Volume 14 Asbestos
1977; 106 pages (*out of print*)

Volume 15 Some Fumigants, The Herbicides 2,4–D and 2,4,5–T, Chlorinated Dibenzodioxins and Miscellaneous Industrial Chemicals
1977; 354 pages;
Sw. fr. 50.–/US $40.00

Volume 16 Some Aromatic Amines and Related Nitro Compounds – Hair Dyes, Colouring Agents and Miscellaneous Industrial Chemicals
1978; 400 pages;
Sw. fr. 50.–/US $40.00

Volume 17 Some N–Nitroso Compounds
1987; 365 pages;
Sw. fr. 50.–/US $40.00

Volume 18 Polychlorinated Biphenyls and Polybrominated Biphenyls
1978; 140 pages;
Sw. fr. 20.–/US $16.00

Volume 19 Some Monomers, Plastics and Synthetic Elastomers, and Acrolein
1979; 513 pages;
Sw. fr. 60.–/US $48.00

Volume 20 Some Halogenated Hydrocarbons
1979; 609 pages (*out of print*)

Volume 21 Sex Hormones (II)
1979; 583 pages;
Sw. fr. 60.–/US $48.00

Volume 22 Some Non–Nutritive Sweetening Agents
1980; 208 pages;
Sw. fr. 25.–/US $20.00

Volume 23 Some Metals and Metallic Compounds
1980; 438 pages (*out of print*)

Volume 24 Some Pharmaceutical Drugs
1980; 337 pages;
Sw. fr. 40.–/US $32.00

Volume 25 Wood, Leather and Some Associated Industries
1981; 412 pages;
Sw. fr. 60.–/US $48.00

Volume 26 Some Antineoplastic and Immunosuppressive Agents
1981; 411 pages;
Sw. fr. 62.–/US $49.60

Volume 27 Some Aromatic Amines, Anthraquinones and Nitroso Compounds, and Inorganic Fluorides Used in Drinking Water and Dental Preparations
1982; 341 pages;
Sw. fr. 40.–/US $32.00

Volume 28 The Rubber Industry
1982; 486 pages;
Sw. fr. 70.–/US $56.00

* A list of WHO sales agents may be obtained from the Distribution of Sales Service, World Health Organization, 1211 Geneva 27, Switzerland

Volume 29 Some Industrial Chemicals and Dyestuffs
1982; 416 pages;
Sw. fr. 60.–/US $48.00

Volume 30 Miscellaneous Pesticides
1983; 424 pages;
Sw. fr. 60.–/US $48.00

Volue 31 Some Food Additives, Feed Additives and Naturally Occurring Substances
1983; 314 pages;
Sw. fr. 60.–/US $48.00

Volume 32 Polynuclear Aromatic Compounds, Part 1: Chemical, Environmental and Experimental Data
1984; 477 pages;
Sw. fr. 60.–/US $48.00

Volume 33 Polynuclear Aromatic Compounds, Part 2: Carbon Blacks, Mineral Oils and Some Nitroarenes
1984; 245 pages;
Sw. fr. 50.–/US $40.00

Volume 34 Polynuclear Aromatic Compounds, Part 3: Industrial Exposures in Aluminium Production, Coal Gasification, Coke Production, and Iron and Steel Founding
1984; 219 pages;
Sw. fr. 48.–/US $38.40

Volume 35 Polynuclear Aromatic Compounds: Part 4: Bitumens, Coal–Tars and Derived Products, Shale–Oils and Soots
1985; 271 pages;
Sw. fr. 70.–/US $56.00

Volume 36 Allyl Compounds, Aldehydes, Epoxides and Peroxides
1985; 369 pages;
Sw. fr. 70.–/US $56.00

Volume 37 Tobacco Habits Other than Smoking; Betel–Quid and Areca–Nut Chewing; and Some Related Nitrosamines
1985; 291 pages;
Sw. fr. 70.–/US $56.00

Volume 38 Tobacco Smoking
1986; 421 pages;
Sw. fr. 75.–/US $60.00

Volume 39 Some Chemicals Used in Plastics and Elastomers
1986; 403 pages;
Sw. fr. 60.–/US $48.00

Volume 40 Some Naturally Occurring and Synthetic Food Components, Furocoumarins and Ultraviolet Radiation
1986; 444 pages;
Sw. fr. 65.–/US $52.00

Volume 41 Some Halogenated Hydrocarbons and Pesticide Exposures
1986; 434 pages;
Sw. fr. 65.–/US $52.00

Volume 42 Silica and Some Silicates
1987; 289 pages;
Sw. fr. 65.–/US $52.00

Volume 43 Man–Made Mineral Fibres and Radon
1988; 300 pages;
Sw. fr. 65.–/US $52.00

Volume 44 Alcohol Drinking
1988; 416 pages;
Sw. fr. 65.–/US $52.00

Volume 45 Occupational Exposures in Petroleum Refining; Crude Oil and Major Petroleum Fuels
1989; 322 pages;
Sw. fr. 65.–/US $52.00

Volume 46 Diesel and Gasoline Engine Exhausts and Some Nitroarenes
1989; 458 pages;
Sw. fr. 65.–/US $52.00

Volume 47 Some Organic Solvents, Resin Monomers and Related Compounds, Pigments and Occupational Exposures in Paint Manufacture and Painting
1990; 536 pages;
Sw. fr. 85.–/US $ 68.00

Volume 48 Some Flame Retardants and Textile Chemicals, and Exposures in the Textile Manufacturing Industry
1990; approx. 350 pages;
Sw. fr. 65.–/US $52.00

Supplement No. 1
Chemicals and industrial processes associated with cancer in humans (IARC Monographs, Volumes 1 to 20)
1979; 71 pages; (*out of print*)

Supplement No. 2
Long–Term and Short–Term Screening Assays for Carcinogens: A critical Appraisal
1980; 426 pages;
Sw. fr. 40.–/US $32.00

Supplement No. 3
Cross index of synonyms and trade names in Volumes 1 to 26
1982; 199 pages (*out of print*)

Supplement No. 4
Chemicals, industrial processes and industries associated with cancer in humans (IARC Monographs, Volumes 1 to 29)
1982; 292 pages (*out of print*)

Supplement No. 5
Cross Index of Synonyms and Trade Names in Volumes 1 to 36
1985; 259 pages;
Sw. fr. 46.–/US $36.80

Supplement No. 6
Genetic and Related Effects: An Updating of Selected IARC Monographs from Volumes 1 to 42
1987; 729 pages;
Sw. fr. 80.–/US $64.00

Supplement No. 7
Overall Evaluations of Carcinogenicity: An
Updating of IARC Monographs Volumes 1–42
1987; 434 pages; Sw. fr. 65.–/US $52.00

Supplement No. 8
Cross Index of Synonyms and Trade Names in
Volumes 1 to 46 of the IARC Monographs
Publ. 1990; 260 pages; Sw. fr. 60.–/US $48.00

IARC TECHNICAL REPORTS*

No. 1 Cancer in Costa Rica
Edited by R. Sierra, R. Barrantes, G. Muñoz
Leiva, D.M. Parkin, C.A. Bieber and N. Muñoz
Calero
1988; 124 pages; Sw. fr. 30.–/US $24.00

**No. 2 SEARCH: A Computer Package to Assist
the Statistical Analysis of Case–Control Studies**
Edited by G.J. Macfarlane, P. Boyle and P.
Maisonneuve (in press)

**No. 3 Cancer Registration in the European
Economic Community**
Edited by M.P. Coleman and E. Démaret
1988; 188 pages; Sw. fr. 30.–/US $24.00

**No. 4 Diet, Hormones and Cancer:
Methodological Issues for Prospective Studies**
Edited by E. Riboli and R. Saracci
1988; 156 pages; Sw. fr. 30.–/US $24.00

No. 5 Cancer in the Philippines
Edited by A.V. Laudico, D. Esteban and D.M.
Parkin
1989; 186 pages; Sw. fr.30.–/US $24.00

INFORMATION BULLETINS ON THE SURVEY OF CHEMICALS BEING
TESTED FOR CARCINOGENICITY*

**No. 8 Edited by M.–J. Ghess, H. Bartsch and
L. Tomatis**
1979; 604 pages; Sw. fr. 40.–

**No. 9 Edited by M.–J. Ghess, J.D. Wilbourn, H.
Bartsch and L. Tomatis**1981; 294 pages; Sw. fr.
41.–

**No. 10 Edited by M.–J. Ghess, J.D. Wilbourn
and H. Bartsch**1982; 362 pages; Sw. fr. 42.–

**No. 11 Edited by M.–J. Ghess, J.D. Wilbourn,
H. Vainio and H. Bartsch**
1984; 362 pages; Sw. fr. 50.–

**No. 12 Edited by M.–J. Ghess, J.D. Wilbourn,
A. Tossavainen and H. Vainio**
1986; 385 pages; Sw. fr. 50.–

**No. 13 Edited by M.–J. Ghess, J.D. Wilbourn
and A. Aitio** 1988; 404 pages; Sw. fr. 43.

NON–SERIAL PUBLICATIONS †

Alcool et Cancer
By A. Tuyns (in French only)
1978; 42 pages; Fr. fr. 35.–

**Cancer Morbidity and Causes of Death Among
Danish Brewery Worker**
By O.M. Jensen 1980; 143 pages; Fr. fr. 75.–

**Directory of Computer Systems Used in Cancer
Registries** By H.R. Menck and D.M. Parkin
1986; 236 pages; Fr. fr. 50.–

*Available from booksellers through the network of WHO sales agents.

† Available directly from IARC.